Image Processing and Analysis for Preclinical and Clinical Applications

Image Processing and Analysis for Preclinical and Clinical Applications

Editors

Alessandro Stefano
Albert Comelli
Federica Vernuccio

MDPI • Basel • Beijing • Wuhan • Barcelona • Belgrade • Manchester • Tokyo • Cluj • Tianjin

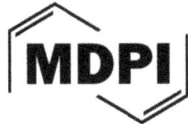

Editors
Alessandro Stefano
National Research Council
(IBFM-CNR)
Italy

Albert Comelli
Ri.MED Foundation
Italy

Federica Vernuccio
University Hospital of
Padova
Italy

Editorial Office
MDPI
St. Alban-Anlage 66
4052 Basel, Switzerland

This is a reprint of articles from the Special Issue published online in the open access journal *Applied Sciences* (ISSN 2076-3417) (available at: https://www.mdpi.com/journal/applsci/special_issues/preclinical_clinical_imaging).

For citation purposes, cite each article independently as indicated on the article page online and as indicated below:

LastName, A.A.; LastName, B.B.; LastName, C.C. Article Title. *Journal Name* **Year**, *Volume Number*, Page Range.

ISBN 978-3-0365-5013-8 (Hbk)
ISBN 978-3-0365-5014-5 (PDF)

© 2022 by the authors. Articles in this book are Open Access and distributed under the Creative Commons Attribution (CC BY) license, which allows users to download, copy and build upon published articles, as long as the author and publisher are properly credited, which ensures maximum dissemination and a wider impact of our publications.

The book as a whole is distributed by MDPI under the terms and conditions of the Creative Commons license CC BY-NC-ND.

Contents

About the Editors vii

Alessandro Stefano, Federica Vernuccio and Albert Comelli
Image Processing and Analysis for Preclinical and Clinical Applications
Reprinted from: *Appl. Sci.* **2022**, *12*, 7513, doi:10.3390/app12157513 1

Albert Comelli, Navdeep Dahiya, Alessandro Stefano, Federica Vernuccio, Marzia Portoghese, Giuseppe Cutaia, Alberto Bruno, Giuseppe Salvaggio and Anthony Yezzi
Deep Learning-Based Methods for Prostate Segmentation in Magnetic Resonance Imaging
Reprinted from: *Appl. Sci.* **2021**, *11*, 782, doi:10.3390/app11020782 7

Nur Banu Albayrak and Yusuf Sinan Akgul
Estimation of the Prostate Volume from Abdominal Ultrasound Images by Image-Patch Voting
Reprinted from: *Appl. Sci.* **2022**, *12*, 1390, doi:10.3390/app12031390 21

Giuseppe Salvaggio, Giuseppe Cutaia, Antonio Greco, Mario Pace, Leonardo Salvaggio, Federica Vernuccio, Roberto Cannella, Laura Algeri, Lorena Incorvaia, Alessandro Stefano, Massimo Galia, Giuseppe Badalamenti and Albert Comelli
Deep Learning Networks for Automatic Retroperitoneal Sarcoma Segmentation in Computerized Tomography
Reprinted from: *Appl. Sci.* **2022**, *12*, 1665, doi:10.3390/app12031665 37

Paulina Vélez, Manuel Miranda, Carmen Serrano and Begoña Acha
Does a Previous Segmentation Improve the Automatic Detection of Basal Cell Carcinoma Using Deep Neural Networks?
Reprinted from: *Appl. Sci.* **2022**, *12*, 2092, doi:10.3390/app12042092 49

Maria Amodeo, Vincenzo Abbate, Pasquale Arpaia, Renato Cuocolo, Giovanni Dell'Aversana Orabona, Monica Murero, Marco Parvis, Roberto Prevete and Lorenzo Ugga
Transfer Learning for an Automated Detection System of Fractures in Patients with Maxillofacial Trauma
Reprinted from: *Appl. Sci.* **2021**, *11*, 6293, doi:10.3390/app11146293 65

Pierpaolo Alongi, Alessandro Stefano, Albert Comelli, Alessandro Spataro, Giuseppe Formica, Riccardo Laudicella, Helena Lanzafame, Francesco Panasiti, Costanza Longo, Federico Midiri, Viviana Benfante, Ludovico La Grutta, Irene Andrea Burger, Tommaso Vincenzo Bartolotta, Sergio Baldari, Roberto Lagalla, Massimo Midiri and Giorgio Russo
Artificial Intelligence Applications on Restaging [^{18}F]FDG PET/CT in Metastatic Colorectal Cancer: A Preliminary Report of Morpho-Functional Radiomics Classification for Prediction of Disease Outcome
Reprinted from: *Appl. Sci.* **2022**, *12*, 2941, doi:10.3390/app12062941 77

Seung Hyun Lee, Joonseok Lim, Jaeseung Shin, Sungwon Kim, and Heasoo Hwang
Pathologic Complete Response Prediction after Neoadjuvant Chemoradiation Therapy for Rectal Cancer Using Radiomics and Deep Embedding Network of MRI
Reprinted from: *Appl. Sci.* **2021**, *11*, 9494, doi:10.3390/app11209494 91

Alessandro Stefano, Antonio Leal, Selene Richiusa, Phan Trang, Albert Comelli, Viviana Benfante, Sebastiano Cosentino, Maria G. Sabini, Antonino Tuttolomondo, Roberto Altieri, Francesco Certo, Giuseppe Maria Vincenzo Barbagallo, Massimo Ippolito and Giorgio Russo
Robustness of PET Radiomics Features: Impact of Co-Registration with MRI
Reprinted from: *Appl. Sci.* **2021**, *11*, 10170, doi:10.3390/app112110170 109

Alessandro Stefano, Pietro Pisciotta, Marco Pometti, Albert Comelli, Sebastiano Cosentino, Francesco Marletta, Salvatore Cicero, Maria G. Sabini, Massimo Ippolito and Giorgio Russo
Early Monitoring Response to Therapy in Patients with Brain Lesions Using the Cumulative SUV Histogram
Reprinted from: *Appl. Sci.* **2021**, *11*, 2999, doi:10.3390/app11072999 . . . . **123**

María J. Carreira, Nicolás Vila-Blanco, Pablo Cabezas-Sainz and Laura Sánchez
ZFTool: A Software for Automatic Quantification of Cancer Cell Mass Evolution in Zebrafish
Reprinted from: *Appl. Sci.* **2021**, *11*, 7721, doi:10.3390/app11167721 . . . . **135**

Wen-Ling Hsu, Shu-Min Chang and Chin-Chuan Chang
Clinical Comparison of the Glomerular Filtration Rate Calculated from Different Renal Depths and Formulae
Reprinted from: *Appl. Sci.* **2022**, *12*, 698, doi:10.3390/app12020698 . . . . **145**

Hana Sheitt, Hansuk Kim, Stephen Wilton, James A White and Julio Garcia
Left Atrial Flow Stasis in Patients Undergoing Pulmonary Vein Isolation for Paroxysmal Atrial Fibrillation Using 4D-Flow Magnetic Resonance Imaging
Reprinted from: *Appl. Sci.* **2021**, *11*, 5432, doi:10.3390/app11125432 . . . . **157**

Roziana Ramli, Khairunnisa Hasikin, Mohd Yamani Idna Idris, Noor Khairiah A. Karim and Ainuddin Wahid Abdul Wahab
Fundus Image Registration Technique Based on Local Feature of Retinal Vessels
Reprinted from: *Appl. Sci.* **2021**, *11*, 11201, doi:10.3390/app112311201 . . . . **165**

Daniele Passaretti, Mukesh Ghosh, Shiras Abdurahman, Micaela Lambru Egito and Thilo Pionteck
Hardware Optimizations of the X-ray Pre-Processing for Interventional Computed Tomography Using the FPGA
Reprinted from: *Appl. Sci.* **2022**, *12*, 5659, doi:10.3390/app12115659 . . . . **195**

About the Editors

Alessandro Stefano

Alessandro Stefano is a Research Scientist at the Institute of Molecular Bioimaging and Physiology, National Research Council (IBFM-CNR) of Cefalu'. He received his BS degree and Ph.D. in Engineering and in Computer Science from the University of Palermo, Italy, in 2005 and 2016, respectively. Currently, his research interests include medical image processing and analysis, in particular for non-invasive imaging techniques, such as positron emission tomography (PET), computerized tomography (CT) and magnetic resonance (MR), radiomics and artificial intelligence in clinical health care applications. He has authored more than 70 scientific papers in peer-reviewed journals and international conference proceedings.

Albert Comelli

Albert Comelli is currently a Researcher/Scientist in Biomedical Image Processing and Analysis at the Ri.MED Foundation, Palermo, Italy. He completed a combined B.Sc/M.Sc degree in Computer Science at the University of Catania and a Ph.D. in Computer Engineering at the University of Palermo. His research interests include biomedical image processing and analysis, radiomics, machine and deep learning to develop personalized predictive and/or prognostic models to support the medical decision process in patients undergoing different imaging methods such as magnetic resonance, computer tomography and positron emission tomography. He is the author of over 45 scientific papers in peer-reviewed journals and international conference proceedings.

Federica Vernuccio

Federica Vernuccio completed a degree in Medicine at the University of Palermo in 2012 and specialization in Radiology in 2018. In 2019, she achieved the Italian scientific certification for Associate Professor in Radiology. She worked as an abdominal radiologist at the University Hospital of Palermo from 2020 to November 2021. Since 15 November 2021, she has been staff radiologist at the Radiology Department of the University Hospital of Padova. She has won over 10 awards at international conferences and authored more than 70 publications as full-length papers in international journals with impact factor, including Radiology, AJR and European Radiology. Her main clinical and research interests are hepato-biliary tumors. She is a strong supporter of equity, diversity and equality in academia.

Editorial

Image Processing and Analysis for Preclinical and Clinical Applications

Alessandro Stefano [1,*], Federica Vernuccio [2] and Albert Comelli [3]

1. Institute of Molecular Bioimaging and Physiology, National Research Council (IBFM-CNR), 90015 Cefalù, Italy
2. Department of Radiology, University Hospital of Padova, Via Nicolò Giustiniani 2, 35128 Padova, Italy; federica.vernuccio@aopd.veneto.it
3. Ri.MED Foundation, Via Bandiera 11, 90133 Palermo, Italy; acomelli@fondazionerimed.com
* Correspondence: alessandro.stefano@ibfm.cnr.it

Preclinical and clinical imaging aims to characterize and measure biological processes and diseases in animals [1] and humans [2]. In recent years, there has been growing interest in the quantitative analysis of clinical images using techniques such as positron emission tomography (PET) [3], computerized tomography (CT) [4], and magnetic resonance imaging (MRI) [5], mainly applied to texture analysis and radiomics. Various image processing and analysis algorithms based on pattern recognition, artificial intelligence, and computer graphics methods have been proposed to extract features from biomedical images. These quantitative approaches are expected to have a positive clinical impact on quantitatively analyzing images, to reveal biological processes and diseases, and to predict response to treatment.

This Special Issue presents a collection of high-quality studies covering state-of-the-art and innovative approaches focusing on image processing and analysis across a variety of imaging modalities as well as the expected clinical applicability of these innovative approaches for personalized patient-tailored medicine.

The topics/keywords covered by this Special Issue includes the following:

- In vivo imaging;
- Therapy response prediction;
- Medical diagnosis support systems;
- Detection, segmentation, and classification of tissues;
- Biomedical image analysis and processing;
- Personalized medicine;
- Artificial intelligence;
- Texture analysis;
- Radiomics.

In response to the call for papers, nineteen papers were submitted to this Special Issue, of which fourteen were accepted for publication. These papers address several research challenges related to image processing and analysis in both preclinical and clinical applications.

Among the published research papers, five of them focus on segmentation and detection applications, including prostate gland segmentation [6,7], retroperitoneal sarcoma segmentation [8], basal cell carcinoma detection [9], and fracture detection in patients with maxillofacial trauma [10].

In one of these papers, the authors estimated prostate volume using ultrasound imaging, which offers many advantages such as portability, low cost, lack of ionizing radiations, and suitability for real-time operation [6]. Since experts usually consider automatic end-to-end volume-estimation procedures as non-transparent and uninterpretable systems, the authors proposed a system that directly estimated the diameter parameters of the standard ellipsoid formula to produce the prostate volume in a dataset of 305 patients. The proposed system detects four diameter endpoints from the transverse images and two diameter endpoints from the sagittal images, as defined by the classical procedure. These endpoints are estimated using a new image-patch voting method to address characteristic problems of ultrasound images. Furthermore, the dataset included 75 MRI images of the initial 305 patients. The results showed optimal performance, confirming that this system can be used in clinical practice.

Another prostate gland segmentation method based on T2-weighted MRI was proposed by Comelli et al. [7]. The authors presented the efficient neural network (ENet) to tackle the fully automated, real-time, and 3D delineation process of the prostate. ENet is mainly applied in self-driving cars to compensate for limited hardware availability while still achieving accurate segmentation. The authors applied this network to a limited set of 85 manual prostate segmentations using the k-fold validation strategy and the Tversky loss function [11] and compared the results with UNet and ERFNet (efficient residual factorized convNet). The results showed that ENet and UNet were more accurate than ERFNet, with ENet much faster than UNet. Specifically, ENet obtains a dice similarity coefficient of 90.89% and a segmentation time of about 6 s using central processing unit (CPU) hardware to simulate real clinical conditions where the graphics processing unit (GPU) is not always available.

In a similar study, Salvaggio et al. [8] used ENet and ERFNet for the automatic segmentation of retroperitoneal sarcoma (RPS) in 94 CT examinations. The volume estimation of RPS is often difficult due to its huge dimensions and irregular shape; thus, it often requires manual segmentation, which is time-consuming and operator-dependent. For this reason, the authors assessed the existence of significant differences between manual segmentation performed by two radiologists and automatic segmentation based on ENet and ERFNet using analysis of variance (ANOVA). A set of performance indicators for the shape comparison were calculated, namely sensitivity, positive predictive value, dice similarity coefficient, volume overlap error, and volumetric differences. There were no significant differences found between the RPS volumes obtained using manual segmentation and deep learning methods. Furthermore, all performance indicators were optimal for both ENet and ERFNet. Finally, ENet took around 15 s for segmentation versus 13 s for ERFNet by using GPU. In the case of CPU, ENet took around 2 min versus 1 min for ERFNet. The manual approach required approximately one hour per segmentation. In conclusion, fully automatic deep learning networks were reliable methods for RPS volume assessment.

Vélez et al. [9] proposed a tool for the detection of basal cell carcinoma (BCC) to provide a prioritization in the tele-dermatology consultation. BCC is the most frequent skin cancer, and its increasing incidence is producing a high overload in dermatology services. The authors analyzed if pre-segmentation of the lesion improved the classification of the lesion. After that, they analyzed three deep neural networks to distinguish between BCC and nevus, or other skin lesions. The best segmentation results were obtained with SegNet with accuracies of 98% and 95% for distinguishing BCC from nevus and other skin lesions, respectively. This method outperformed the winner of the challenge International Skin Imaging Collaboration (ISIC) 2019. Furthermore, the authors concluded that when deep neural networks are used to classify, a pre-segmentation of the lesion does not improve the classification results.

Finally, a novel maxillofacial fracture detection system (MFDS), based on convolutional neural networks and transfer learning, was proposed by Amodeo et al. [10] to detect traumatic fractures in patients. A convolutional neural network pre-trained on non-medical images was re-trained and fine-tuned using 148 CT images to produce a model for the classification of future CTs as fracture or not fracture. The validation and test datasets were characterized by 30 patients: both datasets contained 5 patients without fractures and 25 with fractures. The results showed an accuracy of 80% in classifying the maxillofacial fractures. Consequently, the proposed model can be used as a care support, reducing the risk of human error, preventing patient harm by minimizing diagnostic delays, and reducing the incongruous burden of hospitalization.

Among the other research papers, three of them focus on radiomics applications, including restaging in metastatic colorectal cancer [12], evaluating the robustness of PET radiomics features after MRI co-registration [13], and predicting pathologic complete response after neoadjuvant chemoradiation therapy for rectal cancer [14].

Alongi et al. [12] investigated the application of [18F]FDG PET/CT image-based textural features analysis to early predict disease progression and survival outcome in 52 metastatic colorectal cancer (MCC) patients after first adjuvant therapy. For this purpose, radiomics features from PET and low-dose CT images were extracted. The hybrid descriptive-inferential method [15] was used for feature selection while the discriminant analysis [16] was used for the predictive model implementation. The prediction performance was evaluated for per-lesion analysis, per-patient analysis, and per liver lesions analysis. All results showed that the proposed radiomics model was feasible and potentially useful in the predictive evaluation of disease progression in MCC.

Stefano et al. [13] studied the variability in PET radiomics features under the impact of co-registration with MRI using the difference percentage coefficient and the Spearman's correlation coefficient for three groups of images: (i) original PET, (ii) PET after co-registration with T1-weighted MRI, and (iii) PET after co-registration with FLAIR MRI. For this purpose, 77 patients with brain cancers undergoing [11C]-Methionine PET were considered. Successively, PET images were co-registered with MRI sequences and 107 features were extracted for each mentioned group of images. The variability analysis revealed that shape features, first-order features, and two subgroups of higher-order features possessed a good robustness, unlike the remaining groups of features, which showed large differences in the difference percentage coefficient. Furthermore, using Spearman's correlation coefficient, approximately 40% of the selected features differed from the three mentioned groups of images. This is an important consideration for users conducting radiomics studies with image co-registration constraints to avoid errors in cancer diagnosis, prognosis, and clinical outcome prediction.

Lee et al. [14] evaluated the MRI assessment after neoadjuvant chemoradiotherapy (nCRT) in 912 patients with rectal cancer for staging and treatment planning purposes. They proposed a pathologic complete response (pCR) prediction method based on a novel multi-parametric MRI embedding technique. Specifically, multiple MRI sequences were encapsulated into multi-sequence fusion images (MSFI). Subsequently, radiomics features were extracted and used to predict pCR through a random forest classifier. The results demonstrated that the use of all given MRI sequences is the most effective method regardless of the dimension reduction method. Furthermore, it outperformed four competing baselines in terms of the area under the receiver operating characteristic curve (AUC) and F1-score.

Among the other research papers, four of them focus on biomedical image quantification, including the early monitoring response to therapy in patients with brain lesions [17], the quantification of cancer cell mass evolution in zebrafish [18], the clinical comparison of the glomerular filtration rate calculated from different renal depths and formulae [19], and the assessment of the left atrial flow stasis in patients undergoing pulmonary vein isolation for paroxysmal atrial fibrillation [20].

Stefano et al. [17] evaluated new PET prognostic indices for the early assessment of response to Gamma Knife (GK) treatment. GK is an alternative to traditional brain surgery and whole-brain radiation therapy for the treatment of tumors inaccessible through conventional treatments [21]. Semi-quantitative PET parameters currently used in the clinical setting can be affected by statistical fluctuation errors and/or cannot provide information on tumor extent and heterogeneity. To overcome these limitations, the cumulative standardized uptake value histogram (CSH) and AUC were considered as additional information on the response to GK treatment. Specifically, the absolute level of [11C]-Methionine (MET) uptake was measured and its heterogeneity distribution within PET lesions was evaluated by calculating the CSH and AUC. The results showed good agreement with patient outcomes, and since no relevant correlations were found between CSH and AUC and the indices usually used in PET imaging, these innovative parameters could be a useful tool for assessing patient responses to therapy.

In [18], the authors considered zebrafish as it is a model organism for the study of human cancer and, compared with the murine model, it has several properties that are ideal for personalized therapies. The transparency of the zebrafish embryos and the development of the pigment-deficient "casper" zebrafish line give the capacity to directly observe cancer formation and progression in the living animal. Nevertheless, the automatic quantification of cellular proliferation in vivo is still critical. For this reason, the authors proposed a new tool, namely ZFTool, to automatically quantify the cancer cellular evolution. ZFTool is capable of establishing a base threshold that eliminates the embryo autofluorescence, to automatically measure the area and intensity of green-fluorescent protein marked cells, and to define a proliferation index. As result, the proliferation index computed on different targets demonstrated the efficiency of ZFTool in providing a good automatic quantification of cancer mass evolution in zebrafish, eliminating the influence of its autofluorescence.

In the study proposed by Hsu et al. [19], the authors aimed to compare the differences in renal depths in a camera-based method using Technetium-99 m diethylenetriaminepentaacetic acid (Tc-99 m DTPA). This method is commonly used to calculate the glomerular filtration rate (GFR) as it can easily calculate split renal function. Renal depth is the main factor affecting the measurement of GFR accuracy. For this reason, the difference in renal depths between three formulae (Tonnesen's, Itoh K's, and Taylor's) and a CT scan were compared and used to calculate the GFRs using four methods. For this purpose, 51 patients underwent a laboratory test within one month and a CT scan within two months. The results showed that the renal depths measured using the three formulae were smaller than those measured using the CT scan, and the right renal depth was always larger than the left.

In [20], the authors aimed to demonstrate that left atrial (LA) stasis, derived from 4D-flow, is a useful biomarker of LA recovery in patients with atrial fibrillation (AF). AF is associated with systemic thrombo-embolism and stroke events, which do not appear significantly reduced following successful pulmonary vein (PV) ablation. The authors' hypothesis was that LA recovery was associated with a reduction in LA stasis. For this purpose, 148 subjects with paroxysmal AF and 24 controls were recruited and underwent a cardiac MRI, inclusive of 4D-flow. LA was isolated within the 4D-flow dataset to constrain stasis maps. The results showed that the mean LA stasis in the control was lower than that in the pre-ablation cohort and that the mean LA stasis was reduced in the post-ablation cohort compared with in the pre-ablation cohort. The study demonstrated that 4D flow-derived LA stasis mapping was clinically relevant and revealed stasis changes in the LA body pre- and post-pulmonary vein ablation.

Finally, the last two published studies concern an image registration technique based on local feature of retinal vessels [22], and the hardware optimizations of the X-ray pre-processing using the field programmable gate array (FPGA) [23].

In the first of these two studies [22], an innovative method, namely CURVE, is presented to accurately extract feature points on retinal vessels and throughout the fundus image. The CURVE performance was tested on different datasets and compared with six state-of-the-art feature extraction methods. The results showed that the feature extraction accuracy of CURVE significantly outperformed the existing feature extraction methods. Then, CURVE was paired with a scale-invariant feature transform (SIFT) descriptor to test its registration capability on the fundus image registration (FIRE) dataset. CURVE-SIFT successfully registered 44% of the image pairs while existing feature-based techniques registered less than 27% of the image pairs.

The last study [23] proposed the optimization of the X-ray pre-processing in CT imaging to compute total attenuation projections by avoiding the intermediate step of converting detector data to intensity images. Furthermore, a configurable hardware architecture for data acquisition systems on FPGAs was proposed to fulfill the real-time requirements and with the aim of achieving "on-the-fly" pre-processing of 2D projections. Finally, this architecture was configured for exploring and analyzing different arithmetic representations, such as floating-point and fixed-point data formats. In this way, the best representation and data format that minimized execution time and hardware costs was found without affecting image quality. By comparing the proposed solution with the state-of-the-art pre-processing algorithm, the latency decreased by 4.125× and the resource utilization decreased by ∼6.5×. By using fixed-point representation in the different data precisions, the latency and the resource utilization were further decreased.

In conclusion, this Special Issue covers recent trends in biomedical imaging applications, such as quantification, detection, radiomics, registration, and optimization, constituting a good sample of the current state-of-the-art results in this field.

Author Contributions: Conceptualization, A.S., F.V. and A.C.; methodology, A.S.; resources, F.V. and A.C.; data curation, A.S.; writing—original draft preparation, A.S.; writing—review and editing, A.S.; supervision, A.S.; project administration, A.S., F.V. and A.C.; funding acquisition, A.C. All authors have read and agreed to the published version of the manuscript.

Funding: This research received no external funding.

Institutional Review Board Statement: Not applicable.

Informed Consent Statement: Not applicable.

Data Availability Statement: Not applicable.

Conflicts of Interest: The authors declare no conflict of interest.

References

1. Benfante, V.; Stefano, A.; Comelli, A.; Giaccone, P.; Cammarata, F.P.; Richiusa, S.; Scopelliti, F.; Pometti, M.; Ficarra, M.; Cosentino, S.; et al. A New Preclinical Decision Support System Based on PET Radiomics: A Preliminary Study on the Evaluation of an Innovative 64Cu-Labeled Chelator in Mouse Models. *J. Imaging* **2022**, *8*, 92. [CrossRef] [PubMed]
2. Stefano, A.; Comelli, A. Customized efficient neural network for covid-19 infected region identification in ct images. *J. Imaging* **2021**, *7*, 131. [CrossRef] [PubMed]
3. Banna, G.L.; Anile, G.; Russo, G.; Vigneri, P.; Castaing, M.; Nicolosi, M.; Strano, S.; Gieri, S.; Spina, R.; Patanè, D.; et al. Predictive and Prognostic Value of Early Disease Progression by PET Evaluation in Advanced Non-Small Cell Lung Cancer. *Oncology* **2017**, *92*, 39–47. [CrossRef] [PubMed]
4. Stefano, A.; Gioè, M.; Russo, G.; Palmucci, S.; Torrisi, S.E.; Bignardi, S.; Basile, A.; Comelli, A.; Benfante, V.; Sambataro, G.; et al. Performance of Radiomics Features in the Quantification of Idiopathic Pulmonary Fibrosis from HRCT. *Diagnostics* **2020**, *10*, 306. [CrossRef]
5. Cutaia, G.; la Tona, G.; Comelli, A.; Vernuccio, F.; Agnello, F.; Gagliardo, C.; Salvaggio, L.; Quartuccio, N.; Sturiale, L.; Stefano, A.; et al. Radiomics and prostate MRI: Current role and future applications. *J. Imaging* **2021**, *7*, 34. [CrossRef]
6. Albayrak, N.B.; Akgul, Y.S. Estimation of the Prostate Volume from Abdominal Ultrasound Images by Image-Patch Voting. *Appl. Sci.* **2022**, *12*, 1390. [CrossRef]
7. Comelli, A.; Dahiya, N.; Stefano, A.; Vernuccio, F.; Portoghese, M.; Cutaia, G.; Bruno, A.; Salvaggio, G.; Yezzi, A. Deep learning-based methods for prostate segmentation in magnetic resonance imaging. *Appl. Sci.* **2021**, *11*, 782. [CrossRef]
8. Salvaggio, G.; Cutaia, G.; Greco, A.; Pace, M.; Salvaggio, L.; Vernuccio, F.; Cannella, R.; Algeri, L.; Incorvaia, L.; Stefano, A.; et al. Deep Learning Networks for Automatic Retroperitoneal Sarcoma Segmentation in Computerized Tomography. *Appl. Sci.* **2022**, *12*, 1665. [CrossRef]
9. Vélez, P.; Miranda, M.; Serrano, C.; Acha, B. Does a Previous Segmentation Improve the Automatic Detection of Basal Cell Carcinoma Using Deep Neural Networks? *Appl. Sci.* **2022**, *12*, 2092. [CrossRef]
10. Amodeo, M.; Abbate, V.; Arpaia, P.; Cuocolo, R.; Orabona, G.D.; Murero, M.; Parvis, M.; Prevete, R.; Ugga, L. Transfer learning for an automated detection system of fractures in patients with maxillofacial trauma. *Appl. Sci.* **2021**, *11*, 6293. [CrossRef]
11. Comelli, A.; Dahiya, N.; Stefano, A.; Benfante, V.; Gentile, G.; Agnese, V.; Raffa, G.M.; Pilato, M.; Yezzi, A.; Petrucci, G.; et al. Deep learning approach for the segmentation of aneurysmal ascending aorta. *Biomed. Eng. Lett.* **2021**, *11*, 15–24. [CrossRef] [PubMed]
12. Alongi, P.; Stefano, A.; Comelli, A.; Spataro, A.; Formica, G.; Laudicella, R.; Lanzafame, H.; Panasiti, F.; Longo, C.; Midiri, F.; et al. Artificial Intelligence Applications on Restaging [18F]FDG PET/CT in Metastatic Colorectal Cancer: A Preliminary Report of Morpho-Functional Radiomics Classification for Prediction of Disease Outcome. *Appl. Sci.* **2022**, *12*, 2941. [CrossRef]
13. Stefano, A.; Leal, A.; Richiusa, S.; Trang, P.; Comelli, A.; Benfante, V.; Cosentino, S.; Sabini, M.G.; Tuttolomondo, A.; Altieri, R.; et al. Robustness of pet radiomics features: Impact of co-registration with mri. *Appl. Sci.* **2021**, *11*, 10170. [CrossRef]
14. Lee, S.; Lim, J.; Shin, J.; Kim, S.; Hwang, H. Pathologic Complete Response Prediction after Neoadjuvant Chemoradiation Therapy for Rectal Cancer Using Radiomics and Deep Embedding Network of MRI. *Appl. Sci.* **2021**, *11*, 9494. [CrossRef]
15. Barone, S.; Cannella, R.; Comelli, A.; Pellegrino, A.; Salvaggio, G.; Stefano, A.; Vernuccio, F. Hybrid descriptive-inferential method for key feature selection in prostate cancer radiomics. *Appl. Stoch. Model. Bus. Ind.* **2021**, *37*, 961–972. [CrossRef]

16. Stefano, A.; Comelli, A.; Bravatà, V.; Barone, S.; Daskalovski, I.; Savoca, G.; Sabini, M.G.; Ippolito, M.; Russo, G. A preliminary PET radiomics study of brain metastases using a fully automatic segmentation method. *BMC Bioinform.* **2020**, *21*, 325. [CrossRef] [PubMed]
17. Stefano, A.; Pisciotta, P.; Pometti, M.; Comelli, A.; Cosentino, S.; Marletta, F.; Cicero, S.; Sabini, M.G.; Ippolito, M.; Russo, G. Early monitoring response to therapy in patients with brain lesions using the cumulative SUV histogram. *Appl. Sci.* **2021**, *11*, 2999. [CrossRef]
18. Carreira, M.J.; Vila-Blanco, N.; Cabezas-Sainz, P.; Sánchez, L. Zftool: A software for automatic quantification of cancer cell mass evolution in zebrafish. *Appl. Sci.* **2021**, *11*, 7721. [CrossRef]
19. Hsu, W.L.; Chang, S.M.; Chang, C.C. Clinical Comparison of the Glomerular Filtration Rate Calculated from Different Renal Depths and Formulae. *Appl. Sci.* **2022**, *12*, 698. [CrossRef]
20. Sheitt, H.; Kim, H.; Wilton, S.; White, J.A.; Garcia, J. Left atrial flow stasis in patients undergoing pulmonary vein isolation for paroxysmal atrial fibrillation using 4d-flow magnetic resonance imaging. *Appl. Sci.* **2021**, *11*, 5432. [CrossRef]
21. Stefano, A.; Vitabile, S.; Russo, G.; Ippolito, M.; Marletta, F.; D'Arrigo, C.; D'Urso, D.; Sabini, M.G.; Gambino, O.; Pirrone, R.; et al. An automatic method for metabolic evaluation of gamma knife treatments. In *Lecture Notes in Computer Science, Proceedings of the 18th International Conference, Genoa, Italy, 7–11 September 2015*; Murino, V., Puppo, E., Eds.; International Publishing: Cham, Switzerland, 2015; Volume 9279, pp. 579–589.
22. Ramli, R.; Hasikin, K.; Idris, M.Y.I.; Karim, N.K.A.; Wahab, A.W.A. Fundus image registration technique based on local feature of retinal vessels. *Appl. Sci.* **2021**, *11*, 11201.
23. Passaretti, D.; Ghosh, M.; Abdurahman, S.; Egito, M.L.; Pionteck, T. Hardware Optimizations of the X-ray Pre-Processing for Interventional Computed Tomography Using the FPGA. *Appl. Sci.* **2022**, *12*, 5659.

Short Biography of Authors

Alessandro Stefano is a Research Scientist at the Institute of Molecular Bioimaging and Physiology, National Research Council (IBFM-CNR) of Cefalù. He received his BS degree and his PhD in Engineering in Computer Science from the University of Palermo, Italy, in 2005 and 2016, respectively. Currently, his research interests include medical image processing and analysis, in particular for non-invasive imaging techniques, such as positron emission tomography (PET), computerized tomography (CT), and magnetic resonance (MR); radiomics; and artificial intelligence in clinical health care applications. He is the author of more than 80 scientific papers in peer-reviewed journals and international conference proceedings.

Federica Vernuccio achieved her degree in Medicine at the University of Palermo in 2012 and specialization in Radiology in 2018. In 2019, she achieved an Italian scientific certification for Associate Professor in Radiology. As a radiologist, she worked as an abdominal radiologist at the University Hospital of Palermo from 2020 to November 2021. From November 15, 2021, she became a staff radiologist at the Radiology Department of the University Hospital of Padova. She won more than 10 awards in international conferences and wrote more than 70 publications as full-length papers in international journals with impact factors, including *Radiology*, *AJR* and *European Radiology*. Her main clinical and research interests are hepato-biliary tumors. She is a strong supporter of equity, diversity, and equality in academics.

Albert Comelli is currently a Researcher/Scientist in Biomedical Image Processing and Analysis at the Ri.MED Foundation, Palermo, Italy. He received a combined BSc/MSc degree in Computer Science at the University of Catania and a PhD in Computer Engineering at the University of Palermo. His research interests include biomedical image processing and analysis; radiomics; and machine and deep learning for developing personalized predictive and/or prognostic models to support the medical decision process in patients undergoing different imaging methods such as magnetic resonance, computer tomography, and positron emission tomography. He is the author of over 45 scientific papers in peer-reviewed journals and international conference proceedings.

Article

Deep Learning-Based Methods for Prostate Segmentation in Magnetic Resonance Imaging

Albert Comelli [1,2], Navdeep Dahiya [3], Alessandro Stefano [2,*], Federica Vernuccio [4], Marzia Portoghese [4], Giuseppe Cutaia [4], Alberto Bruno [4], Giuseppe Salvaggio [4] and Anthony Yezzi [3]

1. Ri.MED Foundation, Via Bandiera, 11, 90133 Palermo, Italy; acomelli@fondazionerimed.com
2. Institute of Molecular Bioimaging and Physiology, National Research Council (IBFM-CNR), 90015 Cefalù, Italy
3. Department of Electrical and Computer Engineering, Georgia Institute of Technology, Atlanta, GA 30332, USA; ndahiya3@gatech.edu (N.D.); anthony.yezzi@ece.gatech.edu (A.Y.)
4. Dipartimento di Biomedicina, Neuroscienze e Diagnostica avanzata (BIND), University of Palermo, 90127 Palermo, Italy; federica.vernuccio@unipa.it (F.V.); marzia.portoghese@unipa.it (M.P.); giuseppe.cutaia@community.unipa.it (G.C.); bruno-alberto@hotmail.it (A.B.); p.salvaggio@libero.it (G.S.)
* Correspondence: alessandro.stefano@ibfm.cnr.it; Tel.: +390921920149

Featured Application: The study demonstrates that high-speed deep learning networks could perform accurate prostate delineation facilitating the adoption of novel imaging parameters, through radiomics analyses, for prostatic oncologic diseases.

Abstract: Magnetic Resonance Imaging-based prostate segmentation is an essential task for adaptive radiotherapy and for radiomics studies whose purpose is to identify associations between imaging features and patient outcomes. Because manual delineation is a time-consuming task, we present three deep-learning (DL) approaches, namely UNet, efficient neural network (ENet), and efficient residual factorized convNet (ERFNet), whose aim is to tackle the fully-automated, real-time, and 3D delineation process of the prostate gland on T2-weighted MRI. While UNet is used in many biomedical image delineation applications, ENet and ERFNet are mainly applied in self-driving cars to compensate for limited hardware availability while still achieving accurate segmentation. We apply these models to a limited set of 85 manual prostate segmentations using the k-fold validation strategy and the Tversky loss function and we compare their results. We find that ENet and UNet are more accurate than ERFNet, with ENet much faster than UNet. Specifically, ENet obtains a dice similarity coefficient of 90.89% and a segmentation time of about 6 s using central processing unit (CPU) hardware to simulate real clinical conditions where graphics processing unit (GPU) is not always available. In conclusion, ENet could be efficiently applied for prostate delineation even in small image training datasets with potential benefit for patient management personalization.

Keywords: deep learning; segmentation; prostate; MRI; ENet; UNet; ERFNet; radiomics

1. Introduction

In the biomedical imaging field, target delineation is routinely used as the first step in any automatized disease diagnosis system (i.e., radiotherapy system) and, in the last few years, in radiomics studies [1,2] to obtain a multitude of quantitative parameters from biomedical images [3,4]. These parameters are then used as imaging biomarkers to identify any possible associations with patient outcome. The first task of a radiomics analysis is the automatic and user-independent target (e.g., tumor or organ) delineation to avoid any distortion during the feature extraction process [5]. Manual segmentation might seem like the simplest solution to obtain target boundaries, but it is a time-consuming and user-dependent process that affects the radiomics signature [6]. For this reason, an automatic and operator-independent target delineation method is mandatory. Nevertheless, the segmentation process remains a challenging field of research. Over the years many different

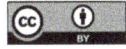

types of segmentation techniques have been developed, for example, [7–9]. Some of the previous techniques include thresholding [10], k-means clustering [11], watersheds [12], followed by more advanced algorithms such as active contour methods [8,13], graph cuts [14], random walks [15], conditional and Markov random fields [16] to name a few. In recent years, particularly the last decade, the field of Machine Learning (ML) and Deep Learning (DL) has seen exponential growth and has produced models that have shown remarkable performance across many benchmark datasets and many different problem domains [17,18]. In general, an artificial intelligence method learns from examples and makes predictions without prior specific programming [19]. In the case of DL, these models implement networked structures to mimic the human brain transforming imaging data in feature vectors. Briefly, between the input and output, a variable number of hidden layers is implemented and the various nodes are connected to others with different weights.

The initial development of DL models was towards image classification problems, followed by object detection and finally, image segmentation, which is seen as a pixel level classification problem where each pixel is classified with one of many possible label classes. For example, in tumor segmentation, every voxel can be classified as either belonging to the class label of the object of interest (target) or the background. Since it is a very common task across many different problem domains, hundreds of different DL based models have been presented for the delineation task over the past several years: fully convolutional [20], encoder-decoder [21], multi-scale and pyramid [22–24], attention [25], recurrent neural [26], generative and adversarial training [27,28] based networks. Even during the current pandemic, DL networks have been widely used to help clinicians diagnose COVID-19 [29,30]. It is beyond the scope of this paper to discuss and describe all these different types of models. Interested readers are directed to recent comprehensive reviews [31,32] of DL based methods/models for image segmentation.

In this study, we deal with the issue of prostate region delineation on magnetic resonance imaging (MRI) studies. Prostatic volume extraction helps in the planning of biopsies, surgeries, focal ablative, radiation, and minimally invasive (e.g., intensity focused ultrasound [33]) treatments. In addition, benign prostatic hyperplasia, also called prostate enlargement, is one of the most common conditions affecting men [34]. A correlation between prostatic volume, and the incidence of prostate cancer, where early tumor identification is crucial to reduce mortality, has been shown in [35]. Since only part of prostate cancer is clinically significant, risk stratification is mandatory to avoid over-diagnosis and over-treatment [36,37]. For this reason, radiomics in MRI has acquired a crucial role in the risk stratification process [19,36]. MRI allows calculating prostatic volume considering the prostate as an ellipsoid. Unfortunately, the shape of the prostate varies and the determination of its volume based on the ellipsoid formula is often incorrect [38]. The presence of prostate cancer may alter the prostate volume as reported, for example, in the study of [39]: the authors reported that shape differences in the prostate gland were consistently observed between patients with or without prostate cancer maybe as the result of cancer localized in the peripheral zone. For this reason, the manual delineation is more accurate than the previously described method but takes time, requires experience, and is highly operator-dependent as noted above. Consequently, several automatic algorithms have been proposed, for example, [40–42]. Due to the lack of large amounts of labeled data for the training process, DL is still far from a widespread application in the biomedical environment. So, there is a need to develop DL networks to obtain accurate delineations with fewer training examples. Then, we explore the efficacy of Efficient Neural Network (ENet) [43] and Efficient Residual Factorized ConvNet (ERFNet) [44] that are mainly applied in self-driving cars to compensate for limited hardware availability while still achieving accurate segmentation, and UNet that is used in many biomedical image delineation applications [45]. Using a limited set of 85 manual prostate segmentation training data, we show that ENet model can be used to obtain accurate, fast and clinically acceptable prostate segmentations.

2. Materials and Methods

2.1. Experimental Setup

To test DL based methods for prostate segmentation, we used prostate studies of patients who underwent MRI examinations using the Achieva scanner (Philips Healthcare, Best, The Netherlands) with a pelvic phased-array coil (8 channel HD Torso XL). Specifically, from September 2019 to May 2020, 202 consecutive patients were referred to our Radiology Department to perform a prostate MRI examination. We excluded patients from the study for (a) incomplete MRI examination due to intolerance, discomfort, or claustrophobia (n = 11); (b) patients with radical prostatectomy (n = 18), subjected to transurethral resection of the prostate (TURP) (n = 20), or radiotherapy (n = 17); (c) lack of median lobe enlargement defined as intra-vesical prostatic protrusion characterized by overgrowth of the prostatic median lobe into the bladder for at least 1 cm (n = 51). So, our final study population consisted of 85 patients (age range 43–75 years, mean age 59 ± 8.4 years) with median lobe enlargement. By reviewing radiological reports, no pathological MRI findings were found in 35 patients (except for median lobe enlargement), while 50 prostate lesions (42 in peripheral zone and 8 in transitional zone) suspected for prostate cancer classified using the Prostate imaging reporting and data system (PI-RADS) 2.1 [46] were found: 18 PI-RADS 3 score, 28 PI-RADS 4 score, and 4 PI-RADS 5 score lesions with size ranged between 0.6 and 1.9 cm (mean 1.052 ± 0.28). In addition, in our study population, by evaluating capsular involvement, 18 patients had capsular abutment and 3 patients had capsular irregularity. It means that the presence of suspected prostate cancer lesions, in our study population, can at least distend the gland boundaries. Consequently, the determination of prostate volume using the above mentioned ellipsoid formula [38] is not suitable, while manual and automatic segmentations are not (or less) affected by this issue.

In this study, axial T2-weighted images with parameters shown in Table 1 were used. However, due to MRI protocol routine update during the study time, datasets had different resolution (2 studies with a matrix resolution of 720 × 720; 45 studies with a matrix resolution of 672 × 672; 23 studies with a matrix resolution of 576 × 576; 15 studies with a matrix resolution of 320 × 320). Consequently, the datasets had different resolutions and sizes. Since DL networks require inputs of the same size for the training process, MRI images were resampled to the isotropic voxel size of 1 × 1 × 1 mm^3 with a matrix resolution of 512 × 512 (matrix resolution in the middle between 720 and 320) using linear interpolation. A set of trained clinical experts (FV, MP, GC, and GS authors) hand segmented the prostate region. The simultaneous ground truth estimation STAPLE tool [47] was used to combine the different segmentations from the clinical experts in a consolidated reference. Finally, manual delineations were resampled using nearest neighbor interpolation and converted to masks with 0 for the background and 1 for the prostate area.

Table 1. Parameter of MRI protocol.

Parameter	Repetition Time (ms)	Echo Time (ms)	Flip Angle (Degrees)	Signal Averages	Signal-to-Noise Ratio
T2w TSE	3091	100	90	3	1

2.2. Deep Learning Models

Three different deep learning models including UNet [45], ENet [43], and ERFNet [44] were investigated to account for accurate prostate segmentation, fast training time, low hardware requirements for inference, and low training data requirements. Specifically, UNet was modified to improve segmentation accuracy, as reported in [48,49]. Briefly, (i) 3 × 3 convolutions were replaced by 5 × 5 convolutions, (ii) zero padding was used to ensure that the size of the output feature maps was the same as the input size, and (iii) an input size of 512 × 512 with 32 filters was used on the first contraction path layer, with doubling of feature maps after each max pool and stopping at 256 feature maps and 2D size of 64 × 64.

Concerning ENet and ERFNet (see Table 1 in [43] and Table 2 in [44] for the description of their architecture), they were mainly applied in self-driving cars to compensate for limited hardware availability maintaining high accuracy and successfully used in two biomedical segmentation issues [48,49], that is, in the segmentation of high resolution computed tomography (HRCT) images characterized by a slice thickness much lower than that of the T2 weighted images of the prostate studies. This means that the number of slices of each patients' study was much greater than in this study.

Table 2. The model parameters and shape output after the first hidden layer in the ENet model for a given provided input image (Patient #7 slice #20).

Layer (Type)	Output Shape	Parameters Number
input_1 (InputLayer)	(None, 512, 512, 1)	0
conv2d_1 (Conv2D)	(None, 256, 256, 15)	150

2.3. Training Methodology

Due to a limited amount of data, the k-fold cross-validation strategy was applied by randomly dividing the dataset into k sub-datasets of equal size (17 patients, k = 5). For each network, we trained k models by combining k-1 folds into the training set and keeping the remaining fold as a holdout test set. Despite the fact that 2D models were considered, slices from the same study were never used for both training and testing purposes. So, there was no cross-contamination between training and test sets.

Moreover, the data augmentation technique was applied in six different modalities to increase the statistic. Additionally, data standardization and normalization were adopted to prevent the weights from becoming too large, to make the model converge faster, and to avoid numerical instability. Regarding loss function, prostate segmentation suffers from the imbalanced data problem because there are very few examples of the positive class compared to the background or negative class. In terms of image segmentation, the target (i.e., the prostatic region) is small compared to the background, which may be composed of many different organs or types of tissue exhibiting a wide range of intensity values. Some slices may have a very small target area compared to the background. This makes it hard for the DL to learn a reliable feature representation of the foreground class. In such cases, the networks tend to simply predict most voxels as belonging to the background class. To deal with this problem, various loss functions have been proposed over the years. These loss functions typically aim to solve the class imbalance problem by providing a larger weight to foreground voxels. This translates to a higher penalty in the loss function for foreground voxels that are misclassified by the network leading to the network being able to learn the foreground object representation more effectively. One such loss function which the authors of this paper have experimentally determined to be better suited for the biomedical image delineation process is the Tversky loss function [50]. Specifically, the Dice similarity coefficient (DSC) between P and G is defined as:

$$\text{DSC} = \frac{2|P \cap G|}{|P| + |G|} \qquad (1)$$

where P and G are the predicted and ground truth labels. DSC measures the overlap between P and G and is used as a loss function in many DL approaches. Nevertheless, DSC is the harmonic mean of false positives and false negatives and weighs both equally. To modify their weights, the Tversky index [51] was proposed as:

$$S(P, G; \alpha, \beta) = \frac{|P \cap G|}{|P \cap G| + \alpha|P \setminus G| + \beta|G \setminus P|} \qquad (2)$$

α and β control the penalty magnitude of false positives and false negatives. Using this index, the Tversky loss [50] is defined as:

$$T(\alpha\ \beta) = \frac{\sum_{i=1}^{N} p_{0i}\ g_{0i}}{\sum_{i=1}^{N} p_{0i}\ g_{0i} + \alpha \sum_{i=1}^{N} p_{0i}\ g_{1i} + \beta \sum_{i=1}^{N} p_{1i}\ g_{0i}} \qquad (3)$$

Additional information about the study design is shown in Figure 1.

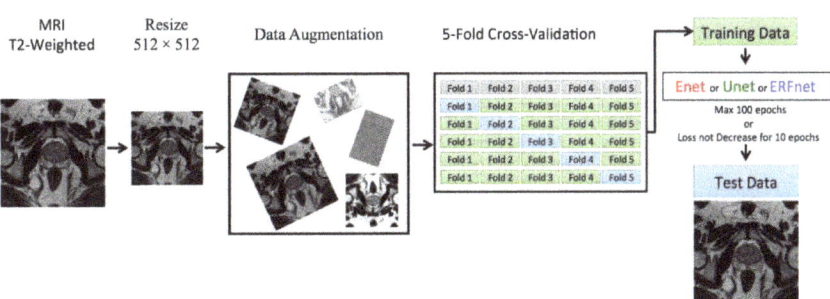

Figure 1. Workflow of the proposed segmentation method.

Starting from 16 patients, the best learning rates for each network were determined experimentally. We used a learning rate of 0.0001 for ENet, 0.00001 for ERFNet, and UNet with Adam optimizer [52]. A batch size of eight slices, α and β of 0.3 and 0.7, respectively for the Tversky loss function, were identified. All the models were allowed to train for a maximum of 100 epochs with an automatic stopping criteria of ending training when the loss did not decrease for 10 epochs continuously. The GEFORCE RTX 2080 Ti with 11GB of RAM (NVIDIA) was used to train DL models and run inference. Table 2 and Figure 2 show the feature representation learned from the first hidden layer in the ENet model.

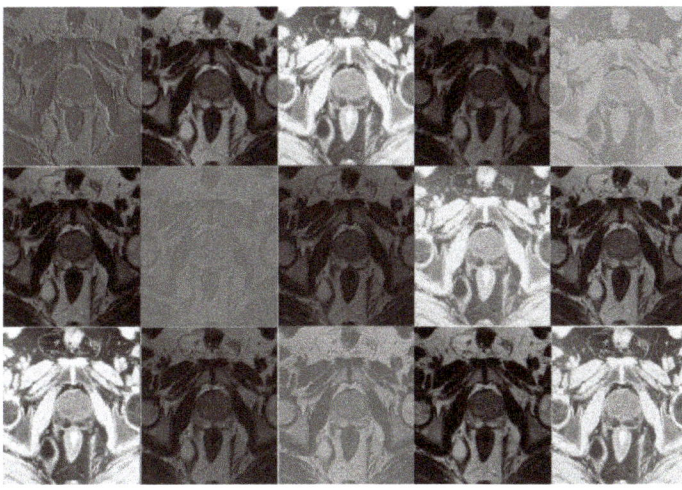

Figure 2. Feature maps (None, 256, 256, 15) extracted from the first hidden layer in the ENet Model for Patient #7 slice #20.

3. Results

Sensitivity, positive predictive value (PPV), DSC, volume overlap error (VOE), and volumetric difference (VD) were used for performance evaluation:

$$\text{Sensitivity} = \frac{TP}{TN + FN} \tag{4}$$

$$\text{PPV} = \frac{TP}{TP + FN} \tag{5}$$

$$\text{DSC} = \frac{2TP}{2TP + FP + FN} \tag{6}$$

$$\text{VOE} = 1 - \frac{TP}{TP + FP + FN} \tag{7}$$

$$\text{DSC} = \frac{2TP}{2TP + FP + FN} \quad \text{DSC} = \frac{2|P \cap G|}{|P| + |G|} \tag{8}$$

Table 3 shows the performance obtained using ENet, UNet, and ERFNet methods. In particular, ENet showed a mean DSC of 90.89 ± 3.87%, UNet of 90.14 ± 4.69%, and ERFNet of 87.18 ± 6.44%.

Table 3. Performance segmentation using the ENet, UNet, and ERFNet methods.

	Sensitivity	PPV	DSC	VOE	VD
	ENet				
Mean	93.06%	89.25%	90.89%	16.50%	4.53%
±std	6.37%	3.94%	3.87%	5.86%	9.43%
±CI (95%)	1.36%	0.84%	0.82%	1.24%	2.00%
	UNet				
Mean	88.89%	91.89%	90.14%	17.66%	3.16%
± std	7.61%	3.31%	4.69%	6.91%	9.36%
±CI (95%)	1.62%	0.70%	1.00%	1.47%	1.99%
	ERFNet				
Mean	89.93%	85.44%	87.18%	22.18%	5.70%
±std	10.92%	5.43%	6.44%	9.61%	14.72%
±CI (95%)	2.32%	1.16%	1.37%	2.04%	3.13%

Analysis of variance (ANOVA) based on DSC was calculated to test statistical differences (a p-value < 0.05 indicates a significant difference) between methods considering all patients (n = 85). Table 4 shows how though ENet and UNet minimized the difference between manual and automated segmentation.

Table 4. ANOVA on the DSC showed statistical differences between segmentation methods.

ANOVA	F Value	F Critic Value	p-Value
ENet vs. ERFNet	20.70407668	3.897407169	0.000010236
ERFNet vs. UNet	11.69135829	3.897407169	0.000788084
ENet vs. UNet	1.301554482	3.897407169	0.255553164

Despite the fact that they were statistically identical, they were computationally different. ENet is much faster than UNet. Specifically, Table 5 shows the comparison of computational complexity and performance of the three models. As both ENet and

ERFNet were developed for real-time applications, these are relatively smaller and faster than UNet. As shown in the table, the ENet model has an order of magnitude with fewer parameters than both ERFNet, and UNet while ERFNet has less than half the number of parameters compared to UNet. Consequently, the size of trained ENet is only 6 MB compared to 65 MB for the UNet model. To estimate the delineation time, we considered one of the trained models during the k-fold strategy for all three architectures and then computed the average. Using a fairly advanced GPU device (GEFORCE RTX 2080 Ti, 11 GB VRAM, 4352 CUDA Cores, NVIDIA), it takes only 1 s for ENet and about 1.5 s for UNet to generate segmentation on a 3D dataset (average 40 slices of 512×512). However, when GPU hardware is not available then computation needs to be done on the CPU. In such a scenario, the size of a model can play a big role. On an AMD Ryzen 2950x processor, ENet only takes about 6 s while UNet takes about 40 s to delineate a study. Soon, this computational advantage of ENet may make it possible to use this model to segment cases on simple hardware like IPads or smartphones for faster clinical workflow. Finally, only the ENet model makes use of batch normalization layers, which have some parameters which are not trained, that is, gradients are not back-propagated during the training process.

Table 5. Computational complexity of the three models.

Model Name	Number of Parameters		Size on Disk	Inference Times/Dataset	
	Trainable	Non-Trainable		CPU	GPU
ENet	362,992	8352	5.8 MB	6.17 s	1.07 s
ERFNet	2,056,440	0	25.3 MB	8.59 s	1.03 s
UNet	5,403,874	0	65.0 MB	42.02 s	1.57 s

In Figure 3, we plot the training DSC and Tversky loss function for each DL network for one fold. DSC and Tversky loss plots indicate that the ENet model converges much faster than both ERFNet and UNet. ENet model reaches a DSC = 0.85 in less than 15 epochs. Consequently, it is much faster to train a new ENet model compared to the other two if more training data become available in the future. Another noticeable feature is that the UNet training loss is much less compared to ENet and ERFNet, indicating the presence of overfitting. It can be concluded that even though ENet and UNet models are not statistically different, it may be advantageous to prefer ENet over UNet. Finally, 2D and 3D segmentation examples of three patient studies are shown in Figures 4 and 5, respectively.

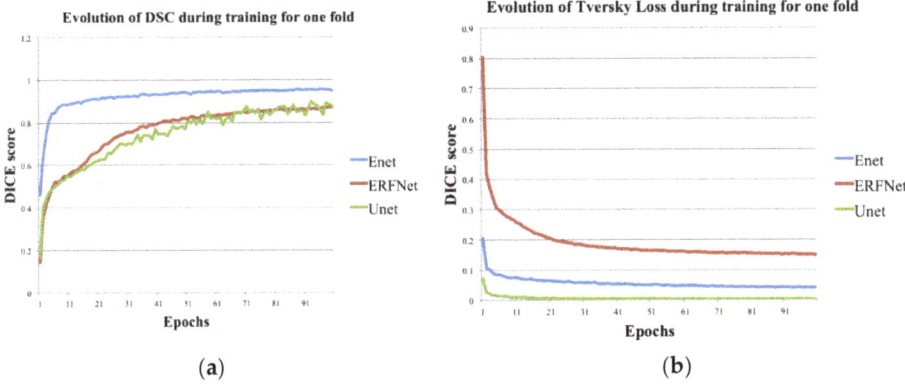

Figure 3. (a) Training DSC and (b) loss function Tversky loss plots for each of the three models for one fold.

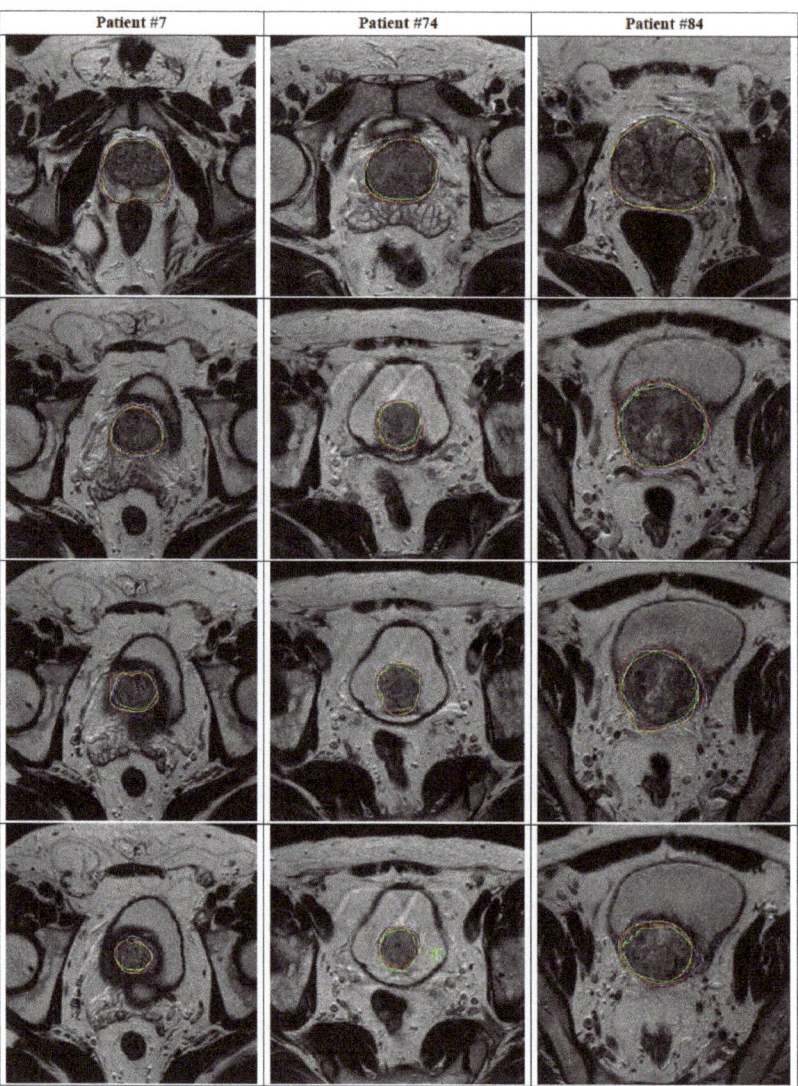

Figure 4. Comparison of segmentation performance for the three Net architectures in #7, #74, and #84 patients (four different slices for each patient). The manual segmentation (yellow), ENet (red), ERFNet (blue), and U-Net (green) are superimposed.

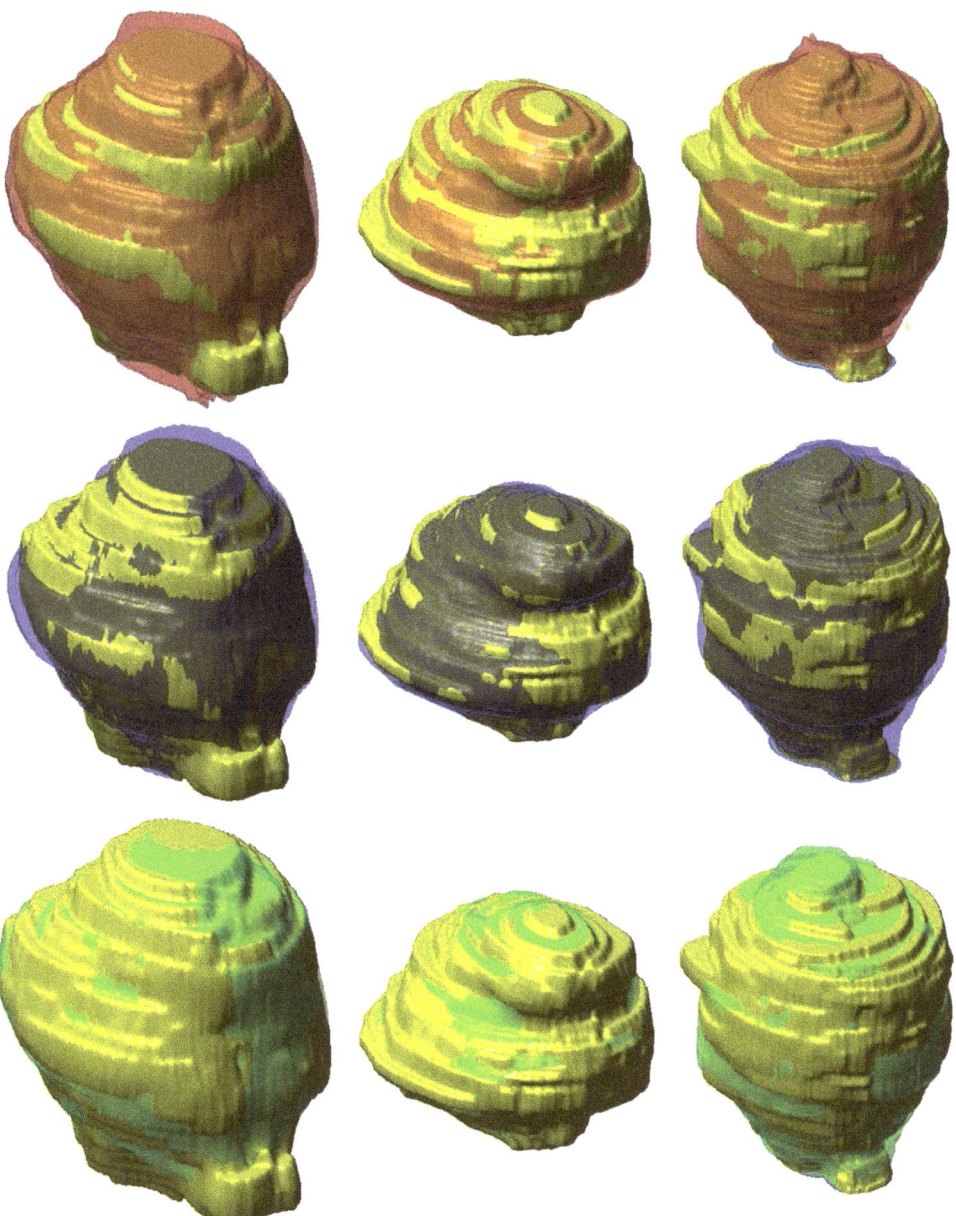

Figure 5. Comparison of 3D segmentation of prostate (patients #7, #74, and #84) for each column using the three Net architectures. The manual segmentation (yellow), ENet (red), ERFNet (blue), and U-Net (green) are superimposed.

4. Discussion

In this paper, we investigate the prostatic region segmentation in MRI studies using three different DL networks (namely UNet, ENet, and ERFNet). The aim is to reduce patient mortality being only a part of prostate cancer that is clinically significant. An accurate and operator-independent segmentation process is needed to obtain a relevant texture-based prediction model. So, the aim of this work was not only just to test the segmentation results of the proposed models, but to evaluate if these models can yield a practical benefit in obtaining accurate and reproducible results. The inclusion of DL models in radiomics analyses will be reserved for a forthcoming paper. The first model considered in this study was UNet, which has been adopted in several image delineation processes [45]. ENet [43], and ERFNet [44] have been implemented for the segmentation process in self-driving cars, and successfully used in lung and aorta segmentation tasks [48,49]. Specifically, they were used for the segmentation of HRCT images characterized by a very high number of slices for each study (about 600 and 450 slices for the lung and aorta studies, respectively). Authors used 32 patients' studies for the parenchyma extraction process [49], and 72 studies for the aorta segmentation process [48]. In this study, only 85 studies were used considering that each patients' image dataset consists of about 40 slices. In addition, to our knowledge, these DL models have never been applied to prostate segmentation before.

In general, a DL approach requires a multitude of labeled data for training and validation purposes. For this reason, DL models are not widely used in clinical practice. As already reported in the Introduction section, there is a need to develop DL networks capable of obtaining accurate segmentations with few training examples. This issue is addressed in some studies, that is, the one-shot learning approach [53], which eliminates the need for iterative sample selection and annotation and the contrastive learning method [29] for the automated diagnosis of COVID-19 with few samples for training. In our study, we applied all three DL models to a small dataset of 85 studies provided with manual prostate segmentation adopting (i) a data augmentation strategy to reduce overfitting, (ii) a data standardization and normalization to prevent too large weights, to make the model converge faster, and to avoid numerical instability, (iii) the five-fold cross-validation strategy to obtain good results despite the few training examples, and (iv) the Tversky loss function [50] to avoid to predict most voxels as belonging to the background class. In the last case, starting from the consideration that DL methods suffer from the imbalanced data problem because the target (i.e., the prostate) is very small compared to the background, we provided a larger weight to target voxels to learn the foreground object representation more effectively. Finally, we compared the obtained performances showing that accurate and clinically acceptable prostate segmentations with few training examples were obtained using indifferently the three DL models (DSC > 87%).

Specifically, results showed that ENet and UNet had better performance in minimizing the difference between automated and manual segmentations than ERFNet. Substantially, ENet and UNet were statistically identical but computationally different; ENet was much faster than UNet (see Figure 3). Also, the training Tversky loss of the UNet was much less compared to ENet. For these reasons, though UNet and ENet were not statistically different, ENet seems to be the best solution. This could justify the time required to include DL networks in radiomics analyses by removing the user-dependence and achieving accurate prostate segmentations (DSC = 90.89%) using a few training examples. In this way, our model can be used to improve prognosis evaluation and prediction of patient outcomes, allowing the personalization of patient management. However, the results presented in this study derive from the performance of DL networks on proprietary imaging datasets; for routine clinical application, it should be mandatory to test and validate the proposed methods in multicenter studies and/or on a large set of publicly released representative training data, such as PROMISE12 [42]. Moreover, in the present study, we test DL networks for the whole prostate gland segmentation, with ENet demonstrating the best performance; however, a main clinical goal is the segmentation of related prostatic structures or substructures such as the prostatic zones (transition, central and peripheral), neurovascular bundles or seminal vesicles. The performance of DL networks, especially ENet, on this topic should play an essential role in many medical imaging and image analysis tasks such as cancer detection, patient management, and treatment planning including surgical planning, and should be analyzed in future works. Automatic segmentation of the whole prostate gland and prostatic zone (transition, central and peripheral) without inter-user variability will lead, in the future, to a correct localization of prostate cancer. This result will increase the reliability of computer-aided design (CAD) algorithms which will help automatically create PI-RADS zone maps to reduce inter-user variability among clinicians when interpreting prostate MRI images. In this scenario, radiomics analysis should be performed automatically providing information that can lead clinicians on the management of patients with prostate cancer.

5. Conclusions

Our study demonstrates that faster and less computationally expensive DL networks can perform accurate prostate delineation and could facilitate the adoption of novel imaging parameters, through radiomics analyses, for prostatic oncologic diseases. Specifically, we assessed the performance of three DL networks using data augmentation, standardization, and normalization, and the five-fold cross-validation strategies, and the Tversky loss function in a small dataset of 85 studies. All DL networks achieved accurate prostate segmentations with a DSC > 87%. Nevertheless, differences related to training time and data requirements were highlighted. ENet and ERFNet, developed for self-driving cars, were much faster than UNet. In addition, ENet had better performance (DSC = 90.89%) than ERFNet (DSC = 87.18%). Future studies with more patients could improve the results.

Author Contributions: Conceptualization, A.C. and G.S.; Data curation, F.V. and G.S.; Formal analysis, A.C.; Funding acquisition, A.S. and A.C.; Investigation, A.S.; Methodology, A.S. and A.C.; Project administration, A.Y.; Resources, F.V., M.P., G.C., A.B., G.S.; Software, A.C. and N.D.; Supervision, A.Y.; Validation, F.V.; Visualization, A.C. and A.S. Writing—original draft, A.C., N.D., A.S., and F.V.; Writing—review and editing, A.C. and A.S. All authors have read and agreed to the published version of the manuscript.

Funding: This research received no external funding.

Informed Consent Statement: This retrospective study was approved by the Institutional Review Board of our Hospital. Informed consent was obtained from all subjects involved in the study.

Data Availability Statement: Data sharing not applicable.

Acknowledgments: This work was partially supported by grant W911NF-18-1-0281, funded by the USA Army Research Office (ARO): "Extending Accelerated Optimization into the PDE Framework", and by grant R01-HL-143350 funded by the National Institute of Health (NIH) "Quantification of myocardial blood flow using Dynamic PET/CTA fused imagery to determine physiological significance of specific coronary lesions".

Conflicts of Interest: The authors declare no conflict of interest. The funders had no role in the design of the study; in the collection, analyses, or interpretation of data; in the writing of the manuscript; or in the decision to publish the results.

References

1. Stefano, A.; Comelli, A.; Bravatà, V.; Barone, S.; Daskalovski, I.; Savoca, G.; Sabini, M.G.; Ippolito, M.; Russo, G. A preliminary PET radiomics study of brain metastases using a fully automatic segmentation method. *BMC Bioinform.* **2020**, *21*, 325. [CrossRef]
2. Cuocolo, R.; Stanzione, A.; Ponsiglione, A.; Romeo, V.; Verde, F.; Creta, M.; La Rocca, R.; Longo, N.; Pace, L.; Imbriaco, M. Clinically significant prostate cancer detection on MRI: A radiomic shape features study. *Eur. J. Radiol.* **2019**, *116*, 144–149. [CrossRef]
3. Baeßler, B.; Weiss, K.; Santos, D.P. Dos Robustness and Reproducibility of Radiomics in Magnetic Resonance Imaging: A Phantom Study. *Investig. Radiol.* **2019**, *54*, 221–228.
4. Gallivanone, F.; Interlenghi, M.; D'Ambrosio, D.; Trifirò, G.; Castiglioni, I. Parameters influencing PET imaging features: A phantom study with irregular and heterogeneous synthetic lesions. *Contrast Media Mol. Imaging* **2018**, *2018*, 12. [CrossRef]
5. Comelli, A.; Stefano, A.; Coronnello, C.; Russo, G.; Vernuccio, F.; Cannella, R.; Salvaggio, G.; Lagalla, R.; Barone, S. *Radiomics: A New Biomedical Workflow to Create a Predictive Model*; Springer: Cham, Switzerland, 2020; pp. 280–293.
6. Comelli, A.; Stefano, A.; Russo, G.; Sabini, M.G.; Ippolito, M.; Bignardi, S.; Petrucci, G.; Yezzi, A. A smart and operator independent system to delineate tumours in Positron Emission Tomography scans. *Comput. Biol. Med.* **2018**, *102*, 1–15. [CrossRef]
7. Dahiya, N.; Yezzi, A.; Piccinelli, M.; Garcia, E. Integrated 3D anatomical model for automatic myocardial segmentation in cardiac CT imagery. *Comput. Methods Biomech. Biomed. Eng. Imaging Vis.* **2019**, *7*, 690–706. [CrossRef]

8. Comelli, A. Fully 3D Active Surface with Machine Learning for PET Image Segmentation. *J. Imaging* **2020**, *6*, 113. [CrossRef]
9. Foster, B.; Bagci, U.; Mansoor, A.; Xu, Z.; Mollura, D.J. A review on segmentation of positron emission tomography images. *Comput. Biol. Med.* **2014**, *50*, 76–96. [CrossRef] [PubMed]
10. Bi, L.; Kim, J.; Wen, L.; Feng, D.; Fulham, M. Automated thresholded region classification using a robust feature selection method for PET-CT. In Proceedings of the International Symposium on Biomedical Imaging, Brooklyn, NY, USA, 16–19 April 2015; Volume 2015-July.
11. Dhanachandra, N.; Manglem, K.; Chanu, Y.J. Image Segmentation Using K-means Clustering Algorithm and Subtractive Clustering Algorithm. In Proceedings of the Procedia Computer Science, Algiers, Algeria, 18–19 October 2015.
12. Chevrefils, C.; Chériet, F.; Grimard, G.; Aubin, C.E. Watershed segmentation of intervertebral disk and spinal canal from MRI images. In Proceedings of the Lecture Notes in Computer Science (including subseries Lecture Notes in Artificial Intelligence and Lecture Notes in Bioinformatics), Redondo Beach, CA, USA, 8–11 July 2007.
13. Comelli, A.; Bignardi, S.; Stefano, A.; Russo, G.; Sabini, M.G.; Ippolito, M.; Yezzi, A. Development of a new fully three-dimensional methodology for tumours delineation in functional images. *Comput. Biol. Med.* **2020**, *120*, 103701. [CrossRef]
14. Boykov, Y.; Veksler, O.; Zabih, R. Fast approximate energy minimization via graph cuts. *Pattern Anal. Mach. Intell. IEEE Trans.* **2001**, *23*, 1222–1239. [CrossRef]
15. Stefano, A.; Vitabile, S.; Russo, G.; Ippolito, M.; Marletta, F.; D'arrigo, C.; D'urso, D.; Gambino, O.; Pirrone, R.; Ardizzone, E.; et al. A fully automatic method for biological target volume segmentation of brain metastases. *Int. J. Imaging Syst. Technol.* **2016**, *26*, 29–37. [CrossRef]
16. Plath, N.; Toussaint, M.; Nakajima, S. Multi-class image segmentation using conditional random fields and global classification. In Proceedings of the 26th International Conference on Machine Learning, ICML 2009, Montreal, QC, Canada, 14–18 June 2009.
17. Dey, D.; Slomka, P.J.; Leeson, P.; Comaniciu, D.; Shrestha, S.; Sengupta, P.P.; Marwick, T.H. Artificial Intelligence in Cardiovascular Imaging: JACC State-of-the-Art Review. *J. Am. Coll. Cardiol.* **2019**, *73*, 1317–1335. [CrossRef] [PubMed]
18. Zhou, T.; Fu, H.; Zhang, Y.; Zhang, C.; Lu, X.; Shen, J.; Shao, L. M2Net: Multi-modal Multi-channel Network for overall survival time prediction of brain tumor patients. *arXiv* **2020**, arXiv:2006.10135.
19. Cuocolo, R.; Cipullo, M.B.; Stanzione, A.; Ugga, L.; Romeo, V.; Radice, L.; Brunetti, A.; Imbriaco, M. Machine learning applications in prostate cancer magnetic resonance imaging. *Eur. Radiol. Exp.* **2019**, *3*, 35. [CrossRef] [PubMed]
20. Long, J.; Shelhamer, E.; Darrell, T. Fully convolutional networks for semantic segmentation. In Proceedings of the IEEE Computer Society Conference on Computer Vision and Pattern Recognition, Boston, MA, USA, 7–12 June 2015.
21. Vincent, P.; Larochelle, H.; Lajoie, I.; Bengio, Y.; Manzagol, P.A. Stacked denoising autoencoders: Learning Useful Representations in a Deep Network with a Local Denoising Criterion. *J. Mach. Learn. Res.* **2010**, *11*, 3371–3408.
22. Zhao, H.; Shi, J.; Qi, X.; Wang, X.; Jia, J. Pyramid scene parsing network. In Proceedings of the 30th IEEE Conference on Computer Vision and Pattern Recognition, CVPR 2017, Honolulu, HI, USA, 21–26 July 2017.
23. Ghiasi, G.; Fowlkes, C.C. Laplacian pyramid reconstruction and refinement for semantic segmentation. In Proceedings of the Lecture Notes in Computer Science (including subseries Lecture Notes in Artificial Intelligence and Lecture Notes in Bioinformatics), Amsterdam, The Netherlands, 8–16 October 2016.
24. He, J.; Deng, Z.; Qiao, Y. Dynamic multi-scale filters for semantic segmentation. In Proceedings of the IEEE International Conference on Computer Vision, Seoul, Korea, 27 October–2 November 2019.
25. Chen, L.C.; Yang, Y.; Wang, J.; Xu, W.; Yuille, A.L. Attention to Scale: Scale-Aware Semantic Image Segmentation. In Proceedings of the IEEE Computer Society Conference on Computer Vision and Pattern Recognition, Las Vegas, NV, USA, 26 June–1 July 2016.
26. Hochreiter, S.; Schmidhuber, J. Long Short-Term Memory. *Neural Comput.* **1997**, *9*, 1735–1780. [CrossRef]
27. Radford, A.; Metz, L.; Chintala, S. Unsupervised representation learning with deep convolutional generative adversarial networks. In Proceedings of the 4th International Conference on Learning Representations, ICLR 2016—Conference Track Proceedings, San Juan, Puerto Rico, 2–4 May 2016.
28. Mirza, M.; Osindero, S. Conditional Generative Adversarial Nets Mehdi. *arXiv* **2018**, arXiv:1411.1784.
29. Chena, X.; Yao, L.; Zhou, T.; Dong, J.; Zhang, Y. Momentum Contrastive Learning for Few-Shot COVID-19 Diagnosis from Chest CT Images. *arXiv* **2020**, arXiv:2006.13276.
30. Chen, X.; Yao, L.; Zhang, Y. Residual attention U-net for automated multi-class segmentation of COVID-19 chest CT images. *arXiv* **2020**, arXiv:2004.05645.
31. Garcia-Garcia, A.; Orts-Escolano, S.; Oprea, S.; Villena-Martinez, V.; Martinez-Gonzalez, P.; Garcia-Rodriguez, J. A survey on deep learning techniques for image and video semantic segmentation. *Appl. Soft Comput. J.* **2018**, *70*, 41–65. [CrossRef]
32. Litjens, G.; Kooi, T.; Bejnordi, B.E.; Setio, A.A.A.; Ciompi, F.; Ghafoorian, M.; van der Laak, J.A.W.M.; van Ginneken, B.; Sánchez, C.I. A survey on deep learning in medical image analysis. *Med. Image Anal.* **2017**, *42*, 60–88. [CrossRef] [PubMed]
33. Borasi, G.; Russo, G.; Alongi, F.; Nahum, A.; Candiano, G.C.; Stefano, A.; Gilardi, M.C.; Messa, C. High-intensity focused ultrasound plus concomitant radiotherapy: A new weapon in oncology? *J. Ther. Ultrasound* **2013**, *1*, 6. [CrossRef] [PubMed]
34. Langan, R.C. Benign Prostatic Hyperplasia. *Prim. Care Clin. Off. Pract.* **2019**, *361*, 1359–1367. [CrossRef] [PubMed]
35. Zhang, L.; Wang, Y.; Qin, Z.; Gao, X.; Xing, Q.; Li, R.; Wang, W.; Song, N.; Zhang, W. Correlation between prostatitis, benign prostatic hyperplasia and prostate cancer: A systematic review and meta-analysis. *J. Cancer* **2020**, *11*, 177–189. [CrossRef]

36. Giambelluca, D.; Cannella, R.; Vernuccio, F.; Comelli, A.; Pavone, A.; Salvaggio, L.; Galia, M.; Midiri, M.; Lagalla, R.; Salvaggio, G. PI-RADS 3 Lesions: Role of Prostate MRI Texture Analysis in the Identification of Prostate Cancer. *Curr. Probl. Diagn. Radiol.* **2019**. In press. [CrossRef]
37. Cuocolo, R.; Stanzione, A.; Ponsiglione, A.; Verde, F.; Ventimiglia, A.; Romeo, V.; Petretta, M.; Imbriaco, M. Prostate MRI technical parameters standardization: A systematic review on adherence to PI-RADSv2 acquisition protocol. *Eur. J. Radiol.* **2019**, *120*, 108662. [CrossRef]
38. Turkbey, B.; Fotin, S.V.; Huang, R.J.; Yin, Y.; Daar, D.; Aras, O.; Bernardo, M.; Garvey, B.E.; Weaver, J.; Haldankar, H.; et al. Fully automated prostate segmentation on MRI: Comparison with manual segmentation methods and specimen volumes. *Am. J. Roentgenol.* **2013**, *201*, W720–W729. [CrossRef]
39. Rusu, M.; Purysko, A.S.; Verma, S.; Kiechle, J.; Gollamudi, J.; Ghose, S.; Herrmann, K.; Gulani, V.; Paspulati, R.; Ponsky, L.; et al. Computational imaging reveals shape differences between normal and malignant prostates on MRI. *Sci. Rep.* **2017**, *7*, 1–11. [CrossRef]
40. Comelli, A.; Terranova, M.C.; Scopelliti, L.; Salerno, S.; Midiri, F.; Lo Re, G.; Petrucci, G.; Vitabile, S. A kernel support vector machine based technique for Crohn's disease classification in human patients. In Proceedings of the Advances in Intelligent Systems and Computing, Torino, Italy, 10–12 July 2017; Springer: Cham, Switzerland, 2018; Volume 611, pp. 262–273.
41. Ghose, S.; Oliver, A.; Martí, R.; Lladó, X.; Vilanova, J.C.; Freixenet, J.; Mitra, J.; Sidibé, D.; Meriaudeau, F. A survey of prostate segmentation methodologies in ultrasound, magnetic resonance and computed tomography images. *Comput. Methods Programs Biomed.* **2012**, *108*, 262–287. [CrossRef]
42. Litjens, G.; Toth, R.; van de Ven, W.; Hoeks, C.; Kerkstra, S.; van Ginneken, B.; Vincent, G.; Guillard, G.; Birbeck, N.; Zhang, J.; et al. Evaluation of prostate segmentation algorithms for MRI: The PROMISE12 challenge. *Med. Image Anal.* **2014**, *18*, 359–373. [CrossRef]
43. Paszke, A.; Chaurasia, A.; Kim, S.; Culurciello, E. ENet: A Deep Neural Network Architecture for Real-Time Semantic Segmentation. *arXiv* **2016**, arXiv:1606.02147.
44. Romera, E.; Alvarez, J.M.; Bergasa, L.M.; Arroyo, R. ERFNet: Efficient Residual Factorized ConvNet for Real-Time Semantic Segmentation. *IEEE Trans. Intell. Transp. Syst.* **2018**, *19*, 263–272. [CrossRef]
45. Ronneberger, O.; Fischer, P.; Brox, T. U-net: Convolutional networks for biomedical image segmentation. In Proceedings of the Lecture Notes in Computer Science (Including Subseries Lecture Notes in Artificial Intelligence and Lecture Notes in Bioinformatics), Fuzhou, China, 13–15 November 2015.
46. Prostate Imaging Reporting & Data System (PI-RADS). Available online: https://www.acr.org/Clinical-Resources/Reporting-and-Data-Systems/PI-RADS (accessed on 17 February 2019).
47. Warfield, S.K.; Zou, K.H.; Wells, W.M. Simultaneous truth and performance level estimation (STAPLE): An algorithm for the validation of image segmentation. *IEEE Trans. Med. Imaging* **2004**, *23*, 903–921. [CrossRef] [PubMed]
48. Comelli, A.; Dahiya, N.; Stefano, A.; Benfante, V.; Gentile, G.; Agnese, V.; Raffa, G.M.; Pilato, M.; Yezzi, A.; Petrucci, G.; et al. Deep learning approach for the segmentation of aneurysmal ascending aorta. *Biomed. Eng. Lett.* **2020**, 1–10. [CrossRef]
49. Comelli, A.; Coronnello, C.; Dahiya, N.; Benfante, V.; Palmucci, S.; Basile, A.; Vancheri, C.; Russo, G.; Yezzi, A.; Stefano, A. Lung Segmentation on High-Resolution Computerized Tomography Images Using Deep Learning: A Preliminary Step for Radiomics Studies. *J. Imaging* **2020**, *6*, 125. [CrossRef]
50. Salehi, S.S.M.; Erdogmus, D.; Gholipour, A. Tversky loss function for image segmentation using 3D fully convolutional deep networks. In Proceedings of the Lecture Notes in Computer Science (Including Subseries Lecture Notes in Artificial Intelligence and Lecture Notes in Bioinformatics), Quebec City, QC, Canada, 10 September 2017; pp. 379–387.
51. Tversky, A. Features of similarity. *Psychol. Rev.* **1977**, *84*, 327. [CrossRef]
52. Kingma, D.P.; Ba, J.L. Adam: A method for stochastic optimization. In Proceedings of the 3rd International Conference on Learning Representations, ICLR 2015—Conference Track Proceedings, San Diego, CA, USA, 7–9 May 2015.
53. Zheng, H.; Yang, L.; Chen, J.; Han, J.; Zhang, Y.; Liang, P.; Zhao, Z.; Wang, C.; Chen, D.Z. Biomedical image segmentation via representative annotation. In Proceedings of the 33rd AAAI Conference on Artificial Intelligence, AAAI 2019, Honolulu, HI, USA, 27 January–1 February 2019; pp. 5901–5908.

Article

Estimation of the Prostate Volume from Abdominal Ultrasound Images by Image-Patch Voting

Nur Banu Albayrak * and Yusuf Sinan Akgul

Department of Computer Engineering, Gebze Technical University, Kocaeli 41400, Turkey; akgul@gtu.edu.tr
* Correspondence: nbalbayrak@gtu.edu.tr

Abstract: Estimation of the prostate volume with ultrasound offers many advantages such as portability, low cost, harmlessness, and suitability for real-time operation. Abdominal Ultrasound (AUS) is a practical procedure that deserves more attention in automated prostate-volume-estimation studies. As the experts usually consider automatic end-to-end volume-estimation procedures as non-transparent and uninterpretable systems, we proposed an expert-in-the-loop automatic system that follows the classical prostate-volume-estimation procedures. Our system directly estimates the diameter parameters of the standard ellipsoid formula to produce the prostate volume. To obtain the diameters, our system detects four diameter endpoints from the transverse and two diameter endpoints from the sagittal AUS images as defined by the classical procedure. These endpoints are estimated using a new image-patch voting method to address characteristic problems of AUS images. We formed a novel prostate AUS data set from 305 patients with both transverse and sagittal planes. The data set includes MRI images for 75 of these patients. At least one expert manually marked all the data. Extensive experiments performed on this data set showed that the proposed system results ranged among experts' volume estimations, and our system can be used in clinical practice.

Keywords: computer-aided diagnosis; medical-image analysis; automated prostate-volume estimation; abdominal ultrasound images; image-patch voting

Citation: Albayrak, N.B.; Akgul, Y.S. Estimation of the Prostate Volume from Abdominal Ultrasound Images by Image-Patch Voting. *Appl. Sci.* 2022, 12, 1390. https://doi.org/10.3390/app12031390

Academic Editors: Alessandro Stefano, Albert Comelli and Federica Vernuccio

Received: 11 December 2021
Accepted: 20 January 2022
Published: 27 January 2022

Publisher's Note: MDPI stays neutral with regard to jurisdictional claims in published maps and institutional affiliations.

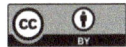

Copyright: © 2022 by the authors. Licensee MDPI, Basel, Switzerland. This article is an open access article distributed under the terms and conditions of the Creative Commons Attribution (CC BY) license (https://creativecommons.org/licenses/by/4.0/).

1. Introduction

Prostate volume is a crucial parameter in many clinical practices. It plays an essential role in the diagnosis of benign prostatic hyperplasia (BPH) [1]. BPH is a widespread prostatic disease that affects most aged men [2]. Clinicians use prostate volume while managing lower urinary tract symptoms (LUTS) [3]. Another critical area for prostate volume is the calculation of the Prostate-Specific Antigen Density (PSAD) value to detect and manage prostate cancer (PCa) [4]. PCa was the second most prevalent cancer for the year 2020 and the most prevalent cancer for the last five years among men [5]. PSAD plays a role as one of the criteria for active surveillance decisions in clinical practice [6]. Combining PSAD with other scores may help to decide biopsies [7].

There are many medical-imaging technologies to estimate prostate volume. Widely used technologies are Magnetic Resonance Imaging (MRI), Computed Tomography (CT), and Ultrasound (US) [8]. US technology differs from others with its portability, low-cost, and harmlessness, and it allows experts to scan the prostate in real-time [9]. Trans Rectal Ultrasound (TRUS) and Abdominal Ultrasound (AUS) technologies are frequently used in prostate applications. As shown in Figure 1, despite its better imaging quality with a higher Signal-to-Noise Ratio (SNR) and a larger view of the prostate with no other anatomic structures, TRUS technology is difficult to use regularly during successive radiotherapy sequences [10] due to patient discomfort [11]. The AUS technique is an easy-to-use alternative US imaging technology and is often used where TRUS is not practical.

Conventionally, a prostate-volume measurement is done manually on medical images by experts. Manual volume estimation results in high intra-expert and inter-expert difference due to factors caused by imaging quality, personal experience, and human error [12], which suggests that the guidance of experts by automatic systems would be beneficial. Automated prostate-volume-estimation systems are also essential to reduce the time spent while measuring the prostate volume.

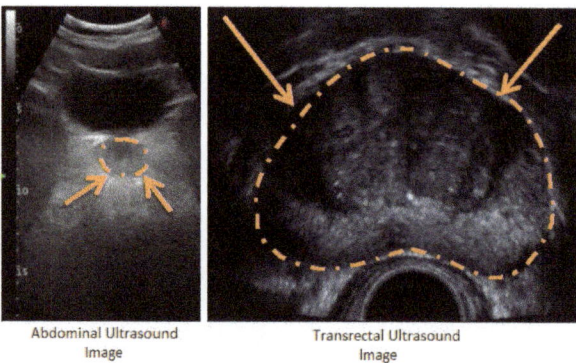

Figure 1. Comparison of AUS and TRUS images of the prostate from transverse plane. While AUS images have lower SNR and contain other anatomical structures, TRUS images have higher SNR, and the prostate is the only anatomical structure contained.

Segmentation and contour extraction methods are used in many studies to infer the prostate volume. However, when AUS images are considered in problems such as low SNR, artifacts and incomplete contours challenge even the state-of-the-art deep-learning techniques. That makes AUS imaging a rarely studied method for automatic prostate-volume measurement systems. This study aimed to demonstrate that an AUS-based automated system for measuring the prostate volume can be an alternative to TRUS, MRI, or CT-based systems.

In our study, we developed a method for estimating prostate volume by following the steps of the standard ellipsoid volume formula, which is not easily applicable in an end-to-end automated system. Our system gives both intermediate and final results, allowing both manual intervention and fully automated employment. To measure prostate volume, we estimated the three major diameters of the ellipsoid representing the prostate. Estimation of diameters was made by detecting four points from transverse and two points from sagittal AUS images. We call these points diameter endpoints. To overcome the characteristic problems of AUS images, we developed a voting-based method to detect points where various locations vote for distance and orientation values relative to each diameter endpoint. We designed a novel network model to carry out the voting process.

We were unable to compare our volume-estimation results with other studies as almost no other studies are available to estimate prostate volume from AUS images. Instead, we evaluated the difference in intra- and inter-expert volume estimates on AUS images and compared these values with our system estimates. Due to the higher SNR values and better image quality compared (Figure 2) to both AUS and TRUS images (Figure 1), MR image annotations are considered the gold standard [13] in prostate applications. Accordingly, we also evaluated the intra- and inter-expert volume estimation difference in MR images and compared these values with our system's volume estimations and expert estimations on AUS images. The results show that our system achieved the volume estimate difference values of human experts.

Our novel data set consists of both transverse and sagittal AUS samples from 305 patients. Of these patients, 75 had corresponding MR images from both the transverse and sagittal planes. These AUS and MR images were annotated by several experts during medical treatments. Two experts marked 251 AUS and 73 MR samples at two marking sessions in our experiments. As one of the contributions of our work, this data set is opened to the academic community. We expect this data set to be particularly useful, as, to our knowledge, there is no AUS data set with corresponding MR markings. Supplementary material for this study is added to https://github.com/nurbalbayrak/prostate_volume_estimation (accessed on 23 January 2022).

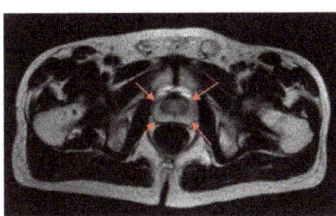
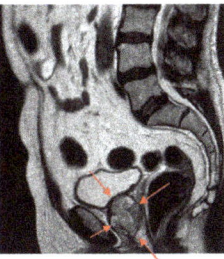

Figure 2. The prostate contours in transverse and sagittal MR images. Due to its high SNR values, MR is accepted as the gold standard in medical image-analysis studies of the prostate.

The rest of this article is organized as follows: Previous work on prostate-segmentation methods on US images is briefly given in Section 2. The proposed method on prostate volume estimation is explained in Section 3. Experiments and results are given in Section 4. The final conclusions and discussions are presented in Section 5.

2. Previous Work

We first briefly review prostate-segmentation methods on US images, as automated prostate volume estimation is primarily performed using segmentation methods. In general, almost all prostate-segmentation studies in the US modality have been performed on TRUS images. To our knowledge, there had been only one study available [10] on AUS images apart from our previous work [14,15]. Therefore, this section will also be a review of prostate segmentation on TRUS images.

Early work on prostate segmentation began with edge-based methods, which often use filters to extract edges from medical images. However, low SNR values in US images caused broken edges, and these algorithms needed to be supported by texture information. Liu et al. [16] used the Radial Bas-Relief (RBR) technique to outline the prostate border. Kwoh et al. [17] used the harmonic method, which eliminates noise and encodes a smooth boundary. Aarnink et al. [18] used the local standard deviation to determine varying homogeneous regions to detect edges. A three-stage method was applied by Pathak et al. [19]. To reduce speckle noise, they first applied a stick filter, then the image was smoothed using an anisotropic diffusion filter, and in the third step, preliminary information such as the shape and the echo model were used. A final step was the manual attachment of the edges, integrating patient-specific anatomical information.

Deformable models were also used in US prostate-segmentation studies and overcame the broken boundary problems in edge-based methods. Deformable models provide a complete contour of the prostate and try to preserve the shape information by internal forces while being placed in the best position representing the prostate border of the image by external forces. Knoll et al. [20] suggested using localized multiscale contour parameterization based on 1D dyadic wavelet transform for elastic deformation constraint to particular object shapes. Ladak et al. [21] required manual initialization of four points from the contour. The estimated contour was then automatically deformed to fit the image better. Ghanei et al. [22] used a 3D deformable model where internal forces were based on local curvature and external forces were based on volumetric data by applying an appropriate edge filter. Shen et al. [23] represented the prostate border using Gabor filter banks to characterize it in a multiscale and multi-orientation fashion. A 3D deformable model was proposed by Hu et al. [24] initialized by considering six manually selected points.

A texture matching-based deformable model for 3D TRUS images was proposed by Zhan et al. [25]. This method used Gabor Support Vector Machines (G-SVMS) on the model surface to capture texture priors for prostate and non-prostate tissues differentiation.

Region-based methods focused on the intensity distributions of the prostate region. Graph-partition algorithms and region-based level sets were used in prostate-segmentation algorithms to overcome the absence of the strong edges problem. A region-based level-set method was used by Fan et al. [26] after a fast-discriminative approach. Zougi et al. [27] used a graph partition scheme where the graph was built with nodes and edges. Nodes were the pixels, and horizontal edges that connect these nodes represented edge-discontinuity penalties.

In classifier-based methods, a feature vector was created for each object (pixels, regions, etc.). A training set was built by assigning each object a class label with supervision. The classifier was trained with the training set and learned to assign a class label to an unseen object. Yang et al. [28] used Gabor filter banks to extract texture features from registered longitudinal images of the same subject. Patient-specific Gabor features were used to train kernel support vector machines and segment newly acquired TRUS images. Akbari et al. [29] trained a set of wavelet support vector machines to adaptively capture features of the US images to differentiate the prostate and non-prostate tissue. The intensity profiles around the boundary were compared to the prostate model. The segmented prostate was updated and compared to the shape model until convergence. Ghose et al. [30] built multiple mean parametric models derived from principal component analysis of shape and posterior probabilities in a multi-resolution framework.

With the development of deep-learning methods, feature-extraction tasks moved from the human side to the algorithm side. This allowed experts in many areas to use deep learning for their studies. Yang et al. [31] formulated the prostate boundary sequentially and explored sequential clues using RNNs to learn the shape knowledge. Lei et al. [32] used a 3D deeply supervised V-Net to deal with the optimization difficulties when training a deep network with limited training data. Karimi et al. [33] trained a CNN ensemble that uses the disagreement among this ensemble to identify uncertain segmentations to estimate a segmentation-uncertainty map. Then uncertain segmentations were improved by utilizing the prior shape information. Wang et al. [34] used attention modules to exploit the complementary information encoded in different layers of CNN. This mechanism suppressed the non-prostate noise at shallow layers and increased more prostate details into features at deep layers of the CNN. Orlando et al. [35] modified the expansion section of the standard U-Net to reduce over-fitting and improve performance.

In our previous work, [14], we implemented a part-based approach to detect the prostate and its bounding box. The system was built on a deformable model of the prostate and adjacent structures. In another previous work, [15], we used concatenated image patches at different scales and trained a model with a single network. There was a voting process for the whole prostate boundary and layers parallel to the boundary. In this study, we extended our previous work to use a new patch mechanism with a new model. Additionally, we have MR annotations corresponding to AUS samples in our experiments, which will be used for comparison with golden volume standard.

Fully automated radiology measurement systems are a topic of discussion in healthcare. Most of these systems are designed in an end-to-end fashion [36,37] that complicates the expert-in-the-loop solutions that are more compatible with experts' normal workflow. Clinicians often need to know how outputs are produced to trust the system [38]. It is not easy to examine the results of end-to-end systems because they are too complex to be understood and explained by many [39]. The operation of these systems should be transparent so that they can be explained and interpreted by experts [40]. The combination of artificial and human intelligence in medical analysis would outperform the analysis of fully automated systems or humans [41], while being faster than traditional systems [42]. Our model addresses these issues by following the classical prostate-volume-estimation process. The resulting system yields intermediate results that allow manual intervention and are explainable for experts. It also produces final results allowing fully automatic use.

3. Proposed Method

Our study aimed to automate the widely used manual prostate-volume-approximation method that uses the standard ellipsoid volume formula,

$$V(W, H, L) = W.H.L.\pi/6, \quad (1)$$

where W, H, and L are the width, the height, and the length of the ellipsoid, respectively. The proposed system detects four diameter endpoints from transverse and two from sagittal planes. These locations provide the ellipsoid diameters to obtain W, H, and L values to estimate the prostate volume. We propose an image-patch voting method in which image patches from different locations vote for diameter endpoints.

In this section, we will first talk about the patching process, then we will explain the learning model and the training phase. Finally, we will explain prostate volume inference by patch voting.

3.1. Patch Extraction

To overcome the characteristic problems of AUS images, we developed an image-patch voting system. Patch-based voting is also useful for augmenting training data. Image-patch voting makes our system robust to noise and prevents it from being affected by unrelated anatomical structures such as the bladder (see Figure 1) by generating a joint solution to the decisions made for patches of many different locations and scales. However, a patch-based system can only extract local information, which may be insufficient for AUS images due to their low SNR values. Therefore, we propose to create multiple patches of different sizes with matching centers to extract information from different scales. As shown in Figure 3, we decided to use four concentric patches, which we call quadruplet patches. The sizes of the patches in our system were 64×64, 128×128, 256×256 and 512×512 pixels. All patches were downsized to 64×64 pixels, except for the smallest scale, which was already 64×64 pixels. The resulting quadruplet patches cast votes for the endpoints of the ellipsoid diameters. For the voting process, we trained a novel neural model explained in Section 3.2.

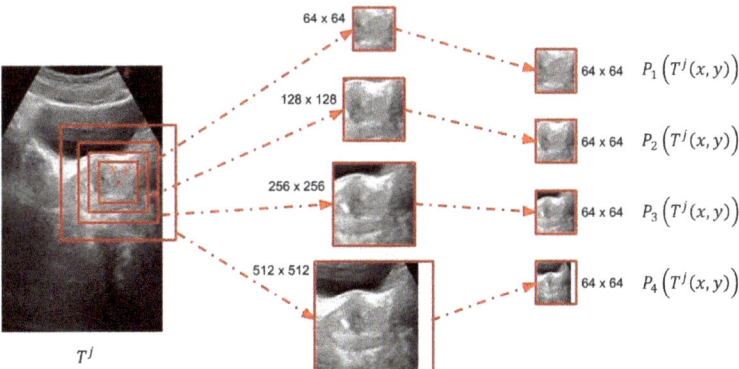

Figure 3. Patch-extraction process. For a given image location $T^j(x, y)$ of patient j, patches from four different scales centering (x, y) were extracted. All of them were downsized to the smallest scale, and the quadruplet patch $PQ(T^j(x, y))$ was obtained.

The locations of the training patches were chosen randomly from a normal distribution around diameter endpoints, while evenly spaced patches were created from test images in a sliding window manner with a stride of 10 pixels. The system extracts 200 patches from each transverse and sagittal image of the training set, which can be considered as an augmentation method that increases size of the training data set. The number of patches extracted from test images changes according to the image size. Sample training patch locations are represented on Figure 4a,b, and test patch locations are represented on Figure 4c,d.

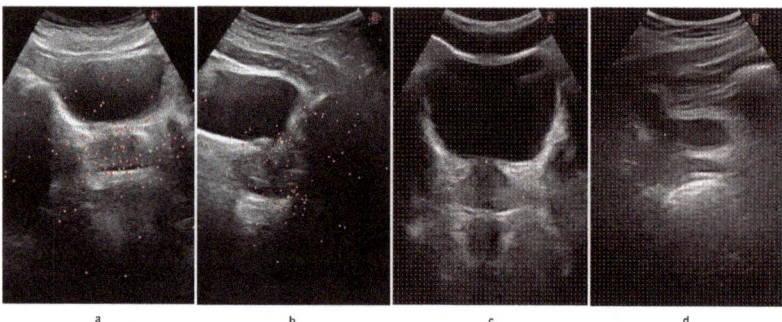

Figure 4. Patch centers are represented on AUS images. Expert marks are shown in green, while patch centers are shown in red. (**a**) Random sample training patch centers on a transverse image. (**b**) Random sample training patch centers on a sagittal image. (**c**) Sample test patch centers on a transverse image. (**d**) Sample test patch centers on a sagittal image.

3.2. Quadruplet Network

The quadruplet patches described in the previous section vote to estimate diameter endpoints through a network we refer to as Quadruplet Deep Convolutional Neural Network (QDCNN), whose structure is shown in Figure 5. QDCNN comprises four ResNet-18 DCNNs with a joint classification layer and a joint loss. Other types of quadruplet networks are very popular in re-identification or similarity learning studies [43], which are trained with four images where two of them are from the same class, and the others are from different classes. Pairs are learned as positive or negative depending on whether they are in the same or different classes. A quadruplet loss is calculated in this way to achieve greater inter-class and less intra-class variation while identifying images. Differently, in our study, each quadruplet patch obtained at different scales is the input of each of the quadruplet networks with a joint classification layer and a joint loss. The first 16 shared layers of these networks were taken as pretrained from the PyTorch/vision library [44] and frozen, and only the last two layers were fine-tuned during the training process. Thanks to this design, QDCNN can retrieve scale-specific information from each scale.

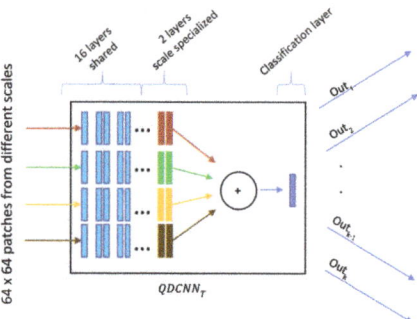

Figure 5. The QDCNN structure is composed of 4 DCNNs with a joint classification layer and a joint loss. The number of outputs k is 8 for transverse and 4 for sagittal images.

Our quadruplet network is actually a multi-task classifier that learns to predict the distance and orientation classes relative to each diameter endpoint for a given quadruplet patch of a location. Figure 6 shows the calculation of distance and orientation class values. The distance values between 0 and 1000 pixels are quantized into 10 classes, and the 11th class is for values greater than 1000. The intervals for distance classes are smaller for small distance values, and they get larger for larger distances. Orientation values $[0, 2\Pi]$ were quantized into eight equal classes.

Consider the jth patient with a transverse image T^j with diameter endpoints e_1, e_2, e_3, e_4 and a sagittal image S^j with diameter endpoints e_5 and e_6, where $e_i \in R^2$. For a given point $T^j(x,y)$ on the transverse image of the patient j, four equal-size patches $P_1(T^j(x,y)), P_2(T^j(x,y)), P_3(T^j(x,y))$, and $P_4(T^j(x,y))$ of different scales were created that composed a quadruplet patch $PQ(T^j(x,y))$ of the transverse image. Quadruplet patch $PQ(S^j(x,y))$ was created similarly for the sagittal image.

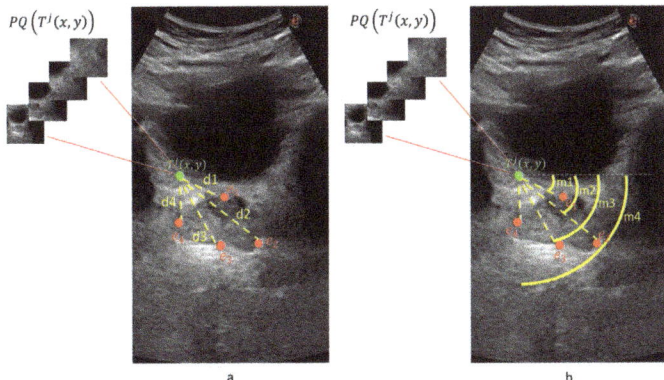

Figure 6. Measurement of the distance (**a**) and the orientation (**b**) class values for a given quadruplet patch $PQ(T^j(x,y))$. For a sample point $T^j(x,y)$ on a transverse image where four diameter end points (e_1, e_2, e_3, e_4) exist, classes for eight different tasks are predicted.

Due to the different structures of transverse and sagittal planes, our system trains two different QDCNN classifiers with a different number of outputs. We defined two functions c_d and c_o to obtain distance (cd) and orientation (co) classes, respectively. For a given point $T^j(x,y)$ on a given transverse image T^j, $cd_i^j(x,y) = c_d(T^j(x,y), e_i)$, and $co_i^j(x,y) = c_o(T^j(x,y), e_i)$ where $i = 1, \ldots, 4$. Similarly, for a given point $S^j(x,y)$ on a given sagittal image S^j, $cd_i^j(x,y) = c_d(S^j(x,y), e_i)$, and $co_i^j(x,y) = c_o(S^j(x,y), e_i)$ where $i = 5, 6$. In other words, the QDCNN classifier for the transverse plane ($QDCNN_T$) has eight classification tasks, and the QDCNN classifier for the sagittal plane ($QDCNN_S$) has four classification tasks.

In the training phase, for each AUS image from transverse or sagittal planes, quadruplet patches are extracted from normally distributed random locations around diameter endpoints. Figure 7 demonstrates this process for transverse training images where n quadruplet patches $PQ(T^j(x_1, y_1)), \ldots, PQ(T^j(x_n, y_n))$ were extracted from each of the m transverse training images $T^1, \ldots, T^m$. Then, these quadruplet patches were fed to the $QDCNN_T$ for the training process. A similar procedure was followed for the training of the $QDCNN_S$ classifier.

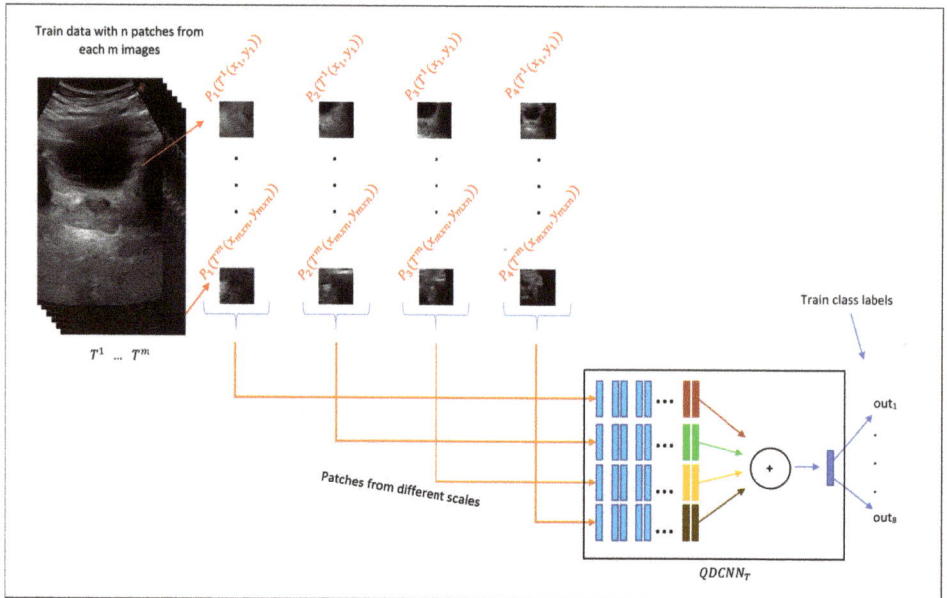

Figure 7. The training process on m transverse images $T^1, \ldots, T^m$. Around the diameter endpoints of each m training image, n quadruplet patches $(PQ(T^1(x_1, y_1))), \ldots, (PQ(T^m(x_{mxn}, y_{mxn})))$ were extracted randomly. The transverse model $QDCNN_T$ was trained to predict eight classes where eight is the $number\_of\_tasks \times number\_of\_diameter\_end\_points$.

3.3. Prostate Volume Inference through Patch Voting

Each quadruplet patch votes for each of the ellipsoid diameter endpoints at the voting space that has the same resolution as the input image. Each quadruplet patch goes through $QDCNN_T$ or $QDCNN_S$ classifier networks (depending on whether it is extracted from a transverse or sagittal image) to produce cd and co values. The actual voting happens along a circular arc where the arc center is the patch center. The arc radius is given by cd and the arc center angle by co. The arc thickness and length are determined by the median and range of the distance and orientation class intervals. This way, a voting map for each diameter endpoint of a given sample is created whose peak gives the location estimation of the diameter endpoint.

Figure 8 shows an example for the voting maps, arcs, and detected diameter endpoints. In Figure 8a, the arcs are drawn in red with the detected diameter endpoints in green. This sample image does not show the thickness to represent the locations of the arcs better. Figure 8b shows the detected points with red dots, while the manually annotated points are shown with green dots. Figure 8c shows the voting maps of each diameter endpoint. A Gaussian smoothing filter convolves these maps to suppress the noise in these images.

In the test phase, for the transverse T^j and the sagittal S^j images of a given unseen patient j, evenly spaced locations vote for the distance and the orientation class values in a sliding window manner. A quadruplet patch was extracted for each voting location where the quadruplet patch centers the location. The voting process proceeds by the classification of the quadruplet patches by the corresponding QDCNN. Figure 9 exemplifies the voting mechanism on an unseen transverse image T^j. For each location (x, y), a quadruplet patch $PQ(T^j(x, y))$ was extracted and given as input to the trained $QDCNN_T$ classifier to produce eight outputs, which are interpreted as cd–co pairs for each of the four endpoints. The final locations of the diameter endpoints were determined as the peaks of the corresponding voting maps. After obtaining the endpoints for the sagittal image S^j similarly, the standard ellipsoid formula was used to estimate the volume.

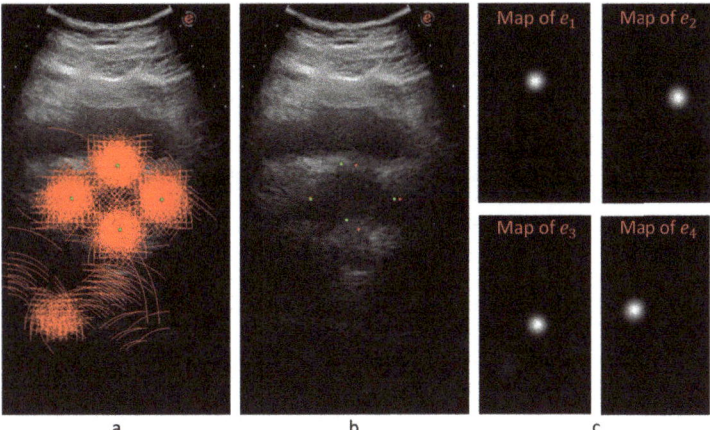

Figure 8. For a given transverse image, (**a**) shows the voting arcs (without thickness); (**b**) shows the detected points (reds are expert marked locations, while greens are the detected locations of the diameter end points); and (**c**) shows the voting maps for e_1, e_2, e_3, and e_4 endpoints.

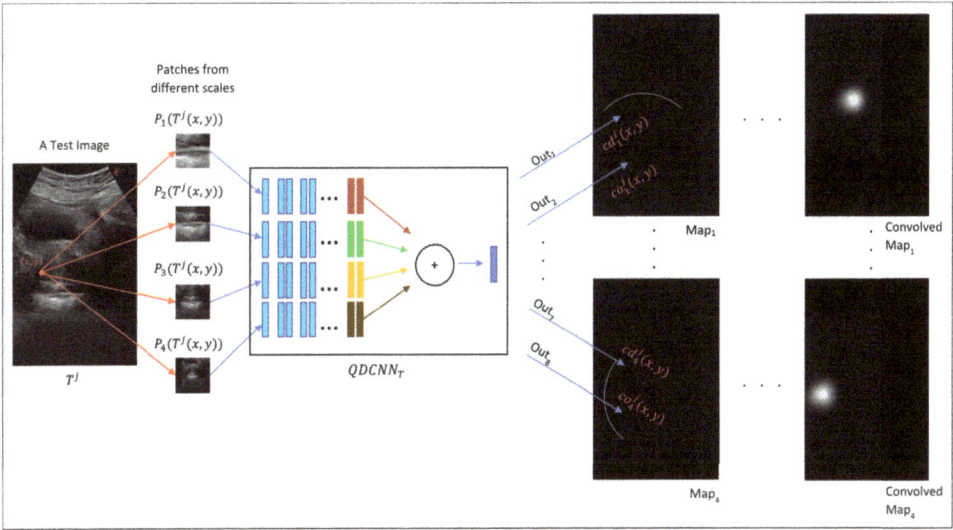

Figure 9. Creation of the voting maps for a given location $T^j(x, y)$ on a transverse image T^j.

4. Experiments and Results

In this section, firstly, we will talk about our data set, then we will explain our experiments and give results.

4.1. Data Set and Manual Annotations on AUS and MR Images

Our data set consisted of 305 AUS patient samples with transverse and sagittal images. Of these samples, 75 also had corresponding MR images from transverse and sagittal planes. Manual annotations of these AUS and MR images were done during medical treatments by several experts. The AUS annotations were used to train and test our system, and MR annotations were used as the gold standard.

Of these 305 AUS and 75 MR images, 251 AUS and 73 MR images were annotated by two different experts (exp1 and exp2) at two different marking sessions (mark1 and mark2) within our experiments. These annotations were used to obtain intra-expert and inter-expert volume-estimation differences and to compare expert estimations with our system's estimations. We defined functions $D_W(M(T^j))$, $D_H(M(T^j))$, and $D_L(M(S^j))$ as the diameters of the width, the height, and the length of the ellipsoid, respectively. M represents the measurement by the experts or the computer. T^j represents transverse and S^j represents sagittal images for the patient j. We calculated the Mean Absolute Value Difference (MAVD) between two different measurements M_1 and M_2 as

$$MAVD(M_1, M_2) = \frac{1}{N} \sum_{j=1}^{N} \left| V_1^j - V_2^j \right|, \tag{2}$$

where

$$V_{k=1,2}^j = V(D_W(M_k(T^j)), D_H(M_k(T^j)), D_L(M_k(S^j)))$$

and V is defined in Equation (1). $N = 251$ when both of the measurements are from AUS images, and $N = 73$ when at least one of the measurements is from a MR image. The top eight rows of Table 1 show intra-expert and inter-expert MAVD values of manual prostate-volume-estimations from AUS and MR images. The respective standard deviation values are shown in Table 2. The column and the row headings of the top part are defined as IT_e^k and represent the modality or the image type ($IT = AUS, MR$), the expert ID ($e = exp1, exp2$), and the annotation session ID ($k = mark1, mark2$).

Table 1. Top part shows intra-expert and inter-expert MAVD values in cm³ for AUS and MR modalities and is symmetrical. The MAVD values between experts, our QDCNN system, and the baseline is shown in the bottom part. Green shows the smallest (best), and red shows the highest MAVD. See the text for the explanation of the column and row headings.

MEAN	AUS_{exp1}^{mark1}	AUS_{exp1}^{mark2}	AUS_{exp2}^{mark1}	AUS_{exp2}^{mark2}	MR_{exp1}^{mark1}	MR_{exp1}^{mark2}	MR_{exp2}^{mark1}	MR_{exp2}^{mark2}
AUS_{exp1}^{mark1}		3.46	5.19	5.44	7.70	7.20	6.36	7.12
AUS_{exp1}^{mark2}	3.46		4.76	4.89	8.67	7.96	6.43	7.06
AUS_{exp2}^{mark1}	5.19	4.76		4.01	9.53	9.08	7.15	8.05
AUS_{exp2}^{mark2}	5.44	4.89	4.01		9.68	9.26	6.93	7.38
MR_{exp1}^{mark1}	7.70	8.67	9.53	9.68		2.63	4.96	5.48
MR_{exp1}^{mark2}	7.20	7.96	9.08	9.26	2.63		4.79	4.92
MR_{exp2}^{mark1}	6.36	6.43	7.15	6.93	4.96	4.79		3.00
MR_{exp2}^{mark2}	7.12	7.06	8.05	7.38	5.48	4.92	3.00	
AUS_{QN}	4.86	4.52	5.08	5.37	7.10	6.55	5.37	5.86
AUS_{BL}	6.62	6.13	5.79	6.46	7.92	7.27	5.97	5.77

Table 2. The corresponding SDAVD values of Table 1.

MEAN	AUS_{exp1}^{mark1}	AUS_{exp1}^{mark2}	AUS_{exp2}^{mark1}	AUS_{exp2}^{mark2}	MR_{exp1}^{mark1}	MR_{exp1}^{mark2}	MR_{exp2}^{mark1}	MR_{exp2}^{mark2}
AUS_{exp1}^{mark1}		3.67	5.38	8.35	6.97	6.29	5.32	5.33
AUS_{exp1}^{mark2}	3.67		5.03	7.70	8.05	7.21	5.88	5.75
AUS_{exp2}^{mark1}	5.38	5.03		7.56	10.51	9.68	7.49	6.73
AUS_{exp2}^{mark2}	8.35	7.70	7.56		10.68	9.71	6.92	6.50
MR_{exp1}^{mark1}	6.97	8.05	10.51	10.68		2.63	6.01	5.92
MR_{exp1}^{mark2}	6.29	7.21	9.68	9.71	2.63		4.83	5.16
MR_{exp2}^{mark1}	5.32	5.88	7.49	6.92	6.01	4.83		2.60
MR_{exp2}^{mark2}	5.33	5.75	6.73	6.50	5.92	5.16	2.60	
AUS_{QN}	5.70	5.05	5.46	8.12	9.15	7.88	6.51	5.25
AUS_{BL}	7.46	7.12	5.98	8.90	11.17	10.07	7.36	7.09

Table 1 shows that the average intra-expert MAVD values for MR images was 2.81 ($\frac{2.63+3.00}{2}$) cm^3, while it was 3.73 ($\frac{3.46+4.01}{2}$) cm^3 for AUS images. These results show that human experts' volume estimations can vary at different marking sessions, even for the MR modality, which is the gold standard. It is expectedly normal that there is a greater intra-expert MAVD for the AUS modality due to lower SNR values and other image-quality problems.

The average intra-expert MAVD was 7.63 ($\frac{7.70+7.20+8.67+7.96+7.15+8.05+6.93+7.38}{8}$) cm^3 between the modalities MR and AUS. Considering MR annotations as the gold standard, we can see that manual AUS annotations cause greater MAVD values.

When examining inter-expert MAVD values, we encountered greater values for both intra-modality and inter-modality comparisons. As shown in Table 1, we obtained average values of 5.03 ($\frac{4.96+5.48+4.79+4.92}{4}$) and 5.07 ($\frac{5.19+5.44+4.76+4.89}{4}$) cm^3 inter-expert MAVD for MR-MR and AUS-AUS comparisons, respectively. That shows us that manual annotations by different experts cause greater MAVD for both MR and AUS modalities. When we considered different modalities for inter-expert MAVD, we obtained an average of 8.06 ($\frac{6.36+7.12+6.43+7.06+9.53+9.08+9.68+9.26}{8}$) cm^3 value from which we inferred that manual annotations have a high MAVD between AUS images and the gold standard.

The comparison of the manually marked images shows that there is always a difference between different experts. Similarly, the same expert will mark different positions at different marking sessions. As a result, besides other benefits mentioned before, the guidance of the automated system is expected to enhance the consistency and the stability of the volume-estimation results by the experts. The following section shows our system's guidance ability, comparing the system and the expert volume estimations.

4.2. Comparison of the Experts, Baseline, and the QDCNN Results

We evaluated our system by 10-fold cross-validation on our data of 305 AUS images. To eliminate any scale differences between images, we re-sampled each image to a 40 pixel/cm scale using the pixel sizes that are always available from the US device.

The second row from the bottom of Table 1 (AUS_{QN}) shows the MAVD values between our QDCNN system and the experts. Comparing our system volume estimations with expert volume estimations on AUS images, we obtained a 4.95 ($\frac{4.86+4.52+5.08+5.37}{4}$) cm^3 average MAVD value, which is smaller than the average inter-expert MAVD value (5.09 cm^3) on AUS images. Overall, we can see that our system's volume estimations rank among inter-expert comparisons on AUS images. Table 2 shows the Standard Deviation of Absolute Value Difference (SDAVD) values, respectively. We observe from this table that generally for small absolute-value differences, we see smaller standard deviation values for both manual and automated measurements. In other words, our system's estimations can be considered as stable as the manual estimations.

To evaluate our system's volume estimations with respect to the gold standard, we compared our system's volume estimations with expert volume estimations on MR images and obtained 6.22 ($\frac{7.10+6.55+5.37+5.86}{4}$) cm^3 average MAVD, which is less than both the intra-expert (7.63 cm^3) and inter-expert (8.06 cm^3) average MAVD between different modalities (AUS versus MR). We can conclude that experts could possibly produce more consistent and accurate volume estimations under the guidance of our system than the complete manual-annotation method.

In order to compare our system's performance against the more traditional deep-learning systems, we implemented a baseline system that accepts 300 × 600 pixels AUS images as input and produces the diameter endpoint location estimations as the output. We modified state-of-the-art DenseNet121 [45] to produce the endpoint locations. The baseline system differs from our QDCNN with its single-network non-voting structure. The training data set for the baseline system was augmented by random cropping. The comparison between our system and the baseline model shows the advantages of our image-patch voting numerically, which is demonstrated by Table 1's last row (AUS_{BL}). We obtained an average of 6.73 ($\frac{7.92+7.27+5.97+5.77}{4}$) cm^3 MAVD between the baseline system and experts on MR images. Similarly, an average of 6.25 ($\frac{6.62+6.13+5.79+6.46}{4}$) cm³ MAVD was observed between the baseline system and experts on AUS images. Comparing these MAVD values with the values of our system, one can conclude that the image-patch voting technique improves the overall results.

4.3. Ablation Study

We performed an ablation experiment with a subset of our data set. Instead of using all four patch scales, we used patches with pixel sizes (64×64) and (128×128). For each patch size, we trained a ResNet-18 network for the transverse and another one for the sagittal plane. In addition, we trained a Twin Deep Convolutional Neural Network (TDCNN) for the transverse and another one for the sagittal plane. A TDCNN is similar to the QDCNN but contains two DCNNs and gets two patches as inputs with sizes (64×64) and (128×128) pixels. The model outputs were the *cd* and the *co* values for each endpoint.

The patch sizes we used for the ablation study were smaller than the prostate sizes in our data set. Thus, these patch sizes allow us to observe the effect of the quadruplet patch structure, which consists of patches both smaller and larger than the prostate.

We compared the volume estimations of these individual ResNet-18 networks and TDCNN with the volume estimations of experts on AUS images. The average MAVD between experts and these models were 13.5 cm³ for the 64×64 ResNet-18 network, 11.4 cm³ for the 128×128 ResNet-18 network, and 8.92 cm³ for the TDCNN. Figure 10 shows a bar chart where each group of bars show MAVD values between two different markings of two experts and a model. The first three models are the models of the ablation study. The fourth model is the baseline model, and the last model is the model of the proposed system. The proposed system, QDCNN, has the best MAVD values, which shows the effect of the quadruplet patches and the quadruplet model. TDCNN has better MAVD values than single networks, but it cannot achieve the MAVD values of the baseline system. These MAVD values of the TDCNN show us that using patches only smaller than the prostate is not enough to obtain results ranging among experts.

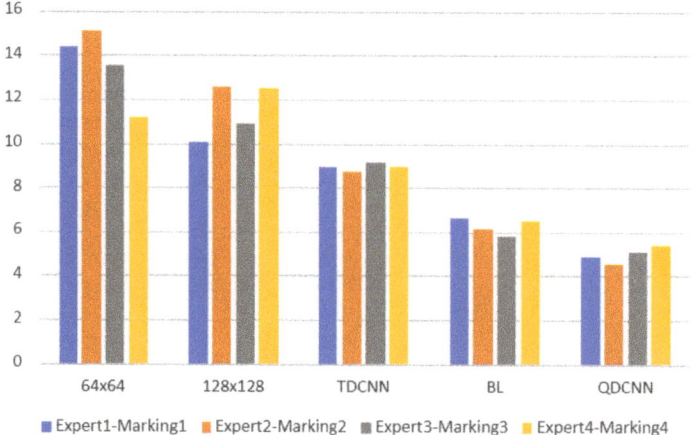

Figure 10. MAVD values between five models and the markings of two experts on AUS images at two different times.

Feature extraction is one of the usage areas of convolutional neural networks [46]. It is known that good deep classifiers can also be used as good feature extractors because good classification results can only come from good features. Thus, we examined the feature-extraction ability of the proposed QDCNN by visualizing the outputs of the last layer before the classification layer of our network as a feature vector. We visualized the feature vectors of the distance tasks for the QDCNN, the individual 64×64 ResNet-18, and the individual

128 × 128 ResNet-18. We used t-SNE graphs [47] for 2D visualization, and Figure 11 shows two examples of distance tasks for each network. Each color represents a distance class, and each colored point represents a feature vector. The color charts in each graph shows colors associated with class numbers. Smaller numbers show shorter distances, while larger numbers show longer distances. We observed that the class values, especially for the small distances, are nicely separated and grouped together for the quadruplet network. The same grouping cannot be observed for the single-scale networks. These visual results indicate the quality of the features extracted by our network.

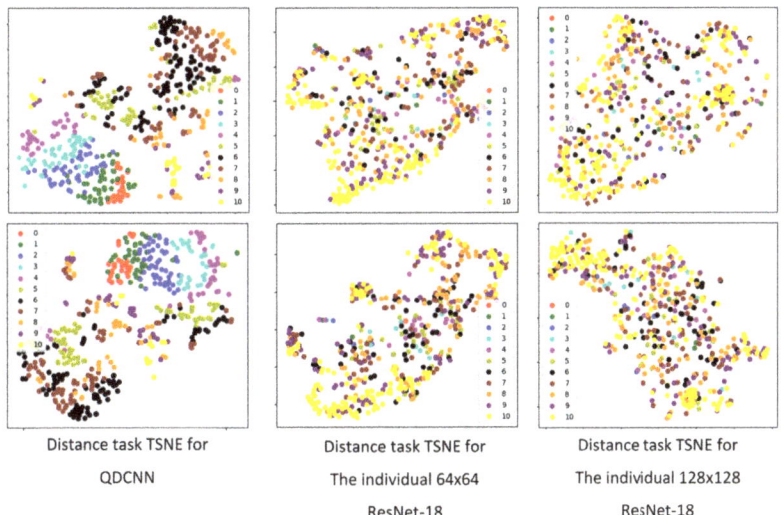

Figure 11. Examples of t-SNE graphs of the feature vectors from the QDCNN, the 64 × 64 pixels ResNet-18, and the 128 × 128 pixels ResNet-18 for the distance tasks.

5. Conclusions

Radiologists often desire computerized radiology systems with an expert-in-the-loop structure in their everyday workflow, but the popular end-to-end systems are difficult to adapt for such employment. We proposed an image-patch voting system to automate the commonly used ellipsoid formula-based prostate-volume-estimation method. Experts can see the detected endpoints of the ellipsoid diameters and change the endpoint positions if necessary, providing explainability and confidence in the final measurement results. We verified the effectiveness of the image-patch voting method against a common baseline model.

Since some of our sample patients had both AUS and MR images, we had the chance to compare our system's AUS volume estimations with the gold standard. By comparing both our system and experts to the gold standard, we showed that our system's volume estimations fall within the expert estimations. The markings made by two experts in two different marking sessions showed unignorable intra-expert and inter-expert MAVD values in the estimations made on both the same and different modalities. On the other hand, the MAVD values of our system, which were less than inter-expert MAVD values on AUS images and intra- and inter-expert MAVD values on different modalities, indicate the good level of guidance ability of the proposed method. Our system can help to enhance expert volume estimations' stability and consistency.

The new data set we created is valuable for further work on AUS images in automated medical-image analysis. To our knowledge, the data set is the first to include expert markings on both AUS and MR images of sample patients in two different marking sessions. Supplementary material, including the data set, the expert markings, and the project code, is available for public use at https://github.com/nurbalbayrak/prostate_volume_estimation (accessed on 23 January 2022).

Future work might apply the proposed model and patch structure to other modalities. Hybrid modalities [48] might be a good supply of data for a multi-patch system like the proposed one. Statistical analysis might be done to test statistical MAVD differences among different groups.

Author Contributions: Writing—original draft preparation, N.B.A.; writing—review and editing, Y.S.A. All authors have read and agreed to the published version of the manuscript.

Funding: This study was supported by TUBITAK project 114E536.

Institutional Review Board Statement: The study was conducted according to the guidelines of the Declaration of Helsinki and approved by the Ethics Committee of MALTEPE UNIVERSITY (protocol code 14 and date of approval 19 March 2014).

Informed Consent Statement: Informed consent was obtained from all subjects involved in the study.

Data Availability Statement: The data set, the expert markings, and the project code, is available for public use at https://github.com/nurbalbayrak/prostate_volume_estimation (accessed on 23 January 2022).

Acknowledgments: We acknowledge Rahmi Çubuk, Orhun Sinanoğlu, Kübra Murzoğlu Altıntoprak, Esra Ümmühan Mermi, and Alev Günaldı from Maltepe University the Hospital of Medical School; Ayşe Betül Oktay from Istanbul Medeniyet University; and Tunahan Refik Dumlu from Kartal Lutfi Kırdar City Hospital for providing data and annotations.

Conflicts of Interest: The authors declare no conflict of interest.

References

1. Roehrborn, C. Pathology of benign prostatic hyperplasia. *Int. J. Impot. Res.* **2008**, *20*, S11–S18. [CrossRef] [PubMed]
2. Liu, D.; Shoag, J.E.; Poliak, D.; Goueli, R.S.; Ravikumar, V.; Redmond, D.; Vosoughi, A.; Fontugne, J.; Pan, H.; Lee, D.; et al. Integrative multiplatform molecular profiling of benign prostatic hyperplasia identifies distinct subtypes. *Nat. Commun.* **2020**, *11*, 1987. [CrossRef] [PubMed]
3. Nickel, J.C. Benign prostatic hyperplasia: Does prostate size matter? *Rev. Urol.* **2003**, *5*, S12. [PubMed]
4. Jue, J.S.; Barboza, M.P.; Prakash, N.S.; Venkatramani, V.; Sinha, V.R.; Pavan, N.; Nahar, B.; Kanabur, P.; Ahdoot, M.; Dong, Y.; et al. Re-examining prostate-specific antigen (PSA) density: Defining the optimal PSA range and patients for using PSA density to predict prostate cancer using extended template biopsy. *Urology* **2017**, *105*, 123–128. [CrossRef]
5. Sung, H.; Ferlay, J.; Siegel, R.L.; Laversanne, M.; Soerjomataram, I.; Jemal, A.; Bray, F. Global cancer statistics 2020: GLOBOCAN estimates of incidence and mortality worldwide for 36 cancers in 185 countries. *CA Cancer J. Clin.* **2021**, *71*, 209–249. [CrossRef]
6. Carroll, P.H.; Mohler, J.L. NCCN guidelines updates: Prostate cancer and prostate cancer early detection. *J. Natl. Compr. Cancer Netw.* **2018**, *16*, 620–623. [CrossRef]
7. Mottet, N.; van den Bergh, R.C.; Briers, E.; Van den Broeck, T.; Cumberbatch, M.G.; De Santis, M.; Fanti, S.; Fossati, N.; Gandaglia, G.; Gillessen, S.; et al. EAU-EANM-ESTRO-ESUR-SIOG guidelines on prostate cancer—2020 update. Part 1: Screening, diagnosis, and local treatment with curative intent. *Eur. Urol.* **2021**, *79*, 243–262. [CrossRef]
8. Turkbey, B.; Pinto, P.A.; Choyke, P.L. Imaging techniques for prostate cancer: Implications for focal therapy. *Nat. Rev. Urol.* **2009**, *6*, 191–203. [CrossRef]
9. Ghose, S.; Oliver, A.; Martí, R.; Lladó, X.; Vilanova, J.C.; Freixenet, J.; Mitra, J.; Sidibé, D.; Meriaudeau, F. A survey of prostate segmentation methodologies in ultrasound, magnetic resonance and computed tomography images. *Comput. Methods Programs Biomed.* **2012**, *108*, 262–287. [CrossRef]
10. Betrouni, N.; Vermandel, M.; Pasquier, D.; Maouche, S.; Rousseau, J. Segmentation of abdominal ultrasound images of the prostate using a priori information and an adapted noise filter. *Comput. Med. Imaging Graph.* **2005**, *29*, 43–51. [CrossRef]
11. De Sio, M.; D'armiento, M.; Di Lorenzo, G.; Damiano, R.; Perdonà, S.; De Placido, S.; Autorino, R. The need to reduce patient discomfort during transrectal ultrasonography-guided prostate biopsy: What do we know? *BJU Int.* **2005**, *96*, 977–983. [CrossRef] [PubMed]
12. Choi, Y.J.; Kim, J.K.; Kim, H.J.; Cho, K.S. Interobserver variability of transrectal ultrasound for prostate volume measurement according to volume and observer experience. *Am. J. Roentgenol.* **2009**, *192*, 444–449. [CrossRef] [PubMed]
13. Wasserman, N.F.; Niendorf, E.; Spilseth, B. Measurement of prostate volume with MRI (a guide for the perplexed): biproximate method with analysis of precision and accuracy. *Sci. Rep.* **2020**, *10*, 575. [CrossRef] [PubMed]

14. Albayrak, N.B.; Oktay, A.B.; Akgul, Y.S. Prostate detection from abdominal ultrasound images: A part based approach. In Proceedings of the 2015 IEEE International Conference on Image Processing (ICIP), Quebec City, QC, Canada, 27–30 September 2015; pp. 1955–1959.
15. Albayrak, N.B.; Yildirim, E.; Akgul, Y.S. Prostate Size Inference from Abdominal Ultrasound Images with Patch Based Prior Information. In Proceedings of the International Conference on Advanced Concepts for Intelligent Vision Systems, Antwerp, Belgium, 18–21 September 2017; pp. 249–259.
16. Liu, Y.; Ng, W.; Teo, M.; Lim, H. Computerised prostate boundary estimation of ultrasound images using radial bas-relief method. *Med. Biol. Eng. Comput.* **1997**, *35*, 445–454. [CrossRef] [PubMed]
17. Kwoh, C.; Teo, M.; Ng, W.; Tan, S.; Jones, L. Outlining the prostate boundary using the harmonics method. *Med. Biol. Eng. Comput.* **1998**, *36*, 768–771. [CrossRef] [PubMed]
18. Aarnink, R.; Pathak, S.D.; De La Rosette, J.J.; Debruyne, F.M.; Kim, Y.; Wijkstra, H. Edge detection in prostatic ultrasound images using integrated edge maps. *Ultrasonics* **1998**, *36*, 635–642. [CrossRef]
19. Pathak, S.D.; Haynor, D.; Kim, Y. Edge-guided boundary delineation in prostate ultrasound images. *IEEE Trans. Med. Imaging* **2000**, *19*, 1211–1219. [CrossRef]
20. Knoll, C.; Alcañiz, M.; Grau, V.; Monserrat, C.; Juan, M.C. Outlining of the prostate using snakes with shape restrictions based on the wavelet transform (Doctoral Thesis: Dissertation). *Pattern Recognit.* **1999**, *32*, 1767–1781. [CrossRef]
21. Ladak, H.M.; Mao, F.; Wang, Y.; Downey, D.B.; Steinman, D.A.; Fenster, A. Prostate boundary segmentation from 2D ultrasound images. *Med. Phys.* **2000**, *27*, 1777–1788. [CrossRef]
22. Ghanei, A.; Soltanian-Zadeh, H.; Ratkewicz, A.; Yin, F.F. A three-dimensional deformable model for segmentation of human prostate from ultrasound images. *Med. Phys.* **2001**, *28*, 2147–2153. [CrossRef]
23. Shen, D.; Zhan, Y.; Davatzikos, C. Segmentation of prostate boundaries from ultrasound images using statistical shape model. *IEEE Trans. Med. Imaging* **2003**, *22*, 539–551. [CrossRef] [PubMed]
24. Hu, N.; Downey, D.B.; Fenster, A.; Ladak, H.M. Prostate boundary segmentation from 3D ultrasound images. *Med. Phys.* **2003**, *30*, 1648–1659. [CrossRef] [PubMed]
25. Zhan, Y.; Shen, D. Deformable segmentation of 3-D ultrasound prostate images using statistical texture matching method. *IEEE Trans. Med. Imaging* **2006**, *25*, 256–272. [CrossRef] [PubMed]
26. Fan, S.; Voon, L.K.; Sing, N.W. 3D prostate surface detection from ultrasound images based on level set method. In Proceedings of the International Conference on Medical Image Computing and Computer-Assisted Intervention, Tokyo, Japan, 25–28 September 2002; pp. 389–396.
27. Zouqi, M.; Samarabandu, J. Prostate segmentation from 2-D ultrasound images using graph cuts and domain knowledge. In Proceedings of the 2008 Canadian Conference on Computer and Robot Vision, Windsor, ON, Canada, 28–30 May 2008; pp. 359–362.
28. Yang, X.; Fei, B. 3D prostate segmentation of ultrasound images combining longitudinal image registration and machine learning. In *Medical Imaging 2012: Image-Guided Procedures, Robotic Interventions, and Modeling*; 2012; Volume 8316, p. 83162O.
29. Akbari, H.; Fei, B. 3D ultrasound image segmentation using wavelet support vector machines. *Med. Phys.* **2012**, *39*, 2972–2984. [CrossRef]
30. Ghose, S.; Oliver, A.; Mitra, J.; Martí, R.; Lladó, X.; Freixenet, J.; Sidibé, D.; Vilanova, J.C.; Comet, J.; Meriaudeau, F. A supervised learning framework of statistical shape and probability priors for automatic prostate segmentation in ultrasound images. *Med. Image Anal.* **2013**, *17*, 587–600. [CrossRef]
31. Yang, X.; Yu, L.; Wu, L.; Wang, Y.; Ni, D.; Qin, J.; Heng, P.A. Fine-grained recurrent neural networks for automatic prostate segmentation in ultrasound images. In Proceedings of the AAAI Conference on Artificial Intelligence, San Francisco, CA USA, 4–9 February 2017; Volume 31.
32. Lei, Y.; Tian, S.; He, X.; Wang, T.; Wang, B.; Patel, P.; Jani, A.B.; Mao, H.; Curran, W.J.; Liu, T.; et al. Ultrasound prostate segmentation based on multidirectional deeply supervised V-Net. *Med. Phys.* **2019**, *46*, 3194–3206. [CrossRef]
33. Karimi, D.; Zeng, Q.; Mathur, P.; Avinash, A.; Mahdavi, S.; Spadinger, I.; Abolmaesumi, P.; Salcudean, S.E. Accurate and robust deep learning-based segmentation of the prostate clinical target volume in ultrasound images. *Med. Image Anal.* **2019**, *57*, 186–196. [CrossRef]
34. Wang, Y.; Dou, H.; Hu, X.; Zhu, L.; Yang, X.; Xu, M.; Qin, J.; Heng, P.A.; Wang, T.; Ni, D. Deep attentive features for prostate segmentation in 3d transrectal ultrasound. *IEEE Trans. Med. Imaging* **2019**, *38*, 2768–2778. [CrossRef]
35. Orlando, N.; Gillies, D.J.; Gyacskov, I.; Romagnoli, C.; D'Souza, D.; Fenster, A. Automatic prostate segmentation using deep learning on clinically diverse 3D transrectal ultrasound images. *Med. Phys.* **2020**, *47*, 2413–2426. [CrossRef]
36. Lapa, P.; Castelli, M.; Gonçalves, I.; Sala, E.; Rundo, L. A hybrid end-to-end approach integrating conditional random fields into CNNs for prostate cancer detection on MRI. *Appl. Sci.* **2020**, *10*, 338. [CrossRef]
37. Wang, Z.; Liu, C.; Cheng, D.; Wang, L.; Yang, X.; Cheng, K.T. Automated detection of clinically significant prostate cancer in mp-MRI images based on an end-to-end deep neural network. *IEEE Trans. Med. Imaging* **2018**, *37*, 1127–1139. [CrossRef] [PubMed]
38. Wang, D.; Wang, L.; Zhang, Z.; Wang, D.; Zhu, H.; Gao, Y.; Fan, X.; Tian, F. "Brilliant AI Doctor" in Rural Clinics: Challenges in AI-Powered Clinical Decision Support System Deployment. In Proceedings of the 2021 CHI Conference on Human Factors in Computing Systems, Yokohama, Japan, 8–13 May 2021; pp. 1–18.

39. Murphy, K.; Di Ruggiero, E.; Upshur, R.; Willison, D.J.; Malhotra, N.; Cai, J.C.; Malhotra, N.; Lui, V.; Gibson, J. Artificial intelligence for good health: a scoping review of the ethics literature. *BMC Med. Ethics* **2021**, *22*, 14 [CrossRef] [PubMed]
40. Sunarti, S.; Rahman, F.F.; Naufal, M.; Risky, M.; Febriyanto, K.; Masnina, R. Artificial intelligence in healthcare: opportunities and risk for future. *Gac. Sanit.* **2021**, *35*, S67–S70. [CrossRef] [PubMed]
41. Rundo, L.; Pirrone, R.; Vitabile, S.; Sala, E.; Gambino, O. Recent advances of HCI in decision-making tasks for optimized clinical workflows and precision medicine. *J. Biomed. Inform.* **2020**, *108*, 103479. [CrossRef]
42. Lutnick, B.; Ginley, B.; Govind, D.; McGarry, S.D.; LaViolette, P.S.; Yacoub, R.; Jain, S.; Tomaszewski, J.E.; Jen, K.Y.; Sarder, P. An integrated iterative annotation technique for easing neural network training in medical image analysis. *Nat. Mach. Intell.* **2019**, *1*, 112–119. [CrossRef]
43. Chen, W.; Chen, X.; Zhang, J.; Huang, K. Beyond triplet loss: A deep quadruplet network for person re-identification. In Proceedings of the IEEE Conference on Computer Vision and Pattern Recognition, Honolulu, HI, USA, 21–26 July 2017; pp. 403–412.
44. Paszke, A.; Gross, S.; Massa, F.; Lerer, A.; Bradbury, J.; Chanan, G.; Killeen, T.; Lin, Z.; Gimelshein, N.; Antiga, L.; et al. PyTorch: An Imperative Style, High-Performance Deep Learning Library. In *Advances in Neural Information Processing Systems 32*; Wallach, H., Larochelle, H., Beygelzimer, A., d'Alché-Buc, F., Fox, E., Garnett, R., Eds.; Curran Associates, Inc.: New York, USA , 2019; pp. 8024–8035.
45. Huang, G.; Liu, Z.; Van Der Maaten, L.; Weinberger, K.Q. Densely connected convolutional networks. In Proceedings of the IEEE Conference on Computer Vision and Pattern Recognition, Honolulu, HI, USA, 21–26 July 2017; pp. 4700–4708.
46. Jogin, M.; Madhulika, M.; Divya, G.; Meghana, R.; Apoorva, S. Feature extraction using convolution neural networks (CNN) and deep learning. In Proceedings of the 2018 3rd IEEE International Conference on Recent Trends in Electronics, Information & Communication Technology (RTEICT), Bangalore, India, 18–19 May 2018; pp. 2319–2323.
47. Van der Maaten, L.; Hinton, G. Visualizing data using t-SNE. *J. Mach. Learn. Res.* **2008**, *9*, 2579–2605 .
48. Kothapalli, S.R.; Sonn, G.A.; Choe, J.W.; Nikoozadeh, A.; Bhuyan, A.; Park, K.K.; Cristman, P.; Fan, R.; Moini, A.; Lee, B.C.; et al. Simultaneous transrectal ultrasound and photoacoustic human prostate imaging. *Sci. Transl. Med.* **2019**, *11*, eaav2169 . [CrossRef]

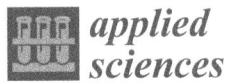

Article

Deep Learning Networks for Automatic Retroperitoneal Sarcoma Segmentation in Computerized Tomography

Giuseppe Salvaggio [1], Giuseppe Cutaia [1,2], Antonio Greco [1], Mario Pace [1], Leonardo Salvaggio [3], Federica Vernuccio [1], Roberto Cannella [1,2], Laura Algeri [4], Lorena Incorvaia [5], Alessandro Stefano [6,*], Massimo Galia [1], Giuseppe Badalamenti [4] and Albert Comelli [7]

1. Section of Radiology, Department of Biomedicine, Neuroscience and Advanced Diagnostics (Bi.N.D.), University of Palermo, 90100 Palermo, Italy; p.salvaggio@libero.it (G.S.); cutaiagiuseppe7@gmail.com (G.C.); antounipa@gmail.com (A.G.); 91mariopace@gmail.com (M.P.); federica.vernuccio@unipa.it (F.V.); rob.cannella89@gmail.com (R.C.); massimo.galia@unipa.it (M.G.)
2. Department of Health Promotion, Mother and Child Care, Internal Medicine and Medical Specialties (PROMISE), University of Palermo, 90100 Palermo, Italy
3. Section of Anaesthesia, Department of Surgical, Oncological and Oral Science (Di.Chir.On.S.), University of Palermo, 90100 Palermo, Italy; leonardosalvaggio95@gmail.com
4. Section of Medical Oncology, Department of Surgical, Oncological and Oral Science, University of Palermo, 90100 Palermo, Italy; lauraw@hotmail.it (L.A.); giuseppe.badalamenti@unipa.it (G.B.)
5. Section of Medical Oncology, Department of Biomedicine, Neuroscience and Advanced Diagnostics (Bi.N.D.), University of Palermo, 90100 Palermo, Italy; lorena.incorvaia@unipa.it
6. Institute of Molecular Bioimaging and Physiology, National Research Council (IBFM-CNR), 90015 Cefalù, Italy
7. Ri.MED Foundation, Via Bandiera 11, 90133 Palermo, Italy; acomelli@fondazionerimed.com
* Correspondence: alessandro.stefano@ibfm.cnr.it

Citation: Salvaggio, G.; Cutaia, G.; Greco, A.; Pace, M.; Salvaggio, L.; Vernuccio, F.; Cannella, R.; Algeri, L.; Incorvaia, L.; Stefano, A.; et al. Deep Learning Networks for Automatic Retroperitoneal Sarcoma Segmentation in Computerized Tomography. *Appl. Sci.* **2022**, *12*, 1665. https://doi.org/10.3390/app12031665

Academic Editors: Qi-Huang Zheng and Fabio La Foresta

Received: 17 December 2021
Accepted: 2 February 2022
Published: 5 February 2022

Publisher's Note: MDPI stays neutral with regard to jurisdictional claims in published maps and institutional affiliations.

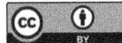

Copyright: © 2022 by the authors. Licensee MDPI, Basel, Switzerland. This article is an open access article distributed under the terms and conditions of the Creative Commons Attribution (CC BY) license (https://creativecommons.org/licenses/by/4.0/).

Featured Application: This study proposes fast and innovative deep learning networks for automatic retroperitoneal sarcoma segmentation in computerized tomography images.

Abstract: The volume estimation of retroperitoneal sarcoma (RPS) is often difficult due to its huge dimensions and irregular shape; thus, it often requires manual segmentation, which is time-consuming and operator-dependent. This study aimed to evaluate two fully automated deep learning networks (ENet and ERFNet) for RPS segmentation. This retrospective study included 20 patients with RPS who received an abdominal computed tomography (CT) examination. Forty-nine CT examinations, with a total of 72 lesions, were included. Manual segmentation was performed by two radiologists in consensus, and automatic segmentation was performed using ENet and ERFNet. Significant differences between manual and automatic segmentation were tested using the analysis of variance (ANOVA). A set of performance indicators for the shape comparison (namely sensitivity), positive predictive value (PPV), dice similarity coefficient (DSC), volume overlap error (VOE), and volumetric differences (VD) were calculated. There were no significant differences found between the RPS volumes obtained using manual segmentation and ENet (p-value = 0.935), manual segmentation and ERFNet (p-value = 0.544), or ENet and ERFNet (p-value = 0.119). The sensitivity, PPV, DSC, VOE, and VD for ENet and ERFNet were 91.54% and 72.21%, 89.85% and 87.00%, 90.52% and 74.85%, 16.87% and 36.85%, and 2.11% and −14.80%, respectively. By using a dedicated GPU, ENet took around 15 s for segmentation versus 13 s for ERFNet. In the case of CPU, ENet took around 2 min versus 1 min for ERFNet. The manual approach required approximately one hour per segmentation. In conclusion, fully automatic deep learning networks are reliable methods for RPS volume assessment. ENet performs better than ERFNet for automatic segmentation, though it requires more time.

Keywords: deep learning; soft tissue sarcoma; volume estimation; segmentation; artificial intelligence

1. Introduction

Soft tissue sarcomas are rare, malignant mesenchymal neoplasms that account for less than 1% of all malignant tumors. Of all sarcomas, the majority occur outside of the retroperitoneum, while around 10% of all sarcomas occur in the retroperitoneum [1], with a mean annual incidence of 2.7 per million [2]. The prognosis for patients with retroperitoneal sarcoma (RPS) is relatively poor, with a 36% to 58% overall 5-year survival rate and a natural history characterized by late recurrence [3]. RPS are frequently underdiagnosed at the early stage, and symptoms appear late, as they are associated with the displacement of adjacent organs and obstructive phenomena. When present, symptoms include abdominal pain, back pain, bowel obstruction, or palpable abdominal mass [1].

A variety of imaging techniques, including computed tomography (CT), positron emission tomography-computed tomography (PET/CT), and magnetic resonance imaging (MRI), may be used to assess RPS. Among them, CT is the most commonly used modality for the identification, localization, and staging of RPS [4]. CT examination allows for tissue components characterization and offers multiplanar reconstructions to easily depict the anatomic site of the origin of a mass, as well as its relationship to adjacent organs and vasculature [5].

RPS is one of the largest tumors of the human body [6]: lesions with a measure of <5 cm are considered rare, while a measure of >20 cm is found in 20 to 50% of masses at the time of resection [7]. Despite RPS's large dimension, the impact of tumor size on the patient's survival remains controversial. Several previous studies have failed to demonstrate any association of tumor size [8–16], while others have found that a size threshold of 10 cm is significant for survival [17,18]. However, these previous studies analyzed just the largest lesion's diameter instead of the volume. RPSs have an irregular shape, and the largest diameter cannot reflect the real tumor volume.

Manual segmentation based on imaging sections could be used for a volume estimation, and it is considered the gold standard for segmentation methods; however it is time-consuming, requires experience, and is strongly operator-dependent. Recently, deep learning methods, especially supervised classification methods based on convolutional neural networks, have been successful in the field of medical imaging for segmenting the anatomy of interest [19,20]. To our knowledge, no prior studies explored deep learning methods for RPS automatic segmentation.

Therefore, the aim of this study is to evaluate fully automated deep learning networks, namely the Efficient Neural Network (ENet) and the Efficient Residual Factorized ConvNet (ERFNet), for RPS segmentation and to compare their results with manual segmentation performed in contrast-enhanced CT examinations of the abdomen.

2. Materials and Methods

The present study is a retrospective study and written informed consent was waived by our ethical committee. All of the patients who underwent CT examination provided written informed consent for the use of their anonymized CT studies for research purposes.

2.1. Population Selection

The tumor registry database of the Department of Oncology of our hospital was queried for patients with RPS between 2013 and 2021. Patients with sarcomas that originated in the gastrointestinal tract (namely gastrointestinal stroma tumors) or in other abdominal visceral organs were excluded from the study due to the different imaging appearances and tumor shapes. The search retrieved 56 patients with histological diagnoses of RPS. From these patients, we identified 20 who underwent contrast-enhanced CT at our hospital. Thirteen of these patients had only CT examinations performed at the time of the diagnosis, while seven patients had CT examinations at the time of diagnosis and after treatments (one patient had three post-treatment CT examinations, two patients had four CTs, two patients had five, one patient had six, and one patient had eight). All CT examinations' images were reviewed by a radiologist (G.S.) with 20 years of experience in abdominal radiology on a Pictures Archiving and Communication System (PACS—Impax, Agfa-Gevaert, Mortsel, Belgium), confirming the presence of RPS and, eventually, the recurrence in post-treatment CT scan examinations. When recurrence was found, post-treatment CT examinations were also included in the present study. Six post-treatment CT examinations were excluded for the lack of recurrence.

2.2. CT Imaging

All patients included in this study performed a standard protocol CT scan at the radiology department of our hospital. Patients underwent an abdominal contrast-enhanced computed tomography scan on a 16-slice CT scanner (General Electric BrightSpeed, Milwaukee, WI, USA). The scanning parameters were a tube current of 100 mAs, a peak tube voltage of 120 KV, a rotation time of 0.6 s, a detector collimation of 16×0.625 mm, a field of view of 350 mm $\times$ 350 mm, and a matrix of 512×512. Contrast-enhanced CT was performed by injecting about 1.5 mL/kg of iodinated contrast agent (400 mg/mL Iomeprol, Iomeron 400, Bracco Imaging, Milan, Italy; 370 mg/dl Iopromide, Ultravist 370, Bayer Pharma, Berlin, Germany; or 350 mg/dL Iobitidrol, Xenetix 350, Guerbet, Roissy, France, depending on the clinical availability) at a flow of 3 mL/s, followed by the infusion of 20 mL of saline solution with a pump injector (Ulrich CT Plus 150, Ulrich Medical, Ulm, Germany). Images were acquired in the non-enhanced scan and portal-venous phase. Portal venous phase was obtained after 70 s of delay after intravenous injection of the contrast agent.

All CT examinations were performed with the patient in a supine position during a single inspiratory breath-hold whenever possible.

2.3. Manual Segmentation

Manual RPS segmentations were performed in consensus by two radiologists (A.G. and M.P.), both with 3 years of experience in abdominal CT. CT portal-venous phase images were used for manual segmentation. Each CT portal-venous examination was anonymized and imported into an open-source DICOM (Digital Imaging and Communication in Medicine), viewer equipped with Horos (LGPL license at Horosproject.org [21]) in order to obtain volume lesion by manual segmentation. Lesion boundaries were manually traced with a contouring tool (pencil), slice by slice. Afterward, the "compute volume" tool was used to obtain the volume rendering of the entire RPS with the volume measurement. The time required by the entire process was dependent on the lesion's dimension. Manual RPS segmentation volumes were used as a reference standard.

2.4. Automatic and User-Independent Segmentation

Deep learning enables automated identification and delineation of regions of interest in biomedical images, and consequently, it is of great interest in radiology. Nevertheless, it requires high computational power and long training times. In order to overcome this issue, ENet [22] and ERFNet [23] have been proposed as fast and lightweight networks capable of obtaining accurate segmentation with low training time and hardware requirements. Indeed, it was developed for fast inference and high accuracy in augmented reality and automotive scenarios where hardware availability is limited.

Specifically, ENet is based on building blocks of residual networks, with each block consisting of 3 convolutional layers. These are a 1×1 projection that reduces dimensionality, a regular convolutional layer, and a 1×1 expansion with batch normalization. ENet has asymmetric convolutions characterized by separable convolutions with sequences of 5×1 and 1×5 convolutions. The 5×5 convolution has 25 parameters, while the corresponding asymmetric convolution has only 10 parameters to reduce the network size. Finally, ENet uses a single starting block in addition to several variations of the bottleneck layer. The bottleneck layer is used to force the network to learn the most salient features present in the input and, consequently, to ignore the irrelevant parts.

ERFNet is optimized over ENet to improve accuracy and efficiency. The basic building block module is a non-bottleneck 1D layer comprised of two sets of factorized (separable or asymmetric) convolutions of a size of 3×1 followed by the 1×3 with rectified linear unit non-linearity. The input feature map of the main convolution path is added element-wise to the output of the convolution path, which represents the input of the next layer after applying the rectified linear unit non-linearity. The size of input is 512×512, while the down-sampler block is similar to that of ENet architecture.

Furthermore, both ENet and ERFNet can be used as an alternative to transfer learning, usually used to compensate for the lack of labeled biomedical images. ENET and ERFNet can learn a lot of information, even from small datasets, as demonstrated in several biomedical segmentation studies [24–27], in which they outperformed other state-of-the-art deep learning approaches, such as UNet.

2.5. Experimental Detail

In the current study, to further overcome the issue related to a limited amount of data, the five-fold cross-validation strategy was adopted by randomly dividing the whole dataset into five folds (9 or 13 studies). Consequently, we trained five models by combining four of the five folds into a training set and by keeping the remaining fold as the validation fold. In our experiments, to avoid including slices from the same patient into the training and validation sets, the patients were firstly split randomly into a training set and validation set and then the slices corresponding to the patients were used to construct the training and validation sets. Therefore, the issue of potential overlap between the training and validation sets does not exist. We used an initial set of 20 lesions to determine the best learning rates experimentally. Specifically, for the training task, the following parameters were used: (i) a learning rate of 0.0001 and 0.00001 with Adam optimizer [28] for ENet and ERFNet, respectively; (ii) a batch size of 8 slices for all studies; (iii) a maximum of 100 epochs with an automatic stopping criterion (if the loss did not decrease for 10 consecutive epochs); and (iv) the Tversky loss function [29] with $\alpha = 0.3$ and $\beta = 0.7$. Data augmentation was obtained by randomly rotating; translating in both the x and y directions; and applying shearing, horizontal flip, and zooming to the input training slices. Consequently, six different types of data augmentation techniques were used to reduce overfitting, while data standardization and normalization were used to help the models converge faster and to avoid numerical instability. A graphics processing unit (GPU), i.e., NVIDIA QUADRO P4000 with 8 GB VRAM and 1792 CUDA Cores, was adopted to train and run inference.

2.6. Evaluation Analyses

Analysis of variance (ANOVA) on the manual and automatic segmentation was used to test the differences (a p-value < 0.05 indicates a significant difference) between the manual and automatic approaches. Specifically, the F-value was calculated to assess if the means between the two populations were significantly different. The F critical value was calculated to compare it with the F-value; if the F-value is larger than the F critical value, the null hypothesis can be rejected. In addition, RPS volumes calculated from the manual and automatic approaches were compared using a correlation graph and Bland Altman plot.

Finally, a set of performance indicators routinely used in the literature for shape comparison [30] were calculated, namely the dice similarity coefficient (DSC), sensitivity, volume overlap error (VOE), volumetric difference (VD), and positive predictive value (PPV):

$$DSC = \frac{2*TP}{2*TP + FP + FN} * 100\% \tag{1}$$

$$Sensitivity = \frac{TP}{TN + FN} * 100\% \tag{2}$$

$$VOE = \frac{1-TP}{TP + FP + FN} * 100\% \tag{3}$$

$$VD = \frac{FN - FP}{2*TP + FP + FN} * 100\% \qquad (4)$$

$$PPV = \frac{TP}{TP + FN} * 100\% \qquad (5)$$

where TP, FP, TN, and FN are the number of true positives, false positives, true negatives, and false negatives, respectively.

3. Results

3.1. Population

The final population consisted of 20 patients (n = 11 women; n = 9 men; mean age, 64 years old; age range, from 40 to 86 years old) with 49 CT examinations and 72 RPS lesions (one lesion in 40 CT examinations, two lesions in eight, three lesions in one, four lesions in one, and nine lesions in one). The most frequent histological subtype of sarcoma was liposarcoma (n = 14), while the remaining patients had leiomyosarcoma (n = 6). All of the liposarcomas and 4 leiomyosarcomas were poorly differentiated (G3; n = 18), while 2 leiomyosarcomas were moderately differentiated (G2).

3.2. ANOVA Analysis

The mean RPS volumes obtained using manual and automatic segmentations were 2697.57 cubic centimeters (cc) (SD = 4075.73 cc) for the manual approach, 2539.88 (SD = ±3464.10 cc) for ENet, and 1701.48 cc (SD = ±1996.71 cc) for ERFNet. Table 1 shows the minimum, 25th percentile, median, 75th percentile, and maximum RPS volume obtained using manual and automatic segmentation.

Table 1. Reference values of manually and automatically segmented RPS volumes from CT examinations in cubic centimeters (cc).

	Minimum	25th Percentile	Median	75th Percentile	Maximum
Manual	227.20 cc	515.30 cc	1108.00 cc	2836.00 cc	13,820.00 cc
ENet	205.90 cc	550.00 cc	1173.00 cc	3024.00 cc	11,780.00 cc
ERFNet	163.10 cc	519.50 cc	605.70 cc	1577.00 cc	6196.00 cc

Table 2 reports no significant difference between the RPS volumes obtained using the manual approach and ENet (p = 0.935), the manual approach and ERFNet (p = 0.544), or ENet and ERFNet (p = 0.119).

Table 2. Analysis of variance (ANOVA) on retroperitoneal sarcoma volumes showed no significant difference between manual and automatic segmentations.

	F-Value	F Critic Value	p-Value
ENet vs. Manual	0.0069	4.494	0.935
ERFNet vs. Manual	0.3854	4.494	0.544
ENet vs. ERFNet	2.3263	4.494	0.119

ENet, Efficient Neural Network; ERFNet, efficient residual factorized ConvNet.

The correlation graph showed a high positive correlation between manual and ENet segmentation [r^2 = 0.99] and a moderate correlation between manual and ERFNet segmentation [r^2 = 0.79], as shown in Figure 1a,c. In the same way, the Bland–Altman plots showed a high consistency between manual and ENet segmentation and a reproducibility coefficient (RPC) of $\leq$ 1400 cc or $\leq$16% of values; values of 0% or 100% indicate a high or low consistency, respectively, and a low consistency between manual and ERFNet segmentation (RPC of $\leq$5200 cc, or $\leq$100% of values), as shown in Figure 1b,d.

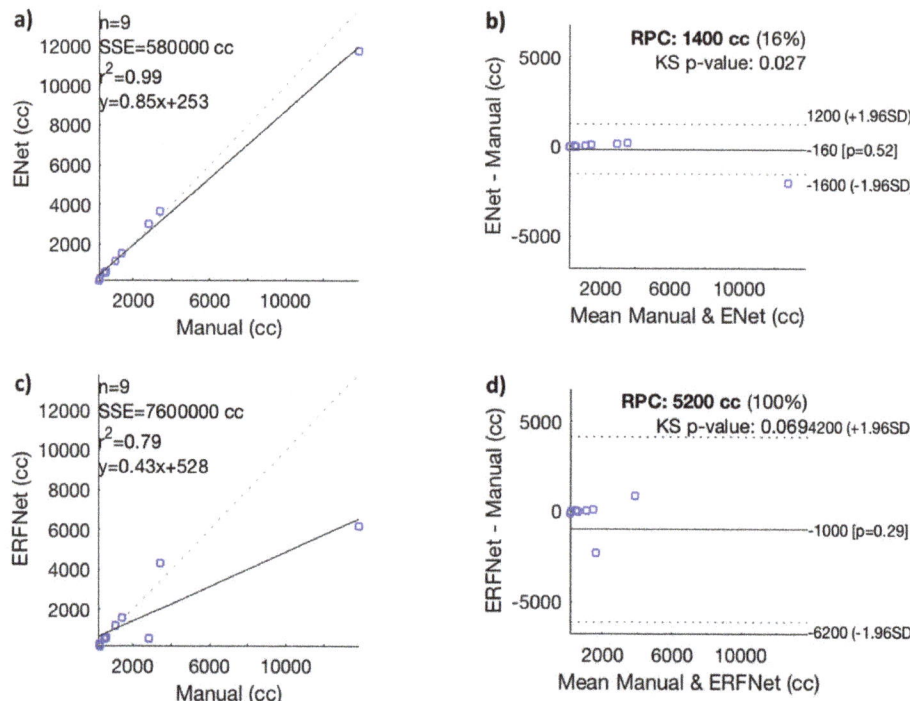

Figure 1. (**a**) Correlation graph, (**b**) Bland–Altman plot between manual and Efficient Neural Network (ENet) volumetric segmentation, (**c**) correlation graph, and (**d**) Bland–Altman plot between manual and Efficient Residual Factorized ConvNet (ERFNet) segmentation. RPC, reproducibility coefficient; SSE, sum of squared error; n, number of data points; p-value, Pearson correlation p-value; r^2, Pearson r-value squared; cc, cubic centimeters; KS, Kolmogorov–Smirnov test; SD, standard deviation.

3.3. Performance Analysis

Table 3 illustrates the performance metrics obtained by comparing the automatic and manual delineations by averaging the results of the five validation folds during the fivefold cross-validation process. A DSC greater than 90% for ENet indicates excellent performances that justify the use of an automatic and independent operator method rather than the manual method, which, although more precise, is very time-consuming, as reported below.

Table 3. Performance results using ENet and ERFNet (fivefold cross-validation strategy).

	Sensitivity	PPV	DSC	VOE	VD
	ENet				
Mean ± SD	91.54 ± 7.49%	89.85 ± 5.66%	90.52 ± 5.49%	16.87 ± 8.81%	2.11 ± 8.53%
±CI (95%)	4.89%	3.70%	3.59%	5.76%	5.58%
	ERFNet				
Mean ± SD	72.21 ± 26.11%	87.00 ± 8.00%	74.85 ± 19.28%	36.85 ± 21.87%	−14.80 ± 33.32%
±CI (95%)	17.06%	5.23%	12.60%	14.29%	21.77%

ENet, Efficient Neural Network; ERFNet, efficient residual factorized ConvNet; PPV, positive predictive value; DSC, dice similarity coefficient; VOE, volume overlap error; VD, volumetric difference; SD, standard deviation; CI, confidence interval.

Figure 2 shows the training DSC and the loss function plots for one fold: a DSC > 90% was achieved in just ~20 iterations for ENet. ERFNet always turns out to be worse than ENet, except for the segmentation speed, as can be seen in Table 4.

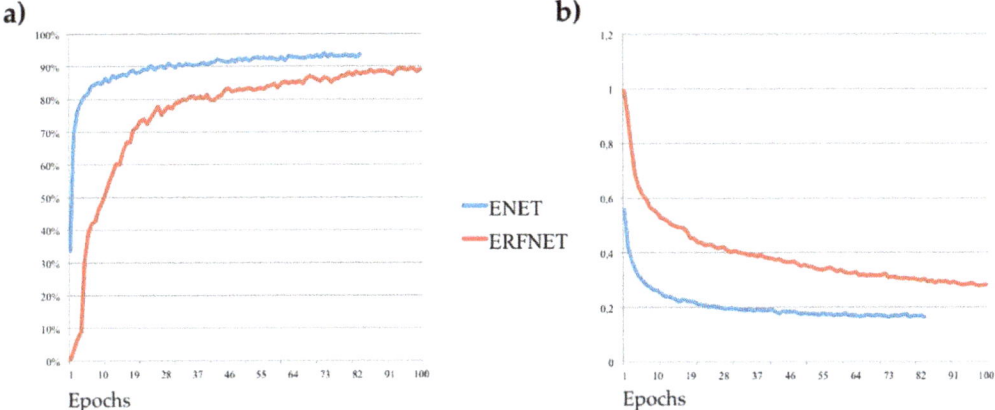

Figure 2. (**a**) Dice similarity coefficient and (**b**) loss function; Tversky loss plots for Efficient Neural Network (ENet) in red lines and Efficient Residual Factorized ConvNet (ERFNet) in blue lines during the training process for one fold.

Table 4. Comparison of computational complexity and performance between the two deep learning models.

	Number of Parameters		Size on Disk	Inference Times (s)/Sataset		Training Times (Days)/Dataset
	Trainable	Non-Trainable		CPU	GPU	GPU
ENet	363,069	8354	5.8 MB	113.10	15.64	5.31
ERFNet	2,056,440	0	25.3 MB	58.08	13.49	4.16

ENet, Efficient Neural Network; ERFNet, efficient residual factorized ConvNet; MB, megabyte; CPU, central processing unit; GPU, graphics processing unit; sec, seconds.

Specifically, using GPU hardware (NVIDIA QUADRO P4000 with 8 GB VRAM and 1792 CUDA Cores), ENet takes about 15 s for a whole segmentation versus 13 s of ERFNet. In the case of a CPU (Intel(R) Xeon(R) W-2125 CPU 4.00GHz processor), ENet takes about 2 min versus 1 min of ERFNet. The manual approach required an average time of 3887 ± 1600 s (approximately one hour per segmentation). Examples of the obtained segmentations are shown in Figure 3 for two patients with abdominal soft tissue sarcomas.

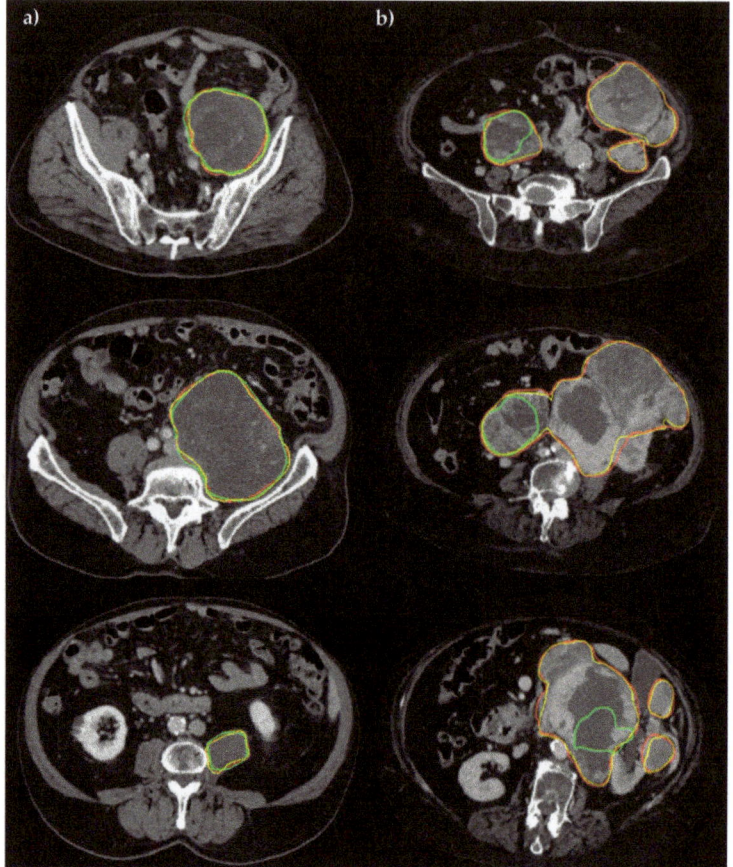

Figure 3. Comparison of segmentation performance in three different slices for (**a**) patient #005, and (**b**) patient #033. Manual (yellow), ENet (red), and ERFNet (green) segmentations are superimposed. In the first study, ENET and ERFNet obtained optimal DSCs (96.69% and 93%, respectively). In the second study, ERFNet showed poor DSC (30.55%) while ENET maintained similar performance compared to the first study (95%).

4. Discussion

4.1. Volume Estimation of Retroperitoneal Sarcoma

Due to the nonspecific presentation of their initial symptoms, RPSs are often seen during an initial evaluation on a CT scan as part of a general abdominal survey [31]. A contrast-enhanced CT allows for confirmation of the site and origin of the mass, and often the tissue composition [32], with the additional benefit of wide availability. An MRI is reserved for patients with an allergy to iodinated contrast agents or problem-solving when some finding is equivocal on a CT scan. It has been reported that different histotypes of RPS can differ widely in terms of both histologic features and clinical behavior; these different histopathologic characteristics may influence glucose metabolism and thus the 18F-FDG uptake in PET examination [33]. Moreover, the difference observed in the maximum standardized uptake value (SUV_{max}) of RPS might be explained by the distinctions in cellularity and necrosis percentage in distinctive histotypes [34]. This different behavior may influence segmentation results. For example, Neabauer et al. [35] reported that the same tumor segmentation yields different results in MRI and PET scans: in an MRI scan, necrosis is considered part of the tumor, but it is not visible on the PET scan, as the necrosis is no longer metabolically active.

The size of the RPS is an important prognostic criterion included in TNM staging (AJCC). Panda et al. [36] reported that size, as measured for the greatest tumor length, was significant in predicting an early relapse. Moreover, in Cox's proportional hazard model, the time-to-event analysis and large size and weight (together with other variables, such as higher age, male sex, incomplete resection, and high grade) become significant, predicting an early recurrence. There is also increasing evidence for the benefits of radiotherapy for RPS to improve local relapse-free survival. Ecker et al. [37] identified size as the only tumor-related variable associated with the use of neoadjuvant radiotherapy. However, all previous studies based their results on tumor size, as measured for the greatest tumor length. An RPS often has a highly irregular shape; therefore, tumors with the same axis length may have a different volume. Further studies are necessary to evaluate whether an overall volume greater than the maximum diameter changes the prognosis and therapy in the era of precision medicine.

4.2. Deep Learning Network and Volume Estimation

This study shows that automatic segmentations with deep learning networks and using portal-venous CT images are reliable methods for the automatic tumor volumetric measurements of RPS. The best performance for automatic segmentation was reached by ENet, with the VD between the automatic and manual segmentation at 2.11% for ENet and at −14.80% for ERFNet. Furthermore, we observed a VOE value of 16.87% for ENet and of 36.85% for ERFNet. These results indicate a low volumetric overlap error between the segmentation results and the manual segmentation, using ENet. To our knowledge, no other studies investigated the role of a deep learning network for RPS segmentation. Our results are concordant with prior investigations exploring the ENet for automatic segmentation in other organs. In a prior study, Lieman-Sifry et al. [38] presented the FastVentricle, an ENet variation, with skip connections for cardiac segmentation. They compared their results to that of the DeepVentricle, the architecture previously cleared by the FDA for clinical use. Both automatic segmentation methods had a median relative absolute error between 5% and 7%. A study involving 103 patients imaged with a prostate MRI [39] used ENet and UNet for the prostate gland segmentation, in comparison with the manual segmentation, which reported a VD of 6.85% and −3.11%. Comelli et al. [40] tested the ENet, UNet, and ERFNet for prostate gland segmentation, which reported mean VDs of 4.53%, 3.16%, and 5.70%, respectively. They obtained the best VOE value with ENet (16.50%), which is similar to the UNet and ERFNet (17.66% and 22.18%, respectively). The DSC is a widely used measure for evaluating medical image segmentation algorithms. It offers a standardized measure of segmentation accuracy, which has proven useful [41]. In the current study, the obtained DCS was 90.52% for ENet and 74.85% for ERFNet. The higher DSC value obtained in our dataset, using ENet, demonstrates a greater similarity to the manual segmentation contour and high-segmentation accuracy.

4.3. Timing Delineation

Our study showed that automatic and user-independent segmentation was much faster than manual segmentation for RPS volumetric analysis. Manual segmentation required an average time of 3887 s, while automatic segmentation required a few seconds. This would suggest good viability for the use of automatic segmentation in clinical practice, where time constraints may restrict which methods are used. ERFNet had better performance than ENet in terms of training times (4.16 days vs. 5.31 days) and in terms of inference times (58.08 s vs. 113.10 s, using a dedicated GPU, and 13.49 s vs. 14.64 s, using CPU). On the other hand, ENet had fewer order-of-magnitude parameters than ERFNet (363,069 vs. 2,056,440, respectively), requiring lower disk space (5.8 MB vs. 25.3 MB, respectively). However, in our experience, both algorithms can be used in a PC equipped with simple hardware and in portable devices, such as a tablet or smartphone.

4.4. Limitations of the Study

Our study has some limitations that need to be reported. We did not consider different tissue components of lesions. RPS are often highly heterogeneous, with variable tissue components that include cellular tumor, macroscopic fat, necrosis, and cystic change depending on the histopathological tumor subtype. These different components have different density values on CT images, which could influence automatic segmentation performances. Further studies with a larger population should be proposed. Moreover, the inter-observer variability for manual segmentation of CT images was not evaluated, as this was beyond the purpose of the current study. Segmentation from radiologists with different experience levels may provide different performances.

5. Conclusions

This study describes two deep learning automatic segmentation methods for RPS volume assessment without the need for user interaction. Starting from the ANOVA test, the results show that ENet and ERFNet obtained automatic segmentations similar to the manual segmentations, with no significant difference found between the two automatic volume estimations. However, ENet seems to perform much better than ERFNet considering the correlation graph and the Bland–Altman plot (Figure 1), the performance scores in Table 3, and the examples in Figure 3. The lack of significant difference is most likely due to the small sample size and high variance in volume size. Furthermore, although ERFNet was faster in the segmentation process using a CPU, ENET and ERFNet obtained similar segmentation times using a GPU. In the future, it would be desirable for the integration of deep learning networks with PACS systems to obtain fast and accurate RPS volume measurements.

Author Contributions: Conceptualization, G.S.; Data curation, A.C.; Formal analysis, A.C.; Investigation; G.B., L.I. and L.A.; Methodology, A.G., M.P. and L.S.; Project administration, M.G.; Resources, G.C.; Software, A.C.; Supervision, F.V. and R.C.; Validation, A.C.; Visualization, A.C.; Writing—original draft, G.S., G.C. and A.S.; Writing—review and editing, G.S., A.C. and A.S. All authors have read and agreed to the published version of the manuscript.

Funding: This research received no external funding.

Institutional Review Board Statement: The proposed research has no implication on patient treatment. Review board approval was not sought: the proposed image analysis was performed offline and thus did not change the current treatment protocol.

Informed Consent Statement: The present study is a retrospective study and written informed consent was waived by our Ethical Committee.

Data Availability Statement: Data sharing not applicable.

Conflicts of Interest: The authors declare no conflict of interest. The funders had no role in the design of the study; in the collection, analyses, or interpretation of data; in the writing of the manuscript; or in the decision to publish the results.

References

1. Choi, J.H.; Ro, J.Y. Retroperitoneal Sarcomas: An Update on the Diagnostic Pathology Approach. *Diagnostics* **2020**, *10*, 642. [CrossRef]
2. Messiou, C.; Moskovic, E.; Vanel, D.; Morosi, C.; Benchimol, R.; Strauss, D.; Miah, A.; Douis, H.; van Houdt, W.; Bonvalot, S. Primary retroperitoneal soft tissue sarcoma: Imaging appearances, pitfalls and diagnostic algorithm. *Eur. J. Surg. Oncol.* **2017**, *43*, 1191–1198. [CrossRef]
3. Porter, G.A.; Baxter, N.N.; Pisters, P.W.T. Retroperitoneal sarcoma: A population-based analysis of epidemiology, surgery, and radiotherapy. *Cancer* **2006**, *106*, 1610–1616. [CrossRef]
4. Varma, D.G. Imaging of soft-tissue sarcomas. *Curr. Oncol. Rep.* **2000**, *2*, 487–490. [CrossRef]
5. Levy, A.D.; Manning, M.A.; Al-Refaie, W.B.; Miettinen, M.M. Soft-tissue sarcomas of the abdomen and pelvis: Radiologic-pathologic features, part 1—Common sarcomas. *Radiographics* **2017**, *37*, 462–483. [CrossRef]
6. Liles, J.S.; Tzeng, C.W.D.; Short, J.J.; Kulesza, P.; Heslin, M.J. Retroperitoneal and Intra-Abdominal Sarcoma. *Curr. Probl. Surg.* **2009**, *46*, 445–503. [CrossRef]

7. Matthyssens, L.E.; Creytens, D.; Ceelen, W.P. Retroperitoneal Liposarcoma: Current Insights in Diagnosis and Treatment. *Front. Surg.* **2015**, *2*. [CrossRef]
8. Singer, S.; Corson, J.M.; Demetri, G.D.; Healey, E.A.; Marcus, K.; Eberlein, T.J. Prognostic factors predictive of survival for truncal and retroperitoneal soft-tissue sarcoma. *Ann. Surg.* **1995**, *221*, 185–195. [CrossRef]
9. Stoeckle, E.; Coindre, J.M.; Bonvalot, S.; Kantor, G.; Terrier, P.; Bonichon, F.; Bui, B.N. Prognostic factors in retroperitoneal sarcoma: A multivariate analysis of a series of 165 patients of the French Cancer Center Federation Sarcoma Group. *Cancer* **2001**, *92*, 359–368. [CrossRef]
10. Heslin, M.J.; Lewis, J.J.; Nadler, E.; Newman, E.; Woodruff, J.M.; Casper, E.S.; Leung, D.; Brennan, M.F. Prognostic factors associated with long-term survival for retroperitoneal sarcoma: Implications for management. *J. Clin. Oncol.* **1997**, *15*, 2832–2839. [CrossRef]
11. Van Dalen, T.; Hennipman, A.; Van Coevorden, F.; Hoekstra, H.J.; Van Geel, B.N.; Slootweg, P.; Lutter, C.F.A.; Brennan, M.F.; Singer, S. Evaluation of a clinically applicable post-surgical classification system for primary retroperitoneal soft-tissue sarcoma. *Ann. Surg. Oncol.* **2004**, *11*, 483–490. [CrossRef]
12. Gronchi, A.; Casali, P.G.; Fiore, M.; Mariani, L.; Lo Vullo, S.; Bertulli, R.; Colecchia, M.; Lozza, L.; Olmi, P.; Santinami, M.; et al. Retroperitoneal soft tissue sarcomas: Patterns of recurrence in 167 patients treated at a single institution. *Cancer* **2004**, *100*, 2448–2455. [CrossRef]
13. Perez, E.A.; Gutierrez, J.C.; Moffat, F.L.; Franceschi, D.; Livingstone, A.S.; Spector, S.A.; Levi, J.U.; Sleeman, D.; Koniaris, L.G. Retroperitoneal and truncal sarcomas: Prognosis depends upon type not location. *Ann. Surg. Oncol.* **2007**, *14*, 1114–1122. [CrossRef]
14. Bonvalot, S.; Rivoire, M.; Castaing, M.; Stoeckle, E.; Le Cesne, A.; Blay, J.Y.; Laplanche, A. Primary retroperitoneal sarcomas: A multivariate analysis of surgical factors associated with local control. *J. Clin. Oncol.* **2009**, *27*, 31–37. [CrossRef]
15. Lewis, J.J.; Leung, D.; Woodruff, J.M.; Brennan, M.F. Retroperitoneal soft-tissue sarcoma: Analysis of 500 patients treated and followed at a single institution. *Ann. Surg.* **1998**, *228*, 355–365. [CrossRef]
16. Gronchi, A.; Lo Vullo, S.; Fiore, M.; Mussi, C.; Stacchiotti, S.; Collini, P.; Lozza, L.; Pennacchioli, E.; Mariani, L.; Casali, P.G. Aggressive surgical policies in a retrospectively reviewed single-institution case series of retroperitoneal soft tissue sarcoma patients. *J. Clin. Oncol.* **2009**, *27*, 24–30. [CrossRef]
17. Haas, R.L.; Baldini, E.H.; Chung, P.W.; van Coevorden, F.; DeLaney, T.F. Radiation therapy in retroperitoneal sarcoma management. *J. Surg. Oncol.* **2018**, *117*, 93–98. [CrossRef]
18. Nathan, H.; Raut, C.P.; Thornton, K.; Herman, J.M.; Ahuja, N.; Schulick, R.D.; Choti, M.A.; Pawlik, T.M. Predictors of survival after resection of retroperitoneal sarcoma: A population-based analysis and critical appraisal of the AJCC Staging system. *Ann. Surg.* **2009**, *250*, 970–976. [CrossRef]
19. Cutaia, G.; La Tona, G.; Comelli, A.; Vernuccio, F.; Agnello, F.; Gagliardo, C.; Salvaggio, L.; Quartuccio, N.; Sturiale, L.; Stefano, A.; et al. Radiomics and Prostate MRI: Current Role and Future Applications. *J. Imaging* **2021**, *7*, 34. [CrossRef]
20. Tian, Z.; Liu, L.; Fei, B. Deep convolutional neural network for prostate MR segmentation. In *Medical Imaging 2017: Image-Guided Procedures, Robotic Interventions, and Modeling*; SPIE: Bellingham, WA, USA, 2017; Volume 10135, p. 101351L.
21. Available online: https://horosproject.org (accessed on 4 February 2021).
22. Paszke, A.; Chaurasia, A.; Kim, S.; Culurciello, E. ENet: A Deep Neural Network Architecture for Real-Time Semantic Segmentation. *arXiv* **2016**, arXiv:1606.02147.
23. Romera, E.; Alvarez, J.M.; Bergasa, L.M.; Arroyo, R. ERFNet: Efficient Residual Factorized ConvNet for Real-Time Semantic Segmentation. *IEEE Trans. Intell. Transp. Syst.* **2018**, *19*, 263–272. [CrossRef]
24. Cuocolo, R.; Comelli, A.; Stefano, A.; Benfante, V.; Dahiya, N.; Stanzione, A.; Castaldo, A.; De Lucia, D.R.; Yezzi, A.; Imbriaco, M. Deep Learning Whole-Gland and Zonal Prostate Segmentation on a Public MRI Dataset. *J. Magn. Reson. Imaging* **2021**, *54*, 452–459.
25. Comelli, A.; Dahiya, N.; Stefano, A.; Benfante, V.; Gentile, G.; Agnese, V.; Raffa, G.M.; Pilato, M.; Yezzi, A.; Petrucci, G.; et al. Deep learning approach for the segmentation of aneurysmal ascending aorta. *Biomed. Eng. Lett.* **2021**, *11*, 15–24. [CrossRef]
26. Comelli, A.; Coronnello, C.; Dahiya, N.; Benfante, V.; Palmucci, S.; Basile, A.; Vancheri, C.; Russo, G.; Yezzi, A.; Stefano, A. Lung Segmentation on High-Resolution Computerized Tomography Images Using Deep Learning: A Preliminary Step for Radiomics Studies. *J. Imaging* **2020**, *6*, 125. [CrossRef]
27. Stefano, A.; Comelli, A. Customized efficient neural network for covid-19 infected region identification in ct images. *J. Imaging* **2021**, *7*, 131. [CrossRef]
28. Kingma, D.P.; Ba, J.L. Adam: A method for stochastic optimization. *arXiv* **2015**, arXiv:1412.6980.
29. Salehi, S.S.M.; Erdogmus, D.; Gholipour, A. Tversky loss function for image segmentation using 3D fully convolutional deep networks. In *Proceedings of the Lecture Notes in Computer Science (Including Subseries Lecture Notes in Artificial Intelligence and Lecture Notes in Bioinformatics)*; Springer: Cham, Switzerland, 2017.
30. Alongi, P.; Stefano, A.; Comelli, A.; Laudicella, R.; Scalisi, S.; Arnone, G.; Barone, S.; Spada, M.; Purpura, P.; Bartolotta, T.V.; et al. Radiomics analysis of 18F-Choline PET/CT in the prediction of disease outcome in high-risk prostate cancer: An explorative study on machine learning feature classification in 94 patients. *Eur. Radiol.* **2021**, *31*, 4595–4605. [CrossRef]
31. Francis, I.R.; Cohan, R.H.; Varma, D.G.K.; Sondak, V.K. Retroperitoneal sarcomas. *Cancer Imaging* **2005**, *5*, 89–94. [CrossRef]

32. Morosi, C.; Stacchiotti, S.; Marchianò, A.; Bianchi, A.; Radaelli, S.; Sanfilippo, R.; Colombo, C.; Richardson, C.; Collini, P.; Barisella, M.; et al. Correlation between radiological assessment and histopathological diagnosis in retroperitoneal tumors: Analysis of 291 consecutive patients at a tertiary reference sarcoma center. *Eur. J. Surg. Oncol.* **2014**, *40*, 1662–1670. [CrossRef]
33. Schwarzbach, M.H.M.; Dimitrakopoulou-Strauss, A.; Willeke, F.; Hinz, U.; Strauss, L.G.; Zhang, Y.M.; Mechtersheimer, G.; Attigah, N.; Lehnert, T.; Herfarth, C. Clinical value of [18-F] fluorodeoxyglucose positron emission tomography imaging in soft tissue sarcomas. *Ann. Surg.* **2000**, *231*, 380–386. [CrossRef]
34. Sambri, A.; Bianchi, G.; Longhi, A.; Righi, A.; Donati, D.M.; Nanni, C.; Fanti, S.; Errani, C. The role of 18F-FDG PET/CT in soft tissue sarcoma. *Nucl. Med. Commun.* **2019**, *40*, 626–631. [CrossRef]
35. Neubauer, T.; Wimmer, M.; Berg, A.; Major, D.; Lenis, D.; Beyer, T.; Saponjski, J.; Bühler, K. Soft Tissue Sarcoma Co-Segmentation in Combined MRI and PET/CT Data. *Lect. Notes Comput. Sci.* **2020**, *12445*, 97–105.
36. Panda, N.; Das, R.; Banerjee, S.; Chatterjee, S.; Gumta, M.; Bandyopadhyay, S.K. Retroperitoneal Sarcoma. Outcome Analysis in a Teaching Hospital in Eastern India- a Perspective. *Indian J. Surg. Oncol.* **2015**, *6*, 99–105. [CrossRef] [PubMed]
37. Ecker, B.L.; Peters, M.G.; McMillan, M.T.; Sinnamon, A.J.; Zhang, P.J.; Fraker, D.L.; Levin, W.P.; Roses, R.E.; Karakousis, G.C. Preoperative radiotherapy in the management of retroperitoneal liposarcoma. *Br. J. Surg.* **2016**, *103*, 1839–1846. [CrossRef] [PubMed]
38. Lieman-Sifry, J.; Le, M.; Lau, F.; Sall, S.; Golden, D. Fastventricle: Cardiac segmentation with ENet. *Lect. Notes Comput. Sci.* **2017**, *10263*, 127–138.
39. Salvaggio, G.; Comelli, A.; Portoghese, M.; Cutaia, G.; Cannella, R.; Vernuccio, F.; Stefano, A.; Dispensa, N.; La Tona, G.; Salvaggio, L.; et al. Deep Learning Network for Segmentation of the Prostate Gland With Median Lobe Enlargement in T2-weighted MR Images: Comparison With Manual Segmentation Method. *Curr. Probl. Diagn. Radiol.* **2021**. [CrossRef] [PubMed]
40. Comelli, A.; Dahiya, N.; Stefano, A.; Vernuccio, F.; Portoghese, M.; Cutaia, G.; Bruno, A.; Salvaggio, G.; Yezzi, A. Deep learning-based methods for prostate segmentation in magnetic resonance imaging. *Appl. Sci.* **2021**, *11*, 782. [CrossRef] [PubMed]
41. Carass, A.; Roy, S.; Gherman, A.; Reinhold, J.C.; Jesson, A.; Arbel, T.; Maier, O.; Handels, H.; Ghafoorian, M.; Platel, B.; et al. Evaluating White Matter Lesion Segmentations with Refined Sørensen-Dice Analysis. *Sci. Rep.* **2020**, *10*, 1–19. [CrossRef] [PubMed]

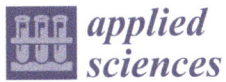

Article

Does a Previous Segmentation Improve the Automatic Detection of Basal Cell Carcinoma Using Deep Neural Networks?

Paulina Vélez *, Manuel Miranda, Carmen Serrano and Begoña Acha

Signal Theory and Communications Department, Universidad de Sevilla, E41092 Seville, Spain; mirandacalixtomanuel@gmail.com (M.M.); cserrano@us.es (C.S.); bacha@us.es (B.A.)
* Correspondence: pauvelnun@alum.us.es

Citation: Vélez, P.; Miranda, M.; Serrano, C.; Acha, B. Does a Previous Segmentation Improve the Automatic Detection of Basal Cell Carcinoma Using Deep Neural Networks? *Appl. Sci.* **2022**, *12*, 2092. https://doi.org/10.3390/app12042092

Academic Editors: Alessandro Stefano, Albert Comelli and Federica Vernuccio

Received: 31 December 2021
Accepted: 15 February 2022
Published: 17 February 2022

Publisher's Note: MDPI stays neutral with regard to jurisdictional claims in published maps and institutional affiliations.

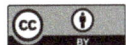

Copyright: © 2022 by the authors. Licensee MDPI, Basel, Switzerland. This article is an open access article distributed under the terms and conditions of the Creative Commons Attribution (CC BY) license (https://creativecommons.org/licenses/by/4.0/).

Abstract: Basal Cell Carcinoma (BCC) is the most frequent skin cancer and its increasing incidence is producing a high overload in dermatology services. In this sense, it is convenient to aid physicians in detecting it soon. Thus, in this paper, we propose a tool for the detection of BCC to provide a prioritization in the teledermatology consultation. Firstly, we analyze if a previous segmentation of the lesion improves the ulterior classification of the lesion. Secondly, we analyze three deep neural networks and ensemble architectures to distinguish between BCC and nevus, and BCC and other skin lesions. The best segmentation results are obtained with a SegNet deep neural network. A 98% accuracy for distinguishing BCC from nevus and a 95% accuracy classifying BCC vs. all lesions have been obtained. The proposed algorithm outperforms the winner of the challenge ISIC 2019 in almost all the metrics. Finally, we can conclude that when deep neural networks are used to classify, a previous segmentation of the lesion does not improve the classification results. Likewise, the ensemble of different neural network configurations improves the classification performance compared with individual neural network classifiers. Regarding the segmentation step, supervised deep learning-based methods outperform unsupervised ones.

Keywords: Basal Cell Carcinoma; deep learning; convolutional neural network; skin lesion; segmentation; classification

1. Introduction

Skin cancer is the most common cancer in the United States and worldwide [1]. Although the majority of the works in the literature are focused on melanoma detection, the most common malign skin lesion is the non-melanoma skin cancer (NMSC). Over 95% of NMSC cases are Basal Cell Carcinoma (BCC) and cutaneous squamous cell carcinoma (SCC) [2]. Specifically, BCC has an incidence higher than 70% [3] among all skin cancer, it has the best validated clinical criteria for its diagnosis [4], and it presents the higher variability in the presence of these dermoscopic criteria.

The detection of NMSC can be performed by visual inspection by a skilled dermatologist, but there are many benign lesions that can be confused with NMSC, leading to unnecessary biopsies, in a proportion of five biopsies versus one actual cancer case [5].

The increase in the incidence of BCC is provoking an overload for dermatologists. In the Andalusian Health System, teledermatology is being implanted. Nowadays, 315 demands of teledermatology consultation per month are received and 210 receive diagnostic criteria of BCC. Thus, a Computer Aided Diagnosis (CAD) tool that assists general practitioner physicians and provides a prioritization in the teledermatology consultation would have great utility.

Different kinds of images have been traditionally used in order to classify NMSC automatically (spectroscopy, optical coherence tomography, etc.). However, the simplest one and most used is the digital dermoscopy, that is, a digital color photograph, enhanced by a dermoscope.

Lately, and due to the availability of databases due to the challenges proposed by ISIC [6], the use of artificial intelligence methods, and in particular, the use of deep learning neural networks, have become very popular in dermatology. In this sense, this paper is focused on machine learning algorithms, in particular, deep learning ones, and using dermatoscopic images from ISIC challenges [6].

Most of the works published have been focused on melanoma segmentation and classification [7,8]. On the contrary, much less work has been devoted to NMSC detection. Marka et al. performed a systematic analysis of existing methods for automatic detection of NMSC in 2019. They came to the conclusion that, although most of the methods attain an accuracy similar to the reported diagnostic accuracy of a dermatologist, all the methods require a clinical study to assess the validity of the methods in a real clinical scenario [9]. There are three methods that attain the best classification metrics according to this study. Wahba et al., in 2017, reached 100% in all the metrics but the test set was only 10 images [10]. The same authors, in 2018, tested their methods with an extended database, obtaining the same results [11]. Møllersen et al. also achieved 100% sensitivity, but their specificity was 12% [12]. Sarkar et al. applied deep neural networks to differentiate between BCC, SCC and benign lesions. They achieved an AUROC score of 0.997, 1 and 0.998, respectively [13]. Pangti et al. analyzed the performance of a deep learning-based application for the diagnosis of BCC, as compared to dermatologist and non-dermatologist physicians [14].

In Han et al., 12 skin diseases were classified, employing a deep learning algorithm. They used three databases and concluded that the tested algorithm performance is comparable to that obtained by 16 dermatologists. One of these skin diseases is BCC [15]. Following this comparison, Carcagni et al. [16] and Zhou et al. [17] also proposed methods based on deep learning to perform a multiclassification of skin diseases. Carcagni et al. proposed an ensemble approach and compared it with the original Densenet-121, obtaining a better performance.

Sies et al. [18] tested two market-approved tools, one employed a Machine Learning (ML) technique and one is based on Convolutional Neural Networks (CNN). Although they tested 1981 skin lesions, only 28 lesions were BCC. The ML algorithm detected only 5 in 28 BCC lesions, whereas the CNN-based algorithm detected 27 in 28 [18]. Dorj et al. use a pre-trained AlexNet convolutional network to extract the features that feed an SVM classifier, in order to classify among four kinds of cancers, including BCC [19].

Recent advances in the field of histopathological and microscopic image analysis, dedicated to the BCC detection, can be found at [20–22], where the authors use deep learning techniques to detect, classify and identify its patterns. However, our approach covers BCC classification, focusing on distinguishing BCC from Nevus, and employing dermoscopic images. From a clinical point of view, it is very interesting to differentiate BCC from nevus, because both represent the most frequent skin lesions appearing at primary health centers, and a good detection of these types of lesions could lead to a more efficient clinical management, performing a first prioritization of the images that arrive from the Primary Health Center by teledermatology.

The main contribution of the paper is that it performs a thorough analysis of deep learning techniques, applied to BCC segmentation and classification.

In addition, to the best of our knowledge, there are no previous works that evaluate the influence of a previous segmentation in the classification of skin lesions with a deep neural network.

2. Materials and Methods

In order to segment and classify the lesion, several experiments have been conducted that try to evaluate how important the segmentation is for an ulterior classification. A comparison between deep learning methods and classical segmentation algorithms is presented.

Regarding the classification task, different deep learning architectures in the following two different classification scenarios are tested: BCC vs. Nevus, BCC vs. All lesions.

2.1. Lesion Segmentation

Skin lesion segmentation becomes a challenging task due to the presence of hair, bubbles, different illumination conditions, blurry boundaries, blood vessels, scars or different skin colors, thus, the segmentation step turns into a very delicate and complex process.

Over the years, many techniques that successfully overcome the segmentation challenges have been developed. Unsupervised segmentation methods, such as thresholding, edge-based, region-based or energy minimization-based ones, and supervised methods, such as support vector machines (SVM), Bayes-based, or deep learning-based segmentation methods (DLBSM) have been successfully tested over any kind of images [23,24].

Lately, regarding dermoscopic images, many works have been focused on deep learning-based methodologies [25]. This kind of segmentation technique combines low-level feature information with high-level semantic information [26] and takes the advantage of its learning capacities, focusing on its learning properties to identify structures that allow us to segment the image. DLBSM allow us to segment images with low contrast, different intensity distribution or images with artifacts [27].

In this paper, we compare unsupervised with supervised segmentation techniques. In fact, we compare the performance of one unsupervised method based on energy minimization, and two segmentation methods based on deep learning. More specifically, the two supervised methods consist of the following: (1) A CNN as feature extractor combined with a classic segmentation method (thresholding), and (2) Semantic neural network (SegNet). These three methods were tested over ISIC-2017 database [28].

2.1.1. Unsupervised Method: Energy Minimization Based Algorithm

Unsupervised methods do not require a labelled training dataset. One of the main advantages they have is the low computational cost [29]. Another one is that they do not need a large database as no training is performed. In contrast, its performance could not be robust for low quality images, or some interaction with the user is needed to achieve a good performance.

There are many state-of-the-art unsupervised algorithms in the literature and some of them have been explored in this paper (edge-based active contour, region-based active contours, segmentation based on convex optimization). However, for the final analysis an energy minimization method was chosen because it is less dependent on the parameter setting. In this kind of algorithm, an energy measure, which includes region and boundary information, is minimized to solve the segmentation problem. Over recent years, energy minimization algorithms based on convex relaxation have been developed [29,30]. This paper presents an algorithm using convex relaxation based on a previous work by the authors [31,32]. The original idea was proposed by Papadakis and Rabin [33]. It consists of posing the problem of segmentation as a problem of minimization of a convex energy function. In this energy function, the distance between the histograms of each region within the image and histogram models is minimized.

Two histogram models were defined for each dermoscopic image, one for the foreground (the lesion) and the other for the background (the skin). To generate these two histogram models, the algorithm requires a manual selection of a partial part of each region (Figure 1).

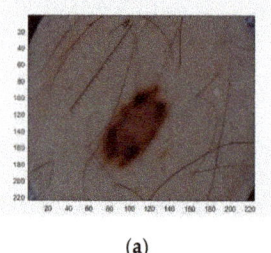 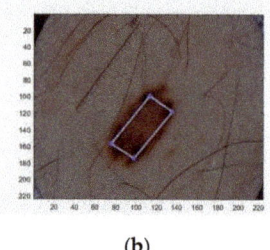 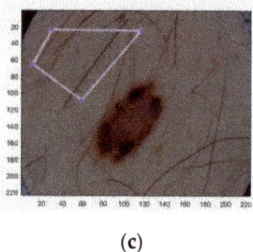

(a)   (b)   (c)

Figure 1. Selected areas of dermoscopic images for calculating the histograms. (**a**) Original image; (**b**) Selected region inside the lesion; (**c**) Selected region in the healthy skin.

2.1.2. Supervised Methods

Supervised methods need a training data set in order to fix the parameters of the classifier. Some of these segmentation methods are based on SVMs, Bayes classifier, decision trees (DTs) or artificial neural networks (ANN) [34].

As supervised algorithms, two different methods were chosen. The first method has been chosen because it segments by employing the information provided by the deep features of a CNN. This fact has the advantage that a small training database is required and even a pre-trained CNN may be utilized. The second supervised segmentation is a fully convolutional neural network, which has been demonstrated to be effective in medical image segmentation. More specifically, SegNet has been chosen because it is state of the art in the field.

Segmentation from Feature Images of a CNN

A CNN possesses convolutional layers that provide a wide information about global and local features of an image. Hence, the deepest convolutional layers contain information of the global, abstract and conceptual features, whereas the lower convolutional layers give information about the local structure, which is relevant for the segmentation process [35]. Likewise, convolutional layers can be used to obtain the image features [36].

We used a VGG-16 pre-trained with ImageNet database. A set of images from the fourth convolutional layer of VGG-16 network was extracted. These images were normalized and filtered by applying a Gaussian filter with standard deviation equal to 2, before being added. Finally, a threshold using Otsu's method and morphological operations (dilation and hole filling) was applied to obtain the final segmentation result. A scheme of this segmentation algorithm is presented in Figure 2.

Semantic Segmentation with SegNet Deep Neural Network

Semantic Segmentation allows us to identify an object in an image by classifying each pixel into a labeled class, which is called pixel-wise labeling. As is described by Badrinarayanan et al. [37], SegNet is a Fully Convolutional Network (FCN) architecture whose encoder is topologically similar to the convolutional layers from VGG-16, but without its fully connected layers. The convolutions are performed with a filter bank. The last layer of the decoder works as a soft-max classifier, which allows us to obtain the predicted segmentation labels for each pixel as output, where each label is associated with an existing class. SegNet admits as input a map of features or an image.

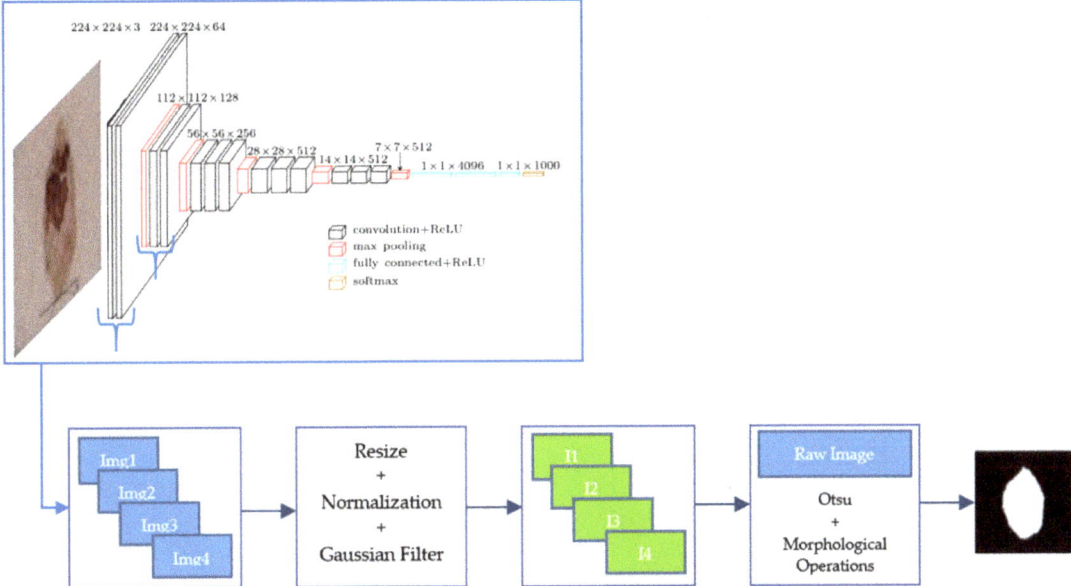

Figure 2. Scheme of this segmentation algorithm from feature images of a CNN.

2.2. Lesion Classification

The classification part of the paper will try to differentiate between different types of skin lesions, being the motivation of the paper, the detection of BCC.

We present the following two types of classifications:

1. BCC vs. Nevus;
2. BCC vs. All, where the term "All" groups the following skin lesions: nevus, benign keratosis, dermatofibroma, melanoma, SCC, actinic keratosis and vascular lesion.

From a clinical point of view, it is very interesting to differentiate BCC from nevus, because both represent the most frequent skin lesions appearing at primary health centers, and a good detection of these types of lesions could lead to a more efficient clinical management.

In the two classification experiments, we have tested how the introduction of previously segmented images could affect the classification.

A wide number of experiments are conducted in order to check which configuration could be better to solve this difficult problem. To this purpose several classification approaches have been proposed, as follows:

1. The use of a VGG-16 neural network. VGG-16 consists of 16 convolutional layers and is very appealing because of its very uniform architecture [38].
2. The use of a ResNet50 neural network. It is a convolutional neural network with 50 layers. It is a type of Residual Network and it first introduced the concept of skip connection [39].
3. The use of an InceptionV3 neural network. InceptionV3 is another type of CNN developed by Google. It is 48 layers deep [40].
4. The use of an ensemble of the three neural networks using the maximum argument. The ArgMax ensemble calculates, for each image, the probability of each class from each neural network, and it selects as the output class the one with highest probability among all the neural networks.
5. The use of an ensemble of the three neural networks using the mean. In this case the average of the three probabilities for each class belonging to each neural network is calculated. The output class selected is the one with the maximum average value.

In Figure 3, the ArgMax ensemble configuration is shown. After training the three DNNs mentioned above, a vector with the probabilities belonging to each class for each DNN is obtained (V_i, $i = 1,2,3$). Each in this vector has dimension $m \times 1$, where m is the number of classes. Finally, a new vector is formed $V = [V_1, V_2, V_3]$ of dimensions $3m \times 1$. The class with the highest probability, denoted by n, is chosen as the predicted class of the lesion.

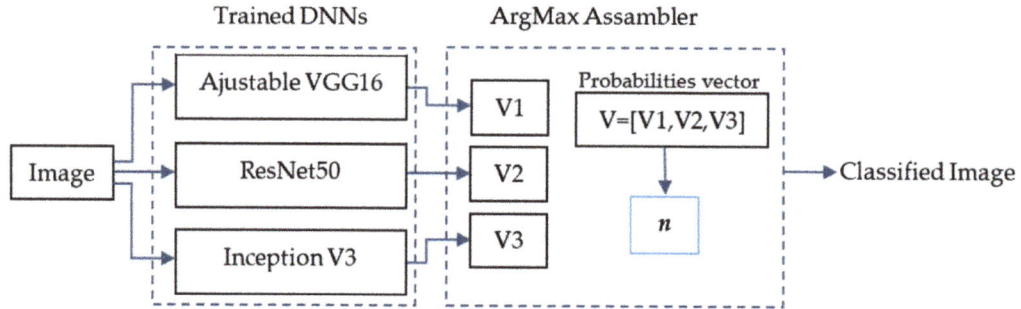

Figure 3. ArgMax ensemble configuration for the skin lesion classification.

3. Results

3.1. Segmentation Results

3.1.1. Database

To perform the comparison among the different segmentation algorithms, the ISIC 2017 database has been used [6,26]. This database provides 2000 images for training and 600 images for testing, with their corresponding ground truth masks. The ISIC 2018 database for the task "Lesion segmentation" does not provide the ground truth masks for the test set, that is why ISIC 2017 database has been chosen for the part of segmentation. The ISIC 2019 challenge [6] does not include a "Lesion segmentation" task.

For the segmentation algorithms based on convolutional neural networks, a data augmentation process was applied. The data augmentation step consists of random rotations between −30 and 30 degrees; random translations on axes x and y within −10 and 10 interval; random horizontal and vertical reflections; scaling with a random scale factor between 0.9 and 1.1. Finally, all images were randomly sheared in horizontal and vertical angles, specified between 0 and 45 degrees. All these operations picked their random values from a continuous uniform distribution.

After data augmentation, the number of training images was 18,000.

3.1.2. Implementation Details

The three methodologies were implemented on a system with an Intel Core I9-3.6 GHz processor, 32 GB of RAM, and NVIDIA TITAN RTX card.

The SegNet neural network was pre-initialized with layers and weights from a VGG-16 pretrained network, with an ImageNet database from the ImageNet Large Scale Visual Recognition Challenge (ILSVRC). The stochastic gradient descent with momentum (SGDM) optimizer was applied and the training parameters were set as follows: momentum of 0.9, mini-batch size of 5, initial learning rate of 0.001, and weight decay (L2Regularization) of 0.005. The model was trained for 200 epochs.

3.1.3. Results

In Figure 4, the results applying the three segmentation methods for four example images are shown.

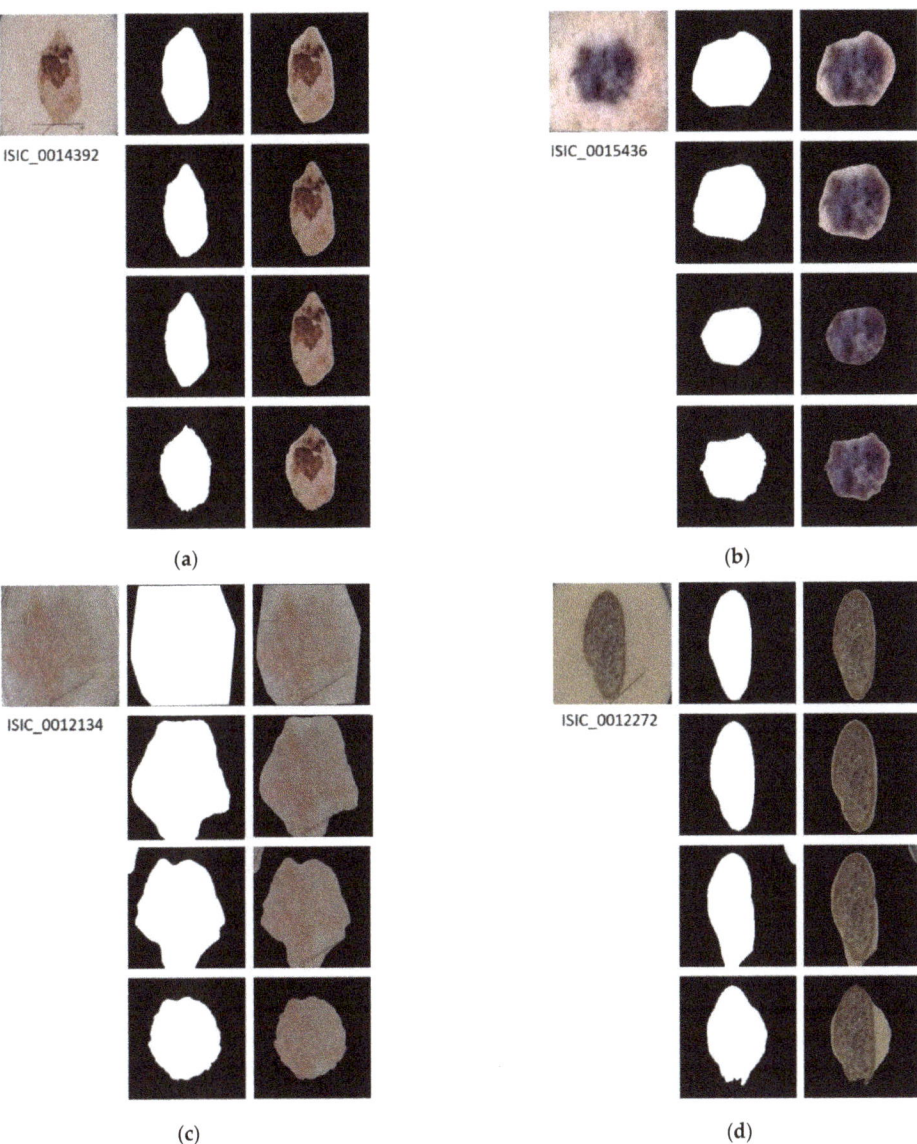

Figure 4. Segmented Images. For images (**a**–**d**): first row shows the original image with its ground truth mask and its corresponding segmentation result; second row shows the results of applying semantic segmentation with SegNet; third row shows the result of energy minimization algorithm via convex optimization; fourth row shows the result of segmentation based on VGG16 feature images.

Table 1 presents the performance parameters for each method, as follows: Dice coefficient (DICE), Jaccard index (JACC), Sensitivity (Se), Specificity (Sp) and Accuracy (Acc). This table presents the results of applying the three methods to the test set of the database, ISIC 2017 (600 images). The best performance is achieved by the SegNet neural network in four out of five parameters.

Table 1. Segmentation results of the tested methods over the Test set (600 images). Numbers represent the average values of the different segmentation performance parameters calculated over the 600 test images.

Methodology	DICE	JACC	Se	Sp	ACC
SegNet	0.8548	0.7730	0.8533	0.9632	0.9357
Energy minimization	0.5937	0.4927	0.6020	0.9131	0.8647
Feature images from VGG16	0.5853	0.4700	0.8627	0.8690	0.8170

Beyond the evaluation parameters, it is relevant to discuss the advantages and drawbacks of each methodology. Although the SegNet neural network obtains the highest performance, the accuracy obtained by the energy minimization algorithm is acceptable, taking into account the resources needed. Nevertheless, SegNet requires a high computational effort for the training but, once the training process has been done, the computational cost of the segmentation process is comparable to the cost required by the other two methods. On the other hand, semantic segmentation via SegNet is an automatic process, which allows us to obtain the segmented lesion without human supervision, as well as the segmentation based on feature images from VGG16. In contrast, energy minimization segmentation requires human intervention, slowing down the segmentation process or making it difficult to use, in the case of large databases.

In Table 2, a comparison with other methods published in the literature is presented. This table shows that the segmentation with SegNet attains competitive results. This justifies that this technique can be chosen as a good segmentation method, in order to evaluate the convenience of including a segmentation step before the classification of the lesions.

Table 2. Segmentation results of benchmark methods over the Test set (600 images). The results obtained with the SegNet neural network have also been included to facilitate the comparison.

Ref.	Methodology	DICE	JACC	Se	Sp	ACC
[41]	FCDN- First Place at Challenge ISBI-2017	0.8490	0.7650	0.8250	0.9750	0.9340
[27]	Separable-UNet model with stochastic weight averaging scheme	0.8693	0.7926	0.8953	0.9632	0.9431
[42]	LinkNet152 model	0.8530	0.7700	–	–	–
[43]	GAN-based model	0.9063	0.8198	0.8781	0.9992	0.9761
[26]	Deep class-specific learning	0.8566	0.7773	0.8620	0.9671	0.9408
	SegNet	0.8548	0.7730	0.8533	0.9632	0.9357

3.2. Classification Results

3.2.1. Database

For the classification step, the ISIC-2019 database has been used [44,45], which contains 25,331 dermoscopic images. This database consists of the following lesions: actinic keratosis (867 images), Basal Cell Carcinoma (3323 images), benign keratosis (2624 images), dermatofibroma (239 images), melanoma (4522 images), nevus (12,875 images), squamous cell carcinoma (628 images), and vascular lesion (253 images). An example of these dermoscopic images is shown in Figure 5.

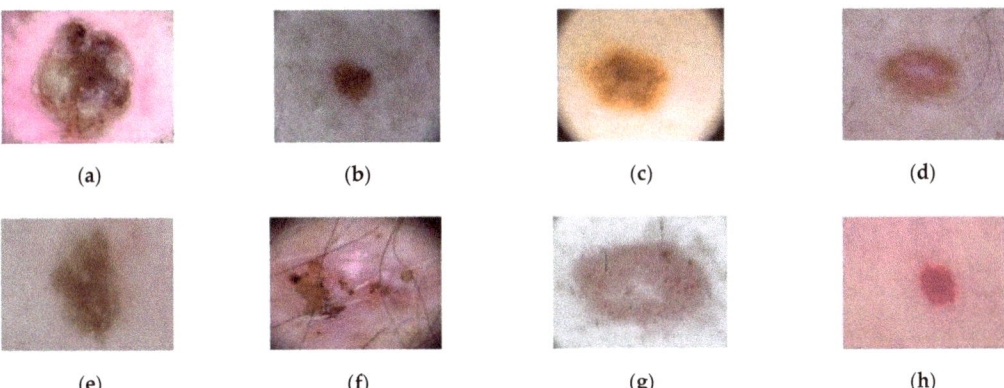

Figure 5. Dermoscopic images from ISIC-2019 database. (**a**) Squamous cell carcinoma; (**b**) Nevus; (**c**) Melanoma; (**d**) Dermofibroma; (**e**) Benign keratosis; (**f**) Basal Cell Carcinoma; (**g**) Actinic keratosis; (**h**) Vascular lesion.

In order to train the convolutional neural networks used to classify the lesions, the database was balanced by a data augmentation process. Data augmentation was carried out by mirror operations and rotations of 36 degrees over each image. The test images were not modified.

As mentioned above, two different experiments were carried out, hence, the database was balanced in two different ways.

For the classification of BCC vs. Nevus, after data augmentation, the following number of images were obtained: 8982 images for training and 1287 for validation, for each class. In this sense, for all the classes, except nevus, the number of images was artificially augmented by the data augmentation process described above. For the nevus class, a downsampling process has been carried out, randomly selecting 10,269 images in total (8982 training + 1287 validation) out of the 12,875 nevus images that the ISIC provides.

For BCC vs. All lesions, the balanced dataset is constituted as follows: 15,419 training images and 2199 validation images, for each of the two classes (BCC and the rest of the types). In this case, data augmentation was applied for the BCC class, increasing the number of nevus images up to 17,618 in total (training and validation set). For each class belonging to the remaining seven classes, the number of images was fixed to 2517 images in total for each class.

3.2.2. Classification Results of BCC vs. Nevus

The database consists of 23,780 images in total, after the data augmentation. The training set consists of 17,964 images, the validation set consists of 2574 images and there are 3242 images for the test process. The results are described in Tables 3 and 4.

Table 3. Performance parameters for the different classifiers without the previous segmentation of the image when classifying BCC vs. Nevus. Se: Sensitivity, Sp: Specificity, Pre: Precision, FPR: False Positive Rate, Acc: Accuracy. The highest values are shown in bold numbers.

Method	Se	Sp	Pre	FPR	Acc
VGG16	0.95	0.97	0.88	**0.99**	0.97
ResNet50	0.95	0.97	0.88	**0.99**	0.96
InceptionV3	0.95	0.97	0.87	0.96	0.94
Ensemble ArgMax	**0.97**	**0.98**	**0.92**	**0.99**	**0.98**
Ensemble Mean	**0.97**	0.97	0.90	**0.99**	0.97

Table 4. Performance parameters for the different classifiers with the previous segmentation of the image by using a SegNet neural network when classifying BCC vs. Nevus. Se: Sensitivity, Sp: Specificity, Pre: Precision, FPR: False Positive Rate, Acc: Accuracy. The highest values are shown in bold numbers.

Method	Se	Sp	Pre	FPR	Acc
VGG16	0.87	**0.97**	0.87	**0.97**	**0.95**
ResNet50	0.88	0.96	0.86	**0.97**	**0.95**
InceptionV3	0.85	**0.97**	0.87	0.96	0.94
Ensemble ArgMax	**0.90**	**0.97**	**0.88**	**0.97**	**0.95**
Ensemble Mean	0.89	**0.97**	**0.88**	**0.97**	**0.95**

Transfer learning has been applied to the pre-trained neural network configurations.

If we denote true positives as TP, true negatives as TN, false positives as FP and false negatives as FN, the classification performance parameters we have used are defined as follows:

Sensitivity, which represents the proportion of people who test positive among all those who actually have the disease: Se = TP/(TP + FN).

Specificity, which is the proportion of people who test negative among all those who actually do not have that disease: Sp = TN/(TN + FP).

Precision, which represents the probability that following a positive test result, that individual will truly have that specific disease: Pre = TP/(TP + FP).

False positive rate, which is calculated as the ratio between the number of negative events wrongly categorized as positive (false positives) and the total number of actual negative events: FPR = FP/(FP + TN).

Accuracy, which represents the proportion of true positive results (both true positive and true negative) in the selected population: Acc = (TN + TP)/(TN + TP + FN + FP).

As shown in Tables 3 and 4, the best configuration is the ensemble ArgMax, without previous segmentation of the image. For this case, the confusion matrix is shown in Figure 6. The confusion matrix shows the classification performed by the specialists (named *True*), versus the predicted classification performed by the ensemble ArgMax classification tool. The larger the numbers in the diagonal are, the better the classification results are.

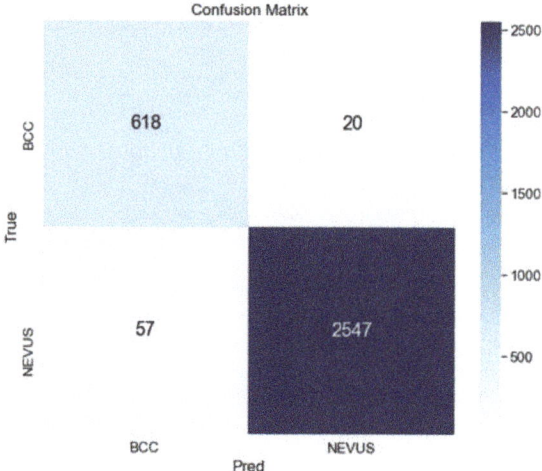

Figure 6. Confusion matrix for the classification of BCC vs. Nevus using the ensemble ArgMax and without previous segmentation.

3.2.3. Classification Results of BCC vs. All Lesions

The total number of images of the database, after data augmentation, was 40,302. The training set was composed of 30,838 images, the validation set, 4398 images, and the test set, 5066 images. The different classes were balanced after applying the data augmentation step. Results are summarized in Tables 5 and 6.

Table 5. Performance metrics for the different classifiers without the previous segmentation of the image when classifying BCC vs. All lesions. Se: Sensitivity, Sp: Specificity, Pre: Precision, FPR: False Positive Rate, Acc: Accuracy. The highest values are shown in bold numbers.

Method	Se	Sp	Pre	FPR	Acc
VGG16	0.84	0.96	0.75	0.97	0.94
ResNet50	0.81	0.95	0.72	0.97	0.93
InceptionV3	0.78	0.95	0.70	0.97	0.93
Ensemble ArgMax	**0.84**	**0.96**	0.78	**0.98**	**0.95**
Ensemble Mean	0.83	**0.96**	0.78	0.97	**0.95**

Table 6. Performance parameters for the different classifiers with the previous segmentation of the image with a SegNet when classifying BCC vs. All lesions. Se: Sensitivity, Sp: Specificity, Pre: Precision, FPR: False Positive Rate, Acc: Accuracy. The highest values are shown in bold numbers.

Method	Se	Sp	Pre	FPR	Acc
VGG16	**0.68**	0.96	0.74	**0.95**	0.94
ResNet50	0.65	0.96	0.70	**0.95**	0.93
InceptionV3	0.60	0.96	0.67	0.94	0.93
Ensemble ArgMax	**0.68**	**0.97**	0.77	**0.95**	**0.95**
Ensemble Mean	**0.68**	**0.97**	0.78	**0.95**	**0.95**

The best result is obtained for the ensemble ArgMax without previous segmentation; the confusion matrix for this case is shown in Figure 7.

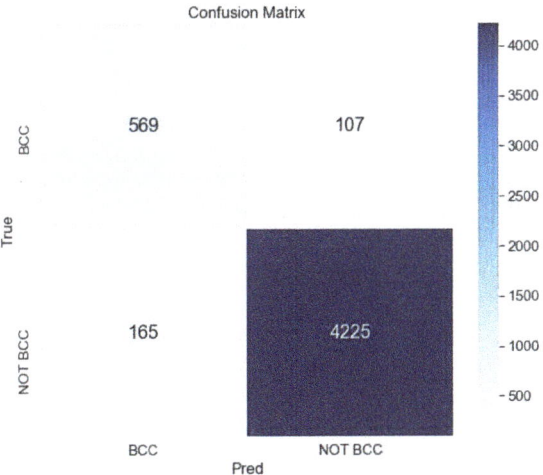

Figure 7. Confusion matrix for the classification BCC vs. All lesions using the ensemble ArgMax without previous segmentation of the lesion.

To the best of our knowledge, there are no published works devoted to classifying BCC vs. non-BCC lesions or BCC vs. nevus. Thus, in order to compare the proposed method with the state of the art, we have performed the classification proposed in the ISIC 2019 Challenge, where eight different lesions are classified. Results are shown in Table 7. We have used as a benchmark algorithm, the winner of the ISIC 2019 Challenge [6,46]. As can be observed, the proposed method outperforms the benchmark algorithm in almost all the metrics.

The reason for these good results may be found in different factors. First of all, the three networks chosen for the ensemble are networks of proven effectiveness (VGG16, ResNet and Inceptionv3 were the winners in the ILSVRC 2014 or ILSVRC 2015 challenges). On the other hand, these networks do not have an excessive number of parameters, which would require a large training database to obtain good classification results. Finally, the ensemble of these three winning networks leads to the obtaining of better results.

Table 7. Performance parameters for the winner of the ISIC Challenge 2019 [46] and for the proposed method (Argmax ensemble without previous segmentation) when classifying into eight types of lesions. Se: Sensitivity, Sp: Specificity, Acc: Accuracy.

	Winner Challenge 2019 [46]		Proposed Method		
	Se	Sp	Se	Sp	Acc
AK	0.48	0.97	0.48	1.00	0.96
BCC	0.72	0.94	0.83	0.98	0.96
BKL	0.39	0.99	0.50	0.99	0.94
DF	0.58	0.98	0.48	1.00	0.99
MEL	0.59	0.96	0.61	0.97	0.91
NEVUS	0.71	0.98	0.97	0.71	0.84
SCC	0.44	0.99	0.43	1.00	0.98
VASC	0.64	0.99	0.79	1.00	1.00

4. Discussion

There are few papers devoted to the detection of BCC in the literature [10–13], and less that apply deep neural networks to solve this problem. One of the main reasons is the lack of public databases with BCC lesions, with contours delineation or with labelled dermoscopic criteria.

From a clinical point of view, it is very convenient to distinguish between BCC and nevus, due to the high incidence of these two types of lesions. Specifically, in primary health centers, it would be desirable to have an automatic tool, in order to help the non-specialist in the diagnosis and to establish a good priority in the attendance at the dermatology services. To the best of our knowledge this is the first time that a classification between BCC and nevus has been performed.

Most works devoted to segment skin lesions claim that an accurate segmentation is necessary to achieve a proper extraction of features and consequent lesion characterization [47]. However, in this paper, we demonstrated that, when using deep learning methods, it is not advantageous to include a segmentation before classifying the lesion. Actually, we get worse results when segmenting the lesion previously to the classification step, showing that, when using a large database, the previous segmentation of the lesion does not improve the classification results. This suggests that the healthy skin surrounding the lesion may contain information significant for the classification. In this sense, other works, such as the one by Teixeira et al., support this statement [48].

The main limitation of our method is the lack of explainability of the classification. An explanation of the classification, by providing the automatic detection of dermoscopic criteria of BCC, would considerably improve the utility of the method for physicians. To this purpose, we are working on developing a database with the dermoscopic criteria of BCC and a system for the automatic detection of these dermoscopic criteria.

As future research, a clinical study to assess the validity of the methods in a real clinical scenario would be desirable.

5. Conclusions

In this paper, two analyses have been performed. Firstly, a comparison between an unsupervised segmentation method and two supervised segmentation methods, based on deep learning, has been carried out. Secondly, the identification of BCC amongst other types of skin lesions has been performed in the following two different scenarios: with a previous segmentation of the lesion and without segmenting the lesion. To this second task, different deep neural networks have been tested.

Experiments to compare the different segmentation methods show that SegNet architecture has attained the best behavior, obtaining 94% accuracy.

The ISIC 2019 public database [6] has been used to carry out the classification task. A 98% accuracy, 0.84% sensitivity and 0.96% specificity, for distinguishing BCC from nevus, and a 95% accuracy, 0.68% sensitivity and 0.97% specificity, classifying BCC vs. all lesions, have been obtained. Furthermore, the proposed algorithm outperforms the winner of the ISIC 2019 challenge in almost all the metrics, when lesions are classified into eight classes.

In summary, this paper adds important comparison studies, applied to the analysis of BCC, that have not been performed previously. These studies are of interest, because BCC is the skin cancer of highest incidence. First, an analysis of the utility of BCC segmentation to improve classification is carried out, driving to the conclusion that previous segmentation does not improve the classification. Secondly, a tool for the discrimination between BCC and nevus, which is the most common pigmented lesion, is provided. Finally, we have demonstrated that an ensemble of well-known CNN can attain results that can compete with the best methods in the ISIC challenge.

Author Contributions: Conceptualization, P.V., C.S. and B.A.; methodology, P.V. and M.M.; software, P.V. and M.M.; validation, P.V., M.M., C.S. and B.A.; resources, C.S. and B.A.; writing—original draft preparation, P.V.; writing—review and editing, C.S. and B.A.; visualization, P.V.; supervision, C.S. and B.A.; funding acquisition, C.S. and B.A. All authors have read and agreed to the published version of the manuscript.

Funding: This work was funded by Project DPI2016-81103-R ("Ministerio de Economía y Competitividad", Spanish Government) and Project US-1381640 (FEDER-US, Regional Government of Andalusia). Manuel Miranda has been hired by "Fondo Social Europeo Iniciativa de Empleo Juvenil" 2019-3-EJ3-83-1 (European Union and Andalusian Government).

Data Availability Statement: Databases employed in this study are available at https://challenge.isic-archive.com/data/ (accessed on 30 December 2021).

Conflicts of Interest: The authors declare no conflict of interest. The funders had no role in the design of the study; in the collection, analyses, or interpretation of data; in the writing of the manuscript, or in the decision to publish the results.

Abbreviation

The following abbreviations are used in this manuscript:

Acc	Accuracy
AK	Actinic Keratosis
ANN	Artificial Neural Networks
AUROC	Area Under the Receiver Operating Characteristic
BCC	Basal Cell Carcinoma
BKL	Bening Keratosis
CAD	Computer Aid Diagnosis
CNN	Convolutional Neural Network
DF	Dermatofibroma
DICE	Dice Coefficient
DLBSM	Deep Learning-Based Segmentation Methods
DNN	Deep Neural Network

DT	Decision Trees
FCN	Fully Convolutional Network
FPR	False Positive Rate
ILSVRC	ImageNet Large Scale Visual Recognition Challenge
ISIC	International Skin Imaging Collaboration
JACC	Jaccard Index
MEL	Melanoma
ML	Machine Learning
NMSC	Non-Melanoma Skin Cancer
Pre	Precision
RAM	Random Access Memory
ResNet	Residual Networks
SCC	Squamous Cell Carcinoma
Se	Sensitivity
SegNet	Semantic Neural Network
SGDM	Stochastic Gradient Descent with Momentum
Sp	Specificity
SVM	Support Vector Machine
VASC	Vascular

References

1. Skin Cancer Foundation. Skin Cancer Facts and Statistics. Available online: https://www.skincancer.org/skin-cancer-information/skin-cancer-facts (accessed on 11 October 2021).
2. Gillard, M.; Wang, T.S.; Johnson, T.M. Nonmelanoma cutaneous malignancies. In *Oncology, An Evidence-Based Approach*; Chang, A.E., Ganz, P.A., Hayes, D.F., Kinsella, T., Pass, H.I., Schiller, J.H., Stone, R.M., et al., Eds.; Springer: New York, NY, USA, 2006; pp. 1102–1118.
3. Ciążyńska, M.; Narbutt, J.; Woźniacka, A.; Lesiak, A. Trends in basal cell carcinoma incidence rates: A 16-year retrospective study of a population in central Poland. *Adv. Dermatol. Allergol.* **2018**, *35*, 47–52. [CrossRef] [PubMed]
4. Peris, K.; Fargnoli, M.C.; Garbe, C.; Kaufman, R.; Bastholt, L.; Basset Seguin, N.; Bataille, V.; Del Marmol, V.; Dummer, R.; Harwood, C.A.; et al. Diagnosis and treatment of basal cell carcinoma: European consensus-based interdisciplinary guidelines. *Eur. J. Cancer* **2019**, *118*, 10–34. [CrossRef] [PubMed]
5. Breitbart, E.W.; Waldmann, A.; Nolte, S.; Capellaro, M.; Greinert, R.; Volkmer, B.; Katalinic, A. Systematic skin cancer screening in northern Germany. *J. Am. Acad. Dermatol.* **2012**, *66*, 201–211. [CrossRef] [PubMed]
6. International Skin Imaging Collaboration. Available online: https://www.isic-archive.com (accessed on 26 October 2020).
7. Kaymak, S.; Esmaili, P.; Serener, A. Deep Learning for Two-Step Classification of Malignant Pigmented Skin Lesions. In Proceedings of the 14th Symposium on Neural Networks and Applications (NEUREL 2018), Belgrade, Serbia, 20–21 November 2018. [CrossRef]
8. Sultana, N.N.; Puhan, N.B. Recent Deep Learning Methods for Melanoma Detection: A Review. In Proceedings of the 4th International Conference Mathematics and Computing (ICMC 2018), Varanasi, India, 9–11 January 2018. [CrossRef]
9. Marka, A.; Carter, J.B.; Toto, E.; Hassanpour, S. Automated detection of nonmelanoma skin cancer using digital images: A systematic review. *BMC Med. Imaging* **2019**, *19*, 21. [CrossRef]
10. Wahba, M.A.; Ashour, A.S.; Napoleon, S.A.; Abd Elnaby, M.M.; Guo, Y. Combined empirical mode decomposition and texture features for skin lesion classification using quadratic support vector machine. *Health Inf. Sci. Syst.* **2017**, *5*, 10. [CrossRef]
11. Wahba, M.A.; Ashour, A.S.; Guo, Y.; Napoleon, S.A.; Elnaby, M.M. A novel cumulative level difference mean based GLDM and modified ABCD features ranked using eigenvector centrality approach for four skin lesion types classification. *Comput. Methods Programs Biomed.* **2018**, *165*, 163–174. [CrossRef]
12. Møllersen, K.; Kirchesch, H.; Zortea, M.; Schopf, T.R.; Hindberg, K.; Godtliebsen, F. Computer-aided decision support for melanoma detection applied on melanocytic and nonmelanocytic skin lesions: A comparison of two systems based on automatic analysis of Dermoscopic images. *Biomed. Res. Int.* **2015**, *2015*, 579282. [CrossRef]
13. Sarkar, R.; Chatterjee, C.C.; Hazra, A. A novel approach for automatic diagnosis of skin carcinoma from dermoscopic images using parallel deep residual networks. In Proceedings of the Third International Conference on Advances in Computing and Data Sciences (ICACDS 2019), Ghaziabad, India, 12–13 April 2019. [CrossRef]
14. Pangti, R.; Chouhan, V.; Mathur, J.; Kumar, S.; Dixit, A.; Gupta, S.; Mahajan, S.; Gupta, A.; Gupta, S. Performance of a deep learning-based application for the diagnosis of BCC in Indian patients as compared to dermatologists and nondermatologists. *Int. J. Dermatol.* **2020**, *60*, e51–e52. [CrossRef]
15. Han, S.S.; Kim, M.S.; Lim, W.; Park, G.H.; Park, I.; Chang, S.E. Classification of the Clinical Images for Benign and Malignant Cutaneous Tumors Using a Deep Learning Algorithm. *J. Investig. Dermatol.* **2018**, *138*, 1529–1538. [CrossRef]

16. Carcagni, P.; Leo, M.; Cuna, A.; Mazzeo, P.; Spagnolo, P.; Celeste, G.; Distante, C. Classification of Skin Lesions by Combining Multilevel Learnings in a DenseNet Architecture. In Proceedings of the 20th International Conference Image Analysis and Processing (ICIAP 2019), Trento, Italy, 9–13 September 2019. [CrossRef]
17. Zhou, H.; Xie, F.; Jiang, Z.; Liu, J.; Wang, S.; Zhu, C. Multi-classification of skin diseases for dermoscopy images using deep learning. In Proceedings of the 2017 IEEE International Conference on Imaging Systems and Techniques (IST 2017), Beijing, China, 18–20 October 2017. [CrossRef]
18. Sies, K.; Winkler, K.; Fink, C.; Bardehle, F.; Toberer, F.; Buhl, T.; Enk, A.; Blum, A.; Rosenberger, A.; Haenssle, H.A. Past and present of computer-assisted dermoscopic diagnosis: Performance of a conventional image analyser versus a convolutional neural network in a prospective data set of 1981 skin lesions. *Eur. J. Cancer* **2020**, *135*, 39–46. [CrossRef]
19. Dorj, U.O.; Lee, K.K.; Choi, J.Y.; Lee, M. The skin cancer classification using deep convolutional neural network. *Multimed. Tools Appl.* **2018**, *77*, 9909–9924. [CrossRef]
20. Cruz-Roa, A.A.; Arevalo Ovalle, J.E.; Madabhushi, A.; González Osorio, F.A. A Deep Learning Architecture for Image Representation, Visual Interpretability and Automated Basal-Cell Carcinoma Cancer Detection. In Proceedings of the International Conference on Medical Image Computing and Computer-Assisted Intervention MICCAI 2013, Nagoya, Japan, 22–26 September 2013. [CrossRef]
21. Campanella, G.; Navarrete-Dechent, C.; Liopyris, K.; Monnier, J.; Aleissa, S.; Minhas, B.; Scope, A.; Longo, C.; Guitera, P.; Pellacani, G.; et al. Deep Learning for Basal Cell Carcinoma Detection for Reflectance Confocal Microscopy. *J. Investig. Dermatol.* **2022**, *142*, 97–103. [CrossRef] [PubMed]
22. Kimeswenger, S.; Tschandl, P.; Noack, P.; Hofmarcher, M.; Rumetshofer, E.; Kindermann, H.; Silye, R.; Hochreiter, S.; Kaltenbrunner, M.; Guenova, E.; et al. Artificial neural networks and pathologists recognize basal cell carcinomas based on different histological patterns. *Mod. Pathol.* **2011**, *34*, 895–903. [CrossRef] [PubMed]
23. Pérez Malla, C.U.; Valdés Hernández, M.D.C.; Rachmadi, M.F.; Komura, T. Evaluation of enhanced learning techniques for segmenting ischaemic stroke lesions in brain magnetic resonance perfusion images using a convolutional neural network scheme. *Front. Neuroinformatics* **2019**, *13*. [CrossRef]
24. Kaur, D.; Kaur, Y. Various image segmentation techniques: A review. *Int. J. Comput. Sci. Mob. Comput.* **2014**, *3*, 809–814. [CrossRef]
25. Sreelatha, T.; Subramanyam, M.V.; Giri Prasad, M.N. Early Detection of Skin Cancer Using Melanoma Segmentation technique. *J. Med. Syst.* **2019**, *43*, 190. [CrossRef] [PubMed]
26. Bi, L.; Jinman, K.; Ahn, E.; Kumar, A.; Feng, D.; Fulham, M. Step-wise integration of deep class-specific learning for dermoscopic image segmentation. *Pattern Recognit.* **2019**, *85*, 78–89. [CrossRef]
27. Tang, P.; Liang, Q.; Yan, X.; Xiang, S.; Sun, W.; Zhang, D.; Coppola, G. Efficient skin lesion segmentation using separable-Unet with stochastic weight averaging. *Comput. Methods Programs Biomed.* **2019**, *178*, 289–301. [CrossRef]
28. Codella, N.C.F.; Gutman, D.; Celebi, M.E.; Helba, B.; Marchetti, M.A.; Dusza, S.W.; Kalloo, A.; Liopyris, K.; Mishra, N.; Kittler, H.; et al. Skin lesion analysis toward melanoma detection. A challenge at the 2017 International symposium on biomedical imaging (ISBI), hosted by the international skin imaging collaboration (ISIC). In Proceedings of the IEEE 15th International Symposium on Biomedical Imaging (ISBI 2018), Washington, DC, USA, 4–7 April 2018. [CrossRef]
29. Punithakumar, K.; Yuan, J. A convex max-flow approach to distribution-based figure-ground separation. *SIAM J. Imaging Sci.* **2012**, *5*, 1333–1354. [CrossRef]
30. Qiu, W.; Yuan, J.; Ukwatta, E.; Sun, Y.; Rajchl, M.; Fenster, A. Prostate segmentation: An efficient convex optimization approach with axial symmetry using 3-D TRUS and MR images. *IEEE Trans. Med. Imaging* **2014**, *33*, 947–960. [CrossRef]
31. Pérez-Carrasco, J.A.; Acha, B.; Suárez-Mejías, C.; López-Guerra, J.L.; Serrano, C. Joint segmentation of bones and muscles using an intensity and histogram-based energy minimization approach. *Comput. Methods Programs Biomed.* **2018**, *156*, 85–95. [CrossRef] [PubMed]
32. Suárez-Mejías, C.; Pérez-Carrasco, J.A.; Serrano, C.; López-Guerra, J.L.; Parra-Calderón, C.; Gómez-Cía, T.; Acha, B. Three-dimensional segmentation of retroperitoneal masses using continuous convex relaxation and accumulated gradient distance for radiotherapy planning. *Med. Biol. Eng. Comput.* **2017**, *55*, 1–15. [CrossRef] [PubMed]
33. Papadakis, N.; Rabin, J. Convex histogram-based joint image segmentation with regularized optimal transport cost. *J. Math. Imaging Vis.* **2017**, *59*, 161–186. [CrossRef]
34. Al-masni, M.A.; Al-antari, M.A.; Choi, M.T.; Han, S.M.; Kim, T.S. Skin lesion segmentation in dermoscopy images via deep full resolution convolutional networks. *Comput. Methods Programs Biomed.* **2018**, *162*, 221–231. [CrossRef]
35. Yu, L.; Chen, H.; Dou, Q.; Qin, J.; Heng, P. Automated melanoma recognition in dermoscopy images via very deep residual networks. *IEEE Trans. Med. Imaging* **2017**, *36*, 994–1004. [CrossRef]
36. Kwasigroch, A.; Mikolajczyk, A.; Grochowski, M. Deep convolutional neural networks as a decision support tool in medical problems—malignant melanoma case study. In Proceedings of the 19th Polish Control Conference (KKA 2014), Kraków, Poland, 12–21 June 2017. [CrossRef]
37. Badrinarayanan, V.; Kendall, A.; Cipolla, R. SegNet: A Deep Convolutional Encoder-Decoder Architecture for Image Segmentation. *IEEE Trans. Pattern Anal. Mach. Intell.* **2017**, *39*, 2481–2495. [CrossRef]
38. Simonyan, K.; Zisserman, A. Very Deep Convolutional Networks for Large-Scale Image Recognition. In Proceedings of the 3rd International Conference on Learning Representations (ICLR 2015), San Diego, CA, USA, 7–9 May 2015.

39. He, K.; Zhang, X.; Ren, S.; Sun, J. Deep Residual Learning for Image Recognition. In Proceedings of the 2016 IEEE Conference on Computer Vision and Pattern Recognition (CVPR 2016), Las Vegas, NV, USA, 27–30 June 2016. [CrossRef]
40. Szegedy, C.; Vanhoucke, V.; Ioffe, S.; Shlens, J. Rethinking the Inception Architecture for Computer Vision. In Proceedings of the 2016 IEEE Conference on Computer Vision and Pattern Recognition (CVPR 2016), Las Vegas, NV, USA, 27–30 June 2016. [CrossRef]
41. Yuan, Y.; Chao, M.; Lo, Y.-C. Automatic skin lesion segmentation with fully convolutional deconvolutional networks. *IEEE J. Biomed. Health Inform.* **2018**, *36*, 1876–1886. [CrossRef]
42. Tschandl, P.; Sinz, C.; Kittler, H. Domain-specific classification pre-trained fully convolutional network encoders for skin lesion segmentation. *Comput. Biol. Med.* **2019**, *104*, 111–116. [CrossRef]
43. Sarker, M.K.; Rashwan, H.A.; Akram, F.; Singh, V.K.; Banu, S.F.; Chowdhury, F.U.H.; Choudhury, K.A.; Chambon, S.; Radeva, P.; Puig, D.; et al. SLSNet: Skin lesion segmentation using a lightweight generative adversarial network. *Expert Syst. Appl.* **2021**, *183*, 115433. [CrossRef]
44. Tschandl, P.; Rosendahl, C.; Kittler, H. The HAM10000 dataset, a large collection of multi-source dermatoscopic images of common pigmented skin lesions. *Sci. Data* **2018**, *5*, 180161. [CrossRef]
45. Combalia, M.; Codella, N.F.C.; Rotemberg, V.; Helba, B.; Vilaplana, V.; Reiter, O.; Halpern, A.C.; Puig, S.; Malvehy, J. BCN20000: Dermoscopic Lesions in the Wild. *arXiv* **2019**, arXiv:1908.02288.
46. Gessert, N.; Nielsen, M.; Shaikh, M.; Werner, R.; Schlaefer, A. Skin lesion classification using ensembles of multi-resolution EfficientNets with meta data. *MethodsX* **2020**, *7*, 100864. [CrossRef] [PubMed]
47. Barata, C.; Celebi, M.E.; Marques, J.S. A survey of feature extraction in dermoscopy image analysis of skin cancer. *IEEE J. Biomed. Health Inform.* **2019**, *23*, 1096–1109. [CrossRef]
48. Teixeira, L.O.; Pereira, R.M.; Bertolini, D.; Oliveira, L.S.; Nanni, L.; Cavalcanti, G.D.C.; Costa, M.G. Impact of lung segmentation on the diagnosis and explanation of COVID-19 in chest X-ray images. *Sensors* **2021**, *21*, 7116. [CrossRef] [PubMed]

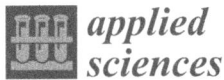

Article

Transfer Learning for an Automated Detection System of Fractures in Patients with Maxillofacial Trauma

Maria Amodeo [1], Vincenzo Abbate [2], Pasquale Arpaia [3,*], Renato Cuocolo [3,4], Giovanni Dell'Aversana Orabona [2], Monica Murero [5,6], Marco Parvis [1], Roberto Prevete [7] and Lorenzo Ugga [8]

1. Department of Electronics and Telecommunications (DET), Polytechnic University of Turin, 10129 Turin, Italy; maria.amodeo@polito.it (M.A.); marco.parvis@polito.it (M.P.)
2. Department of Neurosciences, Reproductive and Odontostomatological Science, University of Naples Federico II, 80131 Naples, Italy; vincenzo.abbate@unina.it (V.A.); dellaversana@unina.it (G.D.O.)
3. Interdepartmental Research Center on Management and Innovation in Healthcare—CIRMIS, University of Naples Federico II, Via Pansini 5, 80138 Naples, Italy; renato.cuocolo@unina.it
4. Department of Clinical Medicine and Surgery, University of Naples Federico II, 80131 Naples, Italy
5. Department of Social Sciences, University of Naples Federico II, 80131 Naples, Italy; monica.murero@unina.it
6. Distributed Artificial Intelligence Lab, Technische Universität, 10587 Berlin, Germany
7. Department of Electrical Engineering and Information Technology (DIETI), University of Naples Federico II, 80100 Naples, Italy; rprevete@unina.it
8. Department of Advanced Biomedical Sciences, University of Naples Federico II, 80131 Naples, Italy; lorenzo.ugga@unina.it
* Correspondence: pasquale.arpaia@unina.it

Abstract: An original maxillofacial fracture detection system (MFDS), based on convolutional neural networks and transfer learning, is proposed to detect traumatic fractures in patients. A convolutional neural network pre-trained on non-medical images was re-trained and fine-tuned using computed tomography (CT) scans to produce a model for the classification of future CTs as either "fracture" or "noFracture". The model was trained on a total of 148 CTs (120 patients labeled with "fracture" and 28 patients labeled with "noFracture"). The validation dataset, used for statistical analysis, was characterized by 30 patients (5 with "noFracture" and 25 with "fracture"). An additional 30 CT scans, comprising 25 "fracture" and 5 "noFracture" images, were used as the test dataset for final testing. Tests were carried out both by considering the single slices and by grouping the slices for patients. A patient was categorized as fractured if two consecutive slices were classified with a fracture probability higher than 0.99. The patients' results show that the model accuracy in classifying the maxillofacial fractures is 80%. Even if the MFDS model cannot replace the radiologist's work, it can provide valuable assistive support, reducing the risk of human error, preventing patient harm by minimizing diagnostic delays, and reducing the incongruous burden of hospitalization.

Keywords: convolutional neural network; transfer learning; maxillofacial fractures; computed tomography images; radiography

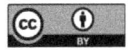

1. Introduction

In recent years, the number of requests for computed tomography (CT), magnetic resonance imaging (MRI), and, in general, radiology services has grown dramatically [1]. Nevertheless, there is a lack of radiologists due to recruitment challenges and many retirements. In this scenario, artificial intelligence (AI) can help radiologists in the time-consuming and challenging medical image analysis task. In any case, the AI-based tools do not replace medical staff, but assistive technologies prioritize, confirm, or validate radiologists' decisions and doubts.

Deep learning, a branch of AI, has recently made substantial progress in analyzing images with a consequent better representation and interpretation of complex data. In particular, various works [2–6] deal with deep learning in orthopedic traumatology. However, the number of studies regarding deep learning on CT scans for fracture detection is low. Furthermore, building and training a neural architecture from scratch requires a huge amount of data. Image classification networks are trained on billions of data in the literature, using multiple servers running for several weeks [7]. This procedure is not feasible for most medical researchers. One way to overcome this obstacle is to use the so-called transfer learning. This process consists of adopting the highly refined characteristics of convolutional neural networks trained on millions of data and using them as a starting point for a new model. For example, to verify the extent of fracture detection on wrist radiographs, Kim and MacKinnon [8] focus on transfer learning from a deep convolutional neural network (CNNs), pre-trained on non-medical images. Using the inception V3 CNN [9], they obtained an area under the receiver operating characteristic curve (AUC-ROC) of 0.95 on the test dataset. This result shows that a CNN pre-trained on non-medical images can be used for medical radiographs successfully. Another study was carried out by Chung et al. [10], based on a CNN to detect and classify proximal humerus fractures using plain anteroposterior shoulder radiographs. The deep neural network showed a similar performance to that of shoulder-specialized orthopedic surgeons, but better than that of the general physicians and the non-shoulder specialized orthopedic surgeons. This result denotes the possibility to diagnose fractures accurately by using plain radiographs automatically. Another study in this field was carried out by Tomita et al. [11], where they focused on detecting osteoporotic vertebral fractures on CT exams. Their system consisted of two blocks: (i) a CNN to extract radiological features from CTs; and (ii) a recurrent neural network (RNN) module to aggregate the previously extracted elements for the final diagnosis. The performance of the proposed system matched the ability of radiologist practitioners. Thus, the system could be used for screening and prioritizing potential fracture cases.

Therefore, although several authors have already described some AI applications in the orthopedic field, the possibility to detect maxillofacial fractures in 3D images (CT scans) of injured patients using artificial neural networks, and in particular a transfer learning approach, has not been explored yet [12–15]. This area's anatomical complexity and the specificity of this type of fracture make radiological diagnosis very often complex with a consistent risk of incongruous hospitalizations. A fracture detection system based on AI able to detect the presence of maxillofacial fractures would be of great use in clinical practice by reducing the costs of treatment and discomfort for patients.

This research aims to develop a fracture detection system, based on the transfer learning approach, able to predict the presence of maxillofacial fractures. The inputs for this system are the CT images of a patient after a trauma. The output of the system indicates the existence or not of a fracture. The block diagram of the system is shown in Figure 1.

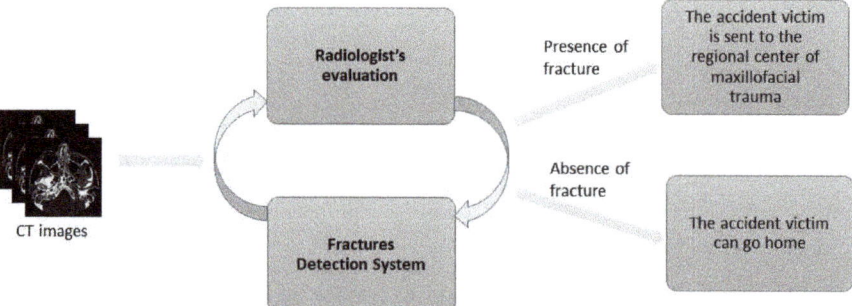

Figure 1. Block diagram of the system for patients with maxillofacial trauma. The fracture detection system assists the radiologist in evaluating the CT images of an injured patient.

The paper is organized as follows. In Section 2, the material and methods are presented, including the description of the dataset and the architecture used. In Section 3, the results are presented in terms of slices and patients. In Section 4, we discuss the results achieved, while in Section 5 the conclusions of the study are presented.

2. Materials and Methods

2.1. Dataset

This retrospective study uses images from CT exams after anonymizing patient personal data. The study was approved by the Ethics Committee of "Federico II" University, Naples, Italy (approval number 81/20). The CT scans were obtained from the internal database of the U.O.C. of Maxillofacial Surgery of the University Hospital "Federico II", which collects examinations conducted from 2000 to 2020. We performed CT investigations of the facial mass on different devices (TC 16–64 slice) with thickness volumetric acquisition (0.5–2 mm) and variable in-plane resolution (0.5 $\times$ 0.5–1 $\times$ 1 mm). For the analysis, we selected only the images we obtained with the bone reconstruction algorithm. Two radiologists (R.C., L.U.) consensually examined, interpreted, and classified each CT image according to fracture rhymes' presence/absence. We also included control CT investigations from patients with the non-traumatic facial mass disorder.

The number of CT scans corresponds to the number of patients (a CT scan for each patient). The total dataset consisted of 208 patients: 170 patients (11,260 slices of CT scans) labeled as with "fracture" and 38 patients (49,762 slices of CT scans) labeled as "noFracture". The total dataset was divided into training, validation, and test datasets. In particular, the training dataset consisted of 148 CT images (120 patients labeled as with "fracture" and 28 patients labeled as with "noFracture"). The validation dataset, used for statistical analysis, was characterized by 30 patients (5 with "noFracture" and 25 with "fracture"), and an additional 30 CT scans, comprising 25 "fracture" and 5 "noFracture" images, were used as a test dataset for final testing. It is worth noting that the total dataset was imbalanced on a patient level with the majority being fractured patients; while on a slice level, the dataset is imbalanced in favor of the slices labeled as "noFracture". Therefore, the dataset overall is not as imbalanced in favor of "fracture" images as can be assumed by only evaluating the patient-level data.

2.2. Experimental Setup Description

The system implementation was carried out through a predictive algorithm written in Python v.3.7.6 (available for different Operating Systems) [16], using PyTorch v.1.4.0 [17] and Fastai v.1.0.60 [18]. We used scikit-learn v.0.22.1 [19] for the neural architecture and Pydicom v.1.4.2 [20] to treat CT images in Dicom format. The implementation of the system is schematized in Figure 2.

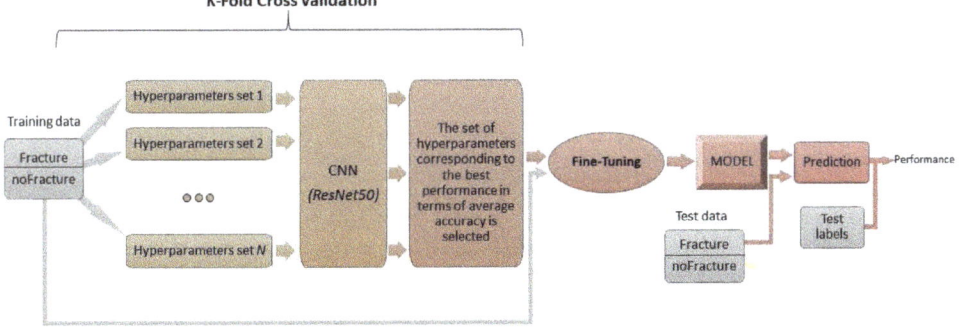

Figure 2. Block diagram of the system's implementation for detecting fractures in patients with maxillofacial trauma.

All the steps can be summarized as follows:

1. K-fold cross validation to identify the hyperparameters (learning rate, weight decay, and drop out) that allow the network to have the highest performance in terms of accuracy;
2. Fine-tuning of the network with the hyperparameters chosen in the previous step:
    2.1 Training only of the last layer;
    2.2 Unfreezing and training the whole model;
3. Evaluation of the network's performance.

All the steps are described in detail in the next paragraphs.

2.2.1. K-Fold Cross Validation

For the implementation of the architecture shown in Figure 2, the first step consists of defining the training dataset for the k-fold cross validation, comprising two classes: "fracture" and "noFracture". In particular, to keep the two classes balanced and reduce the computational times, we considered a reduced dataset, which is a subset of the total dataset described in Section 2.1. In particular, the training dataset used for the k-fold cross validation consists of 359 slices with fracture, belonging to 57 different patients, and 362 slices without fracture, belonging to 59 additional patients. In order to avoid class imbalance in patient-level, from some patients with fractures, we selected only a subset of the "noFracture" slices. Therefore, these patients will become patients with "noFracture" in this phase.

In our case study, we adopted the transfer learning technique to reduce the development burden of the CNN. The pre-trained architecture we used was ResNet50. ResNet is the deep convolutional neural network that won the 2015 ImageNet Large Scale Visual Recognition Challenge (ILSVRC) [21]. ResNet architecture has many variants: the difference between them is not only a different number of layers, but also a novel architecture, such as ResNeXt [22], or densely connected CNN [23]. ResNet50 is trained on more than a million images from the ImageNet database [24]. The network is 50 layers deep and can classify images into 1000 object categories, such as pizza, umbrella, castle, and many animals (tiger, camel, frog, etc.). As a result, the network has learned rich feature representations for a wide range of images. The network has an image input size of 224-by-224.

The architecture of ResNet50 has 4 stages:

1. Initial convolution (kernel size of 7×7) and max-pooling (kernel size of 3×3);
2. Nine convolutional layers: kernel size of 1×1 and 64 different kernels, followed by kernel size of 3×3 and 64 different kernels, followed by kernel size of 1×1 and 256 different kernels. These three layers are repeated 3 times;
3. Twelve convolutional layers: kernel size of 1×1 and 128 different kernels, followed by kernel size of 3×3 and 128 different kernels, followed by kernel size of 1×1 and 512 different kernels. These three layers are repeated 4 times;
4. Eighteen convolutional layers: kernel size of 1×1 and 256 different kernels, followed by kernel size of 3×3 and 256 different kernels, followed by kernel size of 1×1 and 1024 different kernels. These three layers are repeated 6 times;
5. Nine convolutional layers: kernel size of 1×1 and 512 different kernels, followed by kernel size of 3×3 and 512 different kernels, followed by kernel size of 1×1 and 2048 different kernels. These three layers are repeated 3 times;
6. Average pooling layer followed by a fully connected layer with 1000 neurons and a softmax function at the end.

In order to choose the most suitable set of hyperparameters for our case, we used the stratified k-fold cross validation [25] with k = 5. The hyperparameters of interest were the following: learning rate, weight decay, and dropout; we chose them in the following ranges (0.000001; 0.005), (0.0001; 0.0005), (0.1; 0.5). We set the batch size at 50. Specifically, 20 combinations (N = 20 in Figure 2) of the hyperparameters were tested. We used a random search for hyperparameters' optimization. We also chose to adopt a random search compared to a grid search. When there are many hyperparameters, as in our case, the first is more effective from the computational time point of view, while maintaining good performance [26]. Figure 3 describes the procedure of the k-fold cross-validation.

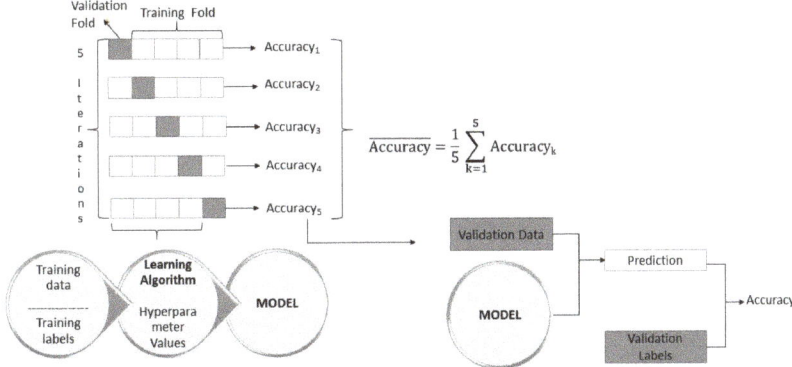

Figure 3. Five-fold cross validation procedure scheme.

Early stopping criteria can be used during the training as a trade-off between generalization ability and computational costs. In our case, we used as early stopping the following criteria: if after three attempts the accuracy does not improve by at least 0.01, the training cycle ends. The number of epochs set for each fold was 6. The images were normalized according to the ImageNet format and resized from 512×512 to 224×224 pixels. An example of Dicom images is shown in Figure 4.

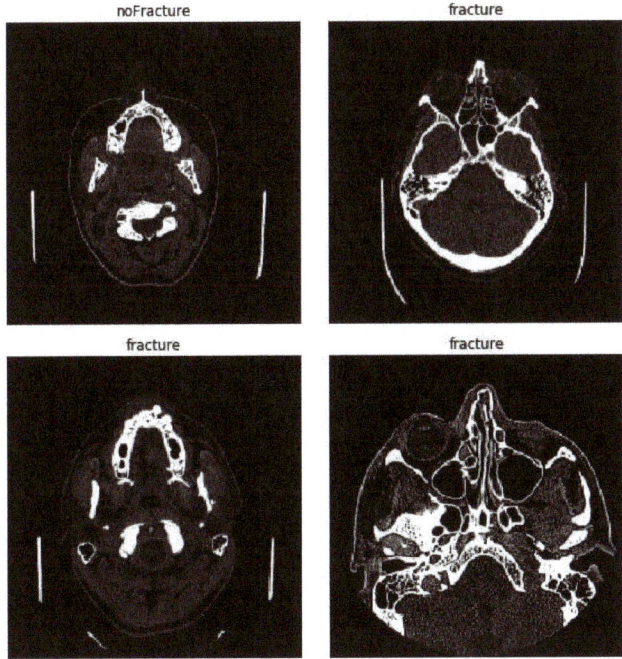

Figure 4. Example of Dicom images (8×8 inches) for both classes (fracture and noFracture).

After carrying out the tests for the 20 configurations, we chose the set of hyperparameters that guaranteed the network to have the highest average accuracy (0.86) and the smallest standard deviation that is the index of little variability (0.05). This set has the following hyperparameters: learning rate of 0.005, weight decay of 0.0005, and drop out of 0.5.

2.2.2. Fine-Tuning of the CNN

Pre-trained networks can be exploited to recognize classes the system is not (initially) trained on, thanks to the fine-tuning process.

The convolutional layers had already learned discriminative filters. After choosing the hyperparameters, described in the previous section (Section 2.2.1), we replaced the final set of fully connected layers of the pre-trained CNN. We introduced a new set of fully-connected layers using random weights. By doing so, the fully connected layers could act entirely randomly. If the gradient backpropagates from these random values and the whole network, the pre-trained network's powerful features risked being destroyed. To avoid this problem, we re-trained the CNN performing the following steps (Figure 5):

1. Training of the last layer: we started with the pre-trained model's weights (pre-trained on ImageNet), freezing all layers in the network's body except the last layer. In this step, we trained only the last layer.
2. Unfreezing and training the whole model: in this step, after the last layer had started to learn patterns of our medical dataset, we unfroze all the weights and trained the entire model with a very small learning rate. We wanted to avoid altering the convolutional filters dramatically.

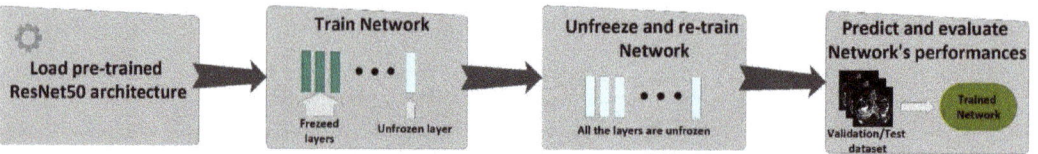

Figure 5. ResNet50 was used as a pre-trained network and, after loading the network, the fine-tuning process was started. We froze all the layers in the network except the fully-connected layers, useful for capturing high-level features on the current dataset. After the fully-connected layers have had a chance to learn patterns from our dataset, we then unfroze all the architecture layers; even the convolutional layers that had initially learned discriminative filters. We allowed each layer to be fine-tuned by performing two training steps and using differential learning rates.

For the fine-tuning of the network, we used the total dataset described in Section 2.1. In particular, the training dataset consisted of 8023 slices labeled as "fracture" and 34,962 labeled as "noFracture", for a total of 148 patients. The training and validation datasets used in the k-fold cross validation were a subset of this total training dataset. Since the two classes were no longer balanced, we used the CrossEntropyLoss as loss function with different weights for the "fracture" and "noFracture" classes (w_f and w_{nf}, respectively):

$$[w_f, w_{nf}] = [\frac{|noFracture|}{|fracture|}, \frac{|noFracture|}{|fracture|}] = [\frac{34,962}{8023}, \frac{34,962}{34,962}] = [4.36, 1.0] \quad (1)$$

The validation dataset, used for the error evaluation, consisted of 1660 slices labeled as "fracture" and 7910 labeled as "noFracture", for a total of 30 patients.

During the second step, we performed an additional fine-tuning, re-training the model twice by changing the learning rate to improve the model's performance. Before each re-train of the model, we loaded the network's weights that gave us the best performance in terms of accuracy. In particular, we used the learning rate finder [27,28] of the Fastai library to choose the learning rate at each step. Since some features remain unchanged (such as the edges and the corners of an image learned in the first layers of the network), we applied the concept of differential learning rates implemented by the Fastai library. Using this approach, we could assign different learning rates to the various layers of our network. In particular, we passed a slice function inside the fit method and: (a) assigned a lower learning rate to the first layer, (b) assigned a higher learning rate to the last layer, and (c) distributed the values for the learning rate among all the other layers in between.

3. Results

The results presented in this section are obtained on the validation dataset and on the test dataset that consists of 1577 slices labeled as "fracture" and 6890 slices labeled as "noFracture", for a total of 30 patients. The partition of the dataset into training, validation, and test dataset was done randomly at level-patient, this means that all the slices for a single patient were considered in one of the three sets (training, validation, and test). Nevertheless, the validation and test datasets were not similar to each other. First, the CT scans were performed on different devices and, therefore, we have substantial differences among them; then, the fracture can affect any part of the splanchnocranium and, since the latter is a very large and complex region, the CT images can be very different from each other. The confusion matrix of the validation and test datasets is shown in Figure 6a,b, respectively; the AUC-ROC for both validation and test datasets is shown in Figure 6c,d, respectively.

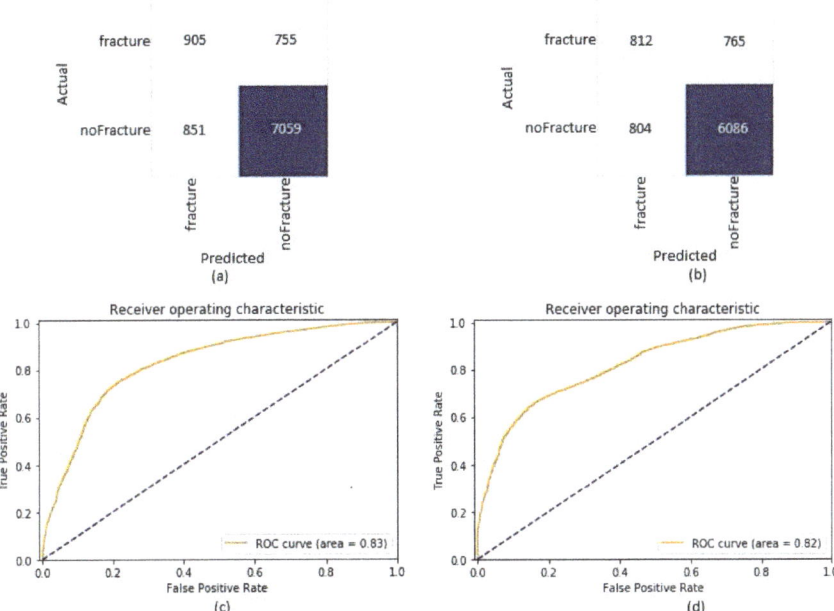

Figure 6. Results in terms of the confusion matrix for the validation (**a**) and test (**b**) datasets and ROC curve for the validation (**c**) and test (**d**) datasets. The corresponding AUC for the validation dataset is 0.83 (0.82, 0.84), while for the test dataset is 0.82 (0.81, 0.83). The 95% confidence intervals for the values of the AUC were calculated with the analytic method of Hanley and McNeil [29], such as described in Ref. [30].

For the evaluation of the performance, we considered the following metrics:
- Accuracy = $\frac{TP+TN}{P+N}$
- Recall (or sensitivity) = $\frac{TP}{TP+FN}$
- Precision (or positive predictive value) = $\frac{TP}{TP+FP}$

The corresponding values for the validation and test datasets are shown in Table 1.

Table 1. Accuracy, recall (sensitivity), and precision (positive predictive value) with the exact (Clopper–Pearson) 95% confidence intervals for the validation and test dataset.

Metric	Validation Dataset	Test Dataset
Accuracy	0.83 (0.82, 0.84)	0.81 (0.81, 0.82)
Recall	0.55 (0.52, 0.57)	0.51 (0.49, 0.54)
Precision	0.52 (0.49, 0.54)	0.50 (0.48, 0.53)

The actual width of the confidence interval is the same for both recall and precision in both validation and test datasets, while it is much smaller for the accuracy in both datasets.

In order to make a prediction in terms of a patient's injury rather than single slices, we performed an evaluation of the neural network. To this aim, the slices were grouped by referring to a single patient according to the following assumption: if two consecutive slices, belonging to the same patient, are classified as "fracture" by the CNN with a probability greater than 0.99, then classify the patient as a patient with a fracture. The confusion matrix we obtained for the test dataset is shown in Figure 7.

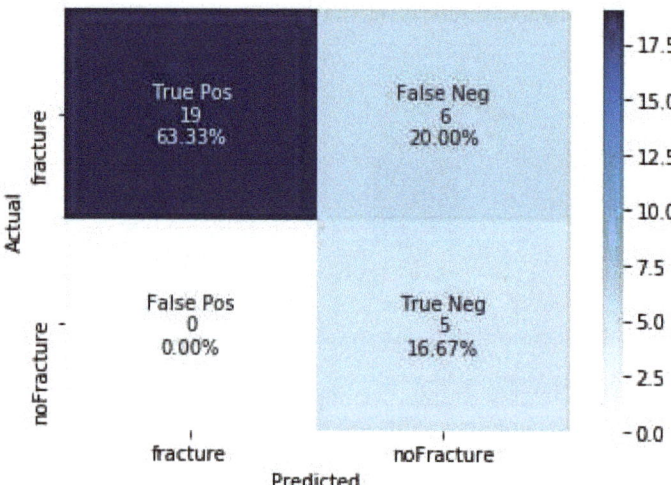

Figure 7. Confusion matrix for the test dataset in terms of patients' fractures.

The measures of diagnostic accuracy (accuracy, recall (sensitivity), and precision (positive predictive value)) with 95% confidence intervals for the test dataset in terms of patients are shown in Table 2.

Table 2. Accuracy, recall (sensitivity), and precision (positive predictive value) with the exact (Clopper–Pearson) 95% confidence intervals for the test dataset in terms of patients.

Metric	Test Dataset
Accuracy	0.80 (0.61, 0.92)
Recall	0.76 (0.55, 0.91)
Precision	1.0 (0.82, 1.00)

4. Discussion

4.1. Statement of Principal Findings

The proposed approach shows the feasibility of using transfer learning techniques to detect maxillofacial fractures in CT images effectively. The results achieved by using the validation and test datasets are of the same order of magnitude. Our trained ResNet50 neural network can distinguish between the fractured and normal bone in CT scans of injured patients with a relatively high accuracy (80%). This result is particularly promising, given the anatomical complexity and thinness of bones in the splanchnocranium, and proves that transfer learning from CNN, pre-trained on non-medical images, can be efficiently applied to the problem of maxillofacial fracture detection on CT images.

4.2. Strengths and Weaknesses of the Study

Although a computer-aided decision system with an AUC of 0.83 (0.82, 0.84) cannot replace human interpretation, this accuracy level may be very useful in assisting radiologists with prompt a diagnosis and treatment. An automated detection system based on our proposed model has the advantages of analyzing the CT image's entire region with equal importance. This reflects in reducing the human errors related to missed readings on the whole region of the 3D image. Furthermore, small fractures are often hardly visible on CT images, and require multiple checks by the radiologists: an automated detection system can also be useful in this context.

4.3. Strengths and Weaknesses in Relation to Other Studies, Discussing Particularly Any Differences in Results

Although several authors have already investigated AI applications in the orthopedic field, the possibility to detect maxillofacial fractures in 3D images of injured patients using deep learning algorithms has not been explored yet. Even if in other studies we can find better results, for example, in terms of AUC-ROC (0.95 [8]), it must be taken into account the complexity of the region of interest, such as the splanchnocranium and the enormous variability of the fracture types that may be present in this anatomically complex district. It is important to remark that the algorithm should be intended as an aid to the radiologist in recognizing facial fractures, more as a second opinion, rather than an independent one.

4.4. Meaning of the Study: Possible Mechanisms and Implications for Clinicians or Policymakers

The assessment of CT images in trauma patients is fundamental to select the appropriate treatment and direct them towards highly specialized units if necessary. When a patient's trauma occurs in an anatomically complex district such as the splanchnocranium, two main difficulties arise from the current clinical practice. The first one is the possible failure to recognize the presence of a bone fracture, and the second is the incorrect classification of normal anatomical structures (i.e., sutures, vascular, and nerve channels) as traumatic injuries. These diagnostic difficulties frequently translate into increased costs for the health system and a burden for the patient due to unnecessary hospitalizations in specialized clinical wards. For example, once the need for urgent treatment is excluded in a craniofacial district trauma, patients are transferred from the emergency room (of first access) to the closest regional reference center specialized in maxillofacial trauma. Here, the clinical case reassessment in specialist settings frequently (about 20% of cases) highlights the incongruity of hospitalization and often the absence of indications for surgical treatment. These patients require only home medical therapy. Although there are several AI applications in the literature of the orthopedic field, they remain still unexplored in the maxillofacial district. An AI-based radiological diagnosis system would allow diagnostic errors to be minimized by providing the radiologist with a support tool to guide therapeutic choices. However, an innovative AI-based radiological system should not replace the radiologist's work but become a valuable assistive technology to reduce medical error risks, unnecessary transportation, hospitalization, and socio-economic burden for society and the public health governance [31].

4.5. Unanswered Questions and Future Research

Future studies can focus on automated fracture detection with tiny fractures, improving the algorithm to detect, for example, the corners of fractured bones to improve the detection sensitivity of the system. Furthermore, to enhance the network's performance, a stage of preprocessing of the CT images could be introduced to remove the region of no interest for the prediction. Another interesting approach could be the investigation of the combination of deep learning models with radiomics [32]. In fact, radiomics [33] is a method for extracting a large amount of advanced quantitative imaging features from radiographic medical images obtained with computed tomography, using data-characterization algorithms. Radiomic data could be integrated into predictive models to hedge against the risk of overfitting the deep learning approach. Another possibility is to use a local feature detector as the speeded-up robust features (SURF) to improve the system's performance. In their work [34], the authors propose a computer-assisted method for automated classification and detection of calcaneus fracture locations in CT images using a deep learning algorithm. In particular, they compared two types of CNNs, a Residual network (ResNet) and a visual geometry group (VGG). Furthermore, the speeded-up robust features (SURF) method was used to determine the exact location and the type of fracture in calcaneal CT scans.

5. Conclusions

This study represents a proof of concept for using transfer learning from CNN, pre-trained on non-medical images, for maxillofacial fracture detection on CT images. In the literature, the use of transfer learning applied to CT scans to detect maxillofacial fractures of injured patients has not yet been explored. Our system proved to be capable of predicting maxillofacial fractures in patients with an accuracy of 80%. MFDC can become a valuable technology in assisting radiologists with prompt diagnosis and treatment that could reduce medical error risks and prevent patient harm and stress by minimizing maxillofacial trauma's diagnostic delays. An AI-based system assisting radiological investigation in non-specialized clinical wards can reduce incongruous hospitalization's socio-economic burden for the patient, society, and health system.

Author Contributions: Conceptualization, V.A., P.A., R.C., G.D.O., R.P. and L.U.; methodology, M.A. and R.P.; software, M.A.; validation, M.A.; investigation, M.A.; data collection, V.A.; data curation, R.C. and L.U.; writing—original draft preparation, M.A.; writing—review and editing, V.A., P.A., R.C., G.D.O., M.M., M.P. and R.P.; visualization, L.U.; supervision, P.A.; project administration, P.A. All authors have read and agreed to the published version of the manuscript.

Funding: This research received no external funding.

Institutional Review Board Statement: The study was conducted according to the guidelines of the Declaration of Helsinki and approved by the Ethics Committee of "Federico II" University, Naples, Italy.

Informed Consent Statement: Informed consent was waived because of the retrospective nature of the study and the analysis used anonymous clinical data.

Data Availability Statement: The data presented in this study are not available due to privacy restrictions.

Acknowledgments: This work was carried out as part of the "ICT for Health" project, which was financially supported by the Italian Ministry of Education, University and Research (MIUR), under the initiative "Departments of Excellence" (Italian Budget Law no. 232/2016), through an excellence grant awarded to the Department of Information Technology and Electrical Engineering of the University of Naples Federico II, Naples, Italy).

Conflicts of Interest: The authors declare no conflict of interest. The funders had no role in the design of the study; in the collection, analyses, or interpretation of data; in the writing of the manuscript, or in the decision to publish the results.

References

1. Kalmet, P.H.S.; Sanduleanu, S.; Primakov, S.; Wu, G.; Jochems, A.; Refaee, T.; Ibrahim, A.; Hulst, L.V.; Lambin, P.; Poeze, M. Deep learning in fracture detection: A narrative review. *Acta Orthop.* **2020**, *91*, 215–220. [CrossRef]
2. Esteva, A.; Kuprel, B.; Novoa, R.A.; Ko, J.; Swetter, S.M.; Blau, H.M.; Thrun, S. Dermatologist-level classification of skin cancer with deep neural networks. *Nature* **2017**, *542*, 115–118. [CrossRef]
3. Gulshan, V.; Peng, L.; Coram, M.; Stumpe, M.C.; Wu, D.; Narayanaswamy, A.; Venugopalan, S.; Widner, K.; Madams, T.; Cuadros, J.; et al. Development and Validation of a Deep Learning Algorithm for Detection of Diabetic Retinopathy in Retinal Fundus Photographs. *JAMA* **2016**, *316*, 2402–2410. [CrossRef]
4. Lee, J.-G.; Jun, S.; Cho, Y.-W.; Lee, H.; Kim, G.B.; Seo, J.B.; Kim, N. Deep Learning in Medical Imaging: General Overview. *Korean J. Radiol.* **2017**, *18*, 570–584. [CrossRef] [PubMed]
5. Olczak, J.; Fahlberg, N.; Maki, A.; Razavian, A.S.; Jilert, A.; Stark, A.; Sköldenberg, O.; Gordon, M. Artificial intelligence for analyzing orthopedic trauma radiographs: Deep learning algorithms—are they on par with humans for diagnosing fractures? *Acta Orthop.* **2017**, *88*, 581–586. [CrossRef] [PubMed]
6. Tang, A.; Tam, R.; Cadrin-Chênevert, A.; Guest, W.; Chong, J.; Barfett, J.; Chepelev, L.; Cairns, R.; Mitchell, J.R.; Cicero, M.D.; et al. Canadian Association of Radiologists White Paper on Artificial Intelligence in Radiology. *Can. Assoc. Radiol. J.* **2018**, *69*, 120–135. [CrossRef] [PubMed]
7. Szegedy, C.; Liu, W.; Jia, Y.; Sermanet, P.; Reed, S.; Anguelov, D.; Erhan, D.; Vanhoucke, V.; Rabinovich, A. Going Deeper with Convolutions. In Proceedings of the IEEE Conference on Computer Vision and Pattern Recognition (CVPR), Boston, MA, USA, 7–12 June 2015; pp. 1–9.
8. Kim, H.D.; MacKinnon, T. Artificial intelligence in fracture detection: Transfer learning from deep convolutional neu-ral networks. *Clin. Radiol.* **2018**, *73*, 439–445. [CrossRef] [PubMed]
9. Szegedy, C.; Vanhoucke, V.; Ioffe, S.; Shlens, J.; Wojna, Z. Rethinking the Inception Architecture for Computer Vision. In Proceedings of the 2016 IEEE Conference on Computer Vision and Pattern Recognition (CVPR) 2016, Las Vegas, NV, USA, 27–30 June 2016.
10. Chung, S.W.; Han, S.S.; Lee, J.W.; Oh, K.-S.; Kim, N.R.; Yoon, J.P.; Kim, J.Y.; Moon, S.H.; Kwon, J.; Lee, H.-J.; et al. Automated detection and classification of the proximal humerus fracture by using deep learning algorithm. *Acta Orthop.* **2018**, *89*, 468–473. [CrossRef]
11. Tomita, N.; Cheung, Y.Y.; Hassanpour, S. Deep neural networks for automatic detection of osteopo-rotic vertebral fractures on CT scans. *Comput. Biol. Med.* **2018**, *98*, 8–15. [CrossRef]
12. Heo, M.-S.; Kim, J.-E.; Hwang, J.-J.; Han, S.-S.; Kim, J.-S.; Yi, W.-J.; Park, I.-W. Artificial intelligence in oral and maxillofacial radiology: What is currently possible? *Dentomaxillofacial Radiol.* **2021**, *50*, 20200375. [CrossRef]
13. Hung, K.; Montalvao, C.; Tanaka, R.; Kawai, T.; Bornstein, M.M. The use and performance of artificial intelligence applications in dental and maxillofacial radiology: A systematic review. *Dentomaxillofacial Radiol.* **2020**, *49*, 20190107. [CrossRef] [PubMed]
14. Litjens, G.; Kooi, T.; Bejnordi, B.E.; Setio, A.A.A.; Ciompi, F.; Ghafoorian, M.; van der Laak, J.A.; van Ginneken, B.; Sánchez, C.I. A survey on deep learning in medical image analysis. *Med. Image Anal.* **2017**, *42*, 60–88. [CrossRef] [PubMed]
15. Nagi, R.; Aravinda, K.; Rakesh, N.; Gupta, R.; Pal, A.; Mann, A.K. Clinical applications and performance of intelligent systems in dental and maxillofacial radiology: A review. *Imaging Sci. Dent.* **2020**, *50*, 81–92. [CrossRef]
16. Python. Available online: https://www.python.org/ (accessed on 24 June 2021).
17. PyTorch. Available online: https://pytorch.org/ (accessed on 3 July 2020).
18. Fastai. Available online: https://docs.fast.ai/ (accessed on 3 February 2021).
19. Scikit-Learn. Available online: https://scikit-learn.org/stable/ (accessed on 6 July 2020).
20. Pydicom. Available online: https://pydicom.github.io/ (accessed on 8 July 2020).
21. He, K.; Zhang, X.; Ren, S.; Sun, J. Deep residual learning for image recognition. In Proceedings of the IEEE Conference on Computer Vision and Pattern Recognition (CVPR), Las Vegas, NV, USA, 26 June–1 July 2016; pp. 770–778.
22. Xie, S.; Girshick, R.; Dollar, P.; Tu, Z.; He, K. Aggregated Residual Transformations for Deep Neural Networks. In Proceedings of the 2017 IEEE Conference on Computer Vision and Pattern Recognition, Honolulu, HI, USA, 21–26 July 2017; pp. 1492–1500.
23. Huang, G.; Liu, Z.; van der Maaten, L.; Weinberger, K.Q. Densely connected convolutional networks. In Proceedings of the IEEE Conference on Computer Vision and Pattern Recognition (CVPR), Honolulu, HI, USA, 22–25 July 2017; pp. 4700–4708.
24. Russakovsky, O.; Deng, J.; Su, H.; Krause, J.; Satheesh, S.; Ma, S.; Huang, Z.; Karpathy, A.; Khosla, A.; Bernstein, M.; et al. ImageNet Large Scale Visual Recognition Challenge. *Int. J. Comput. Vis.* **2015**, *115*, 211–252. [CrossRef]
25. Raschka, S. Model evaluation, model selection, and algorithm selection in machine learning. *arXiv* **2018**, arXiv:1811.12808.
26. Bergstra, J.; Bengio, Y. Random search for hyper-parameter optimization. *J. Mach. Learn. Res.* **2012**, *13*, 281–305.
27. Learning Rate Finder. Available online: https://fastai1.fast.ai/callbacks.lr_finder.html (accessed on 3 February 2021).
28. Howard, J.; Gugger, S. Fastai: A Layered API for Deep Learning. *Information* **2020**, *11*, 108. [CrossRef]
29. Hanley, J.A.; McNeil, B.J. The meaning and use of the area under a receiver operating characteristic (ROC) curve. *Radiology* **1982**, *143*, 29–36. [CrossRef]
30. Nicholls, A. Confidence limits, error bars and method comparison in molecular modeling. Part 1: The calculation of confidence intervals. *J. Comput. Mol. Des.* **2014**, *28*, 887–918. [CrossRef]

31. Murero, M. Building Artificial Intelligence for Digital Health: A socio-tech-med approach and a few surveillance night-mares. *Ethnogr. Qual. Res. Il Mulino* **2020**, *13*, 374–388.
32. Comelli, A.; Coronnello, C.; Dahiya, N.; Benfante, V.; Palmucci, S.; Basile, A.; Vancheri, C.; Russo, G.; Yezzi, A.; Stefano, A. Lung Segmentation on High-Resolution Computerized Tomography Images Using Deep Learning: A Preliminary Step for Radiomics Studies. *J. Imaging* **2020**, *6*, 125. [CrossRef]
33. Gillies, R.J.; Kinahan, P.E.; Hricak, H. Radiomics: Images Are More than Pictures, They Are Data. *Radiology* **2016**, *278*, 563–577. [CrossRef]
34. Pranata, Y.D.; Wang, K.-C.; Wang, J.-C.; Idram, I.; Lai, J.-Y.; Liu, J.-W.; Hsieh, I.-H. Deep learning and SURF for automated classification and detection of calcaneus fractures in CT images. *Comput. Methods Programs Biomed.* **2019**, *171*, 27–37. [CrossRef]

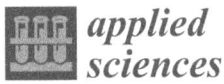

Article

Artificial Intelligence Applications on Restaging [^{18}F]FDG PET/CT in Metastatic Colorectal Cancer: A Preliminary Report of Morpho-Functional Radiomics Classification for Prediction of Disease Outcome

Pierpaolo Alongi [1,2], Alessandro Stefano [3], Albert Comelli [4,*], Alessandro Spataro [5], Giuseppe Formica [5], Riccardo Laudicella [1,4,5,6], Helena Lanzafame [5], Francesco Panasiti [5], Costanza Longo [5], Federico Midiri [7], Viviana Benfante [4,8], Ludovico La Grutta [8], Irene Andrea Burger [6,9], Tommaso Vincenzo Bartolotta [7], Sergio Baldari [5], Roberto Lagalla [7], Massimo Midiri [7] and Giorgio Russo [3]

1. Nuclear Medicine Unit, Fondazione Istituto Giuseppe Giglio, 90015 Cefalù, Italy; alongi.pierpaolo@gmail.com (P.A.); riccardo.laudicella@usz.ch (R.L.)
2. Nuclear Medicine Unit, A.R.N.A.S. Ospedale Civico Di Cristina e Benfratelli, 90127 Palermo, Italy
3. Institute of Molecular Bioimaging and Physiology, National Research Council (IBFM-CNR), 90015 Cefalù, Italy; alessandro.stefano@ibfm.cnr.it (A.S.); giorgio.russo@ibfm.cnr.it (G.R.)
4. Ri.MED Foundation, 90133 Palermo, Italy; vbenfante@Fondazionerimed.com
5. Nuclear Medicine Unit, Department of Biomedical and Dental Sciences and Morpho-Functional Imaging, University of Messina, 98122 Messina, Italy; alessandro.spataro@outlook.it (A.S.); giuseppeformica23@gmail.com (G.F.); helena.lanzafame@gmail.com (H.L.); francesco.panasiti90@gmail.com (F.P.); costanza.longo@virgilio.it (C.L.); sbaldari@unime.it (S.B.)
6. Department of Nuclear Medicine, University Hospital Zurich, University of Zurich, 8091 Zurich, Switzerland; Irene.burger@usz.ch
7. Section of Radiological Sciences, Department of Biomedicine, Neuroscience and Advanced Diagnostics, University of Palermo, 90133 Palermo, Italy; federico.midiri@hotmail.com (F.M.); tommasovincenzo.bartolotta@unipa.it (T.V.B.); roberto.lagalla@unipa.it (R.L.); massimo.midiri@unipa.it (M.M.)
8. Department of Health Promotion, Mother and Child Care, Internal Medicine and Medical Specialties, Molecular and Clinical Medicine, University of Palermo, 90127 Palermo, Italy; ludovico.lagrutta@unipa.it
9. Department of Nuclear Medicine, Kantonsspital Baden, 5404 Baden, Switzerland
* Correspondence: acomelli@fondazionerimed.com

Featured Application: Based on results defined in this study, new investigations might propose morpho-functional-based radiomics algorithms for risk stratification with possible impact on treatment management in colorectal cancer.

Abstract: The aim of this study was to investigate the application of [^{18}F]FDG PET/CT images-based textural features analysis to propose radiomics models able to early predict disease progression (PD) and survival outcome in metastatic colorectal cancer (MCC) patients after first adjuvant therapy. For this purpose, 52 MCC patients who underwent [^{18}F]FDGPET/CT during the disease restaging process after the first adjuvant therapy were analyzed. Follow-up data were recorded for a minimum of 12 months after PET/CT. Radiomics features from each avid lesion in PET and low-dose CT images were extracted. A hybrid descriptive-inferential method and the discriminant analysis (DA) were used for feature selection and for predictive model implementation, respectively. The performance of the features in predicting PD was performed for per-lesion analysis, per-patient analysis, and liver lesions analysis. All lesions were again considered to assess the diagnostic performance of the features in discriminating liver lesions. In predicting PD in the whole group of patients, on PET features radiomics analysis, among per-lesion analysis, only the GLZLM_GLNU feature was selected, while three features were selected from PET/CT images data set. The same features resulted more accurately by associating CT features with PET features (AUROC 65.22%). In per-patient analysis, three features for stand-alone PET images and one feature (i.e., HUKurtosis) for the PET/CT data set were selected. Focusing on liver metastasis, in per-lesion analysis, the same analysis recognized one PET feature (GLZLM_GLNU) from PET images and three features from PET/CT data set. Similarly,

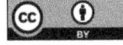

in liver lesions per-patient analysis, we found three PET features and a PET/CT feature (HUKurtosis). In discrimination of liver metastasis from the rest of the other lesions, optimal results of stand-alone PET imaging were found for one feature (SUVbwmin; AUROC 88.91%) and two features for merged PET/CT features analysis (AUROC 95.33%). In conclusion, our machine learning model on restaging [^{18}F]FDGPET/CT was demonstrated to be feasible and potentially useful in the predictive evaluation of disease progression in MCC.

Keywords: colon; cancer; radiomics; artificial intelligence; positron emission tomography-computed tomography; nuclear medicine

1. Introduction

Colorectal cancer (CRC) is the third most common cancer and the second leading cause of death worldwide. Almost 20% of such patients will develop metastatic disease, about one-third of patients already present with liver metastases at the time of diagnosis [1,2]. Alongside traditional imaging (e.g., ultrasonography, CT, MRI), [^{18}F]FDG PET/CT is routinely used as a tool for accurate staging and restaging after therapy in patients with colorectal metastatic disease, and it represents a valuable ally for risk assessment, prognosis evaluation, and treatment strategy decisions making.

Radiomics is that part of artificial intelligence (AI) that aims to provide quantitative characteristics (features) from biomedical images of different nature that cannot be assessed by the human eye, assuming that any smallest image's constituent (i.e., voxel and/or pixel) may encompass features of tumor's phenotypes that may be potentially related to tumor's outcome and patients' response to therapy, reflecting the pathophysiological process and supporting medical decisions. The workflow of radiomics' processes can be simply resumed in five main steps starting with the acquisition of images, pre-processing tasks (registration, deconvolution, denoizing, and so on) and VOI delineation, features extraction, reduction, and selection, and finally, the selection of the predictive model using AI-based classifiers [3]. In the last decade, the use of radiomics in the study of medical images has aroused increasing interest [4,5]. Several studies have demonstrated the correlation between the heterogeneity of the tissues and the radiomics features, which would allow obtaining relevant information through the analysis of the images alone [6].

[^{18}F]FDG PET/CT could be a useful modality for assessing tumor viability and differential diagnosis also for colorectal metastatic cancer and may provide important data regarding the appropriate treatment strategy [7,8]. The further integration of [^{18}F]FDG PET/CT data with radiomics features could reach the provision of new insightful information also regarding tumor biology. In other words, the statistical analysis of the features using methods of increasing complexity (first order, second order, or higher) can be useful in the prognostic evaluation, in therapeutic management, and in characterizing tumor phenotypes [9]. Radiomics' literature in colorectal cancer is highly limited in PET imaging, but it nonetheless holds promise for genetic mutation status assessment [10,11] and the prediction of outcomes.

The present study aimed to investigate the potential application of texture analysis on restaging [^{18}F]FDG PET/CT images in metastatic colorectal patients, proposing a radiomics model able to select PET and CT imaging features for global disease status prediction, liver metastasis evaluation, and survival outcomes.

2. Materials and Methods

Sixty-three metastatic lesions from fifty-two colorectal patients were retrospectively considered. Patients underwent restaging [^{18}F]FDG PET/CT after first adjuvant therapy between November 2008 and December 2018 following these inclusion criteria: (a) pathology confirmed diagnosis of primary colorectal adenocarcinoma; (b) clinical-instrumental (ceCT, MR, histopathology, and/or clinical report) confirmed metastatic disease status;

(c) [^{18}F]FDG PET/CT performed at restaging after first adjuvant therapy (at least 15 days from the last cycle of chemotherapy and three months after RT); (d) [^{18}F]FDG PET/CT positive for lymph-nodal/metastatic disease; (e) minimum follow-up (FU) duration of 12 months after [^{18}F]FDG PET/CT; (f) complete clinical (clinical case notes and multidisciplinary meeting reports), laboratory, pathological and imaging data available (contrast-enhanced CT, MRI); (g) [^{18}F]FDG PET/CT findings retrospectively confirmed at clinical follow-up with biopsy and/or through other imaging modalities. The study was approved by the institutional review board. The internal procedures provide informed consent also regarding the potential scientific use of all nuclear medicine examinations performed at the Fondazione Istituto G.Giglio of Cefalù (Palermo, Italy). Therefore, written informed consent was available for each patient.

2.1. [^{18}F]FDG PET/CT Imaging

According to the standard [^{18}F]FDG PET/CT protocol in use at our institution, the scans were performed following the international clinical recommendations [12]. After six hours of fasting, patients underwent examination on Discovery STE GE Healthcare. The clinical protocol included a full-body PET scan (6–8 beds, 2–3 min per bed position) after 60 min the i.v. administration of 3.7 MBq/kg of [^{18}F]FDG and a co-registered low-dose CT scan (120 kV, 80–120 mA) without contrast enhancement. PET images (256×256 voxel size) were reconstructed with CT-based attenuation correction. The 3D reconstruction was based on the ordered subset expectation maximization (OSEM) algorithm with the two iterative processes. Two nuclear medicine physicians (over 5 years' experience, PA and RL) qualitatively analyze the examinations, being aware of the results of other imaging modalities and clinical data. Following inclusion criteria, [^{18}F]FDG PET/CT positivity was confirmed by the raters after consensus reading if a non-physiological [^{18}F]FDG uptake was moderately (tracer uptake superior to the background at visual assessment) or markedly (tracer uptake superior to physiological liver uptake at visual assessment) increased to the background activity; in case of multiple [^{18}F]FDG uptake foci, the higher qualitative assessed uptake was selected among multiple lesions for each disease location (N and/or M). CT imaging was used to assist the physician in delineating the tumor for local recurrence or lymph node/metastatic disease. Following clinical, laboratory, and CT, MRI, [^{18}F]FDG PET/CT data were recorded. According to such information, the terms disease progression (PD) and stable disease (SD) were used to define the disease status during the follow-up.

2.2. Radiomics Analysis

The volumetric segmentations were performed with the freely available texture analysis LIFEx platform [13] that is the most widely used IBSI (Image Biomarker Standardization Initiative) compliant software in PET imaging to obtain reproducible and robust radiomics features. Specifically, two board-certified nuclear physicians evaluated and segmented PET/CT lesions by consensus and blinded to the purpose of the study and to the pathology information. Signal intensity on PET images was judged as hyperintense when the signal intensity of the tumor was higher than the signal intensity of non-tumoral tissue. SUV_{max} was used as a PET parameter to select the most avid lesion for the global evaluation of disease status and for the most avid liver lesion in every patient. The same volume was transposed in the same region on CT images for extraction of morphological features. Successively, 105 and 66 features were automatically extracted using LifeX starting from the above-mentioned volumes of interest (VOI) from each lesion in PET and CT images, respectively. The extracted features were classified into two categories based on their information type: (I) shape features, which consider the geometric aspects of the VOI, such as shape and volume, (II) statistical features including first-order statistic (histogram-based) features describing intensity values within the target and higher-order statistics (texture) features that are designed to quantify the perceived texture of an image and to provide spatial information of intensities in a VOI. In the last case, five texture classes were considered:

(i) gray-level cooccurrence matrix (GLCM), (ii) gray-level run-length matrix (GLRLM), (iii) gray-level dependence matrix (GLDM), (iv) gray-level zone length matrix (GLZLM), and (v) neigh-boring gray-level dependence matrix (NGLDM). Specifically, (i) GLCM evaluates the incidence of voxels with the same intensities at a predetermined distance along a fixed direction; (ii) GLRLM assesses consecutive voxels with the same intensity along fixed directions; (iii) GLDM counts the number of voxel segments having the same intensity in a given direction; (iv) GLZLM is defined as the number of connected voxels that have equal gray-level intensity; (v) NGTDM assesses the spatial interrelationships between 3 or more voxels [14]. In the work of [13], there is an extensive description of each extracted feature. Successively, the mixed descriptive-inferential sequential approach, as described in two complementary studies [15,16], was used to identify a small set of radiomics features with valuable association with patients' outcomes for better predictive performance, leading to the exclusion of non-reproducible, redundant, and nonrelevant features from the initial feature data set.

After the selection and reduction process, the predictive model was implemented using the discriminant analysis (DA) [17]. The training step was performed only once, and when completed, the DA was capable of classifying new PET lesions. Using the k-fold cross-validation strategy, data were divided into training and validation sets using a random partition. Specifically, data were divided into k-folds: one-fold was used as the validation set while the others folds were used as the training set. The folds were created in such a way that the training and validation sets maintained the same percentage of patient status as the original data set. After applying the trial-and-error methodology, k = 5 was determined as the best value for our analyses (k range: 5–15, step size of 5). Consequently, this process was repeated 5 times, and the mean error was calculated (i) to avoid the over-fitting and asymmetrical sampling by increasing the accuracy of the final results, (ii) to test different models, and (iii) to obtain more robust results [18–22].

The steps between the reduction and selection of features and the implementation of the model were repeated ten times to evaluate different aspects, listed below:

- Four predictive models per-lesion and -patient analysis: Performances of radiomics features extracted from PET and PET/CT, respectively, in assessing the treatment response for each lesion (without considering the patient treatment response) and in assessing the patient treatment response;
- Four models per-patient and -lesion analysis considering the only subset of liver lesions;
- Two models to evaluate the performances of PET and PET/CT radiomics features in discriminating liver metastasis from the rest of the other lesions.

2.3. Diagnostic Performance Evaluation

Sensitivity, specificity, positive predictive value (PPV), accuracy, and receiver operating characteristics (ROC) with 95% confidence intervals (C.I.) and areas under the ROC curve (AUROC; 95% C.I.) were calculated to assess the diagnostic performance on prediction of disease progression (dichotomized evaluation = 1) versus stable disease or partial response or complete response (dichotomized evaluation = 0).

3. Results

Fifty-two patients (mean age 62,28 years ± 11.23) who underwent [^{18}F]FDG PET/CT between November 2008 and December 2018 met the inclusions criteria. The main characteristics are summarized in Table 1. Tumor grading was distributed as follows: G1 in 2/52 (3.85%); G2 in 23/52 (44.23%); G2-3 in 2/52 (3.85%); G3 in 10/52 (19.23%); unknown in 15/52 (28.84%). TNM staging was distributed as follows: Stage I in 4/52 patients (7.69%); Stage II in 9/52 (17.03%); Stage III in 13/52 (25%); Stage IV in 10/52 (19.23%), unknown in 16/52 (30.76%). As first adjuvant therapy, 1 patient (1.92%) was treated by radiotherapy, 49 patients (94.2%) by chemotherapy, and 2 patients (3.85%) by chemotherapy associated with radiotherapy.

Table 1. Patients' main characteristics.

	All Patients (n = 52)
Age (Mean ± SD)	62.28 ± 11.23 y
Sex	
Male	41 (77.35%)
Female	11 (22.65%)
Grading	
G1	2 (3.85%)
G2	23 (44.23%)
G2–G3	2 (3.85%)
G3	10 (19.23%)
Unknown	15 (28.84%)
First Adjuvant Therapy	
Radiotherapy	1 (1.92%)
Chemotherapy	49 (94.2%)
Cht+RT	2 (3.85%)
PET Lesions	
Liver	23 (36.51%)
Lymph nodes	13 (19.05%)
Lungs	8 (12.7%)
Presacral	7 (11.11%)
Peritoneum	4 (6.35%)
Rectum	3 (4.76%)
Spleen	2 (3.17%)
Bones	2 (3.17%)
Thorax	1 (1.59%)
Stages At Diagnosis	
Stage I	4 (7.69%)
Stage II	9 (17.30%)
Stage III	13 (25%)
Stage IV	10 (19.23%)
Unknown	16 (30.76%)

3.1. [^{18}F]FDG PET/CT Findings

At the first [^{18}F]FDG PET/CT scan, 43 patients (82.7%) were PET-positive for a single lesion and 9 (17.3%) for 2 or more lesions. Sites of metastasis were distributed as follows: 23 liver (36.51%), 12 lymph nodes (19.05%), 8 lungs (12.7%), 7 presacral lymph nodes (11.11%), 4 peritoneum (6.35%), 3 rectum (4.76%), 2 spleen (3.17%), 2 bones (3.17%), 1 thorax (1.59%), and 1 anastomosis tissue (1.59%).

3.2. Follow-Up

FU lasted a mean of 22 months (range 13–48 months). We calculated a median progression-free survival (PFS) of 17 months (range 1–105) and a median overall survival of 45 months (range 4–117). At the last FU, 32 (62%) patients showed progression of the disease, 9 (17%) stable disease, and 11 (21%) responded to therapy with a regression of the disease.

3.3. Radiomics Features Analysis

A total of 63 lesions out of 52 patients included in the study were selected. The analysis of the classification model has been divided into three parts, as explained in the "*Radiomics features extraction and Machine-learning features classification*" section, for a total of 10 different radiomics models (Figure 1). In the first case, the prediction disease outcome for each lesion was analyzed (per-lesion analysis) considering the features extracted from PET and PET/CT images, respectively; then, the same analysis was developed of considering each patient (per-patient analysis) considering all the features extracted from the same images for a total of four different radiomics models.

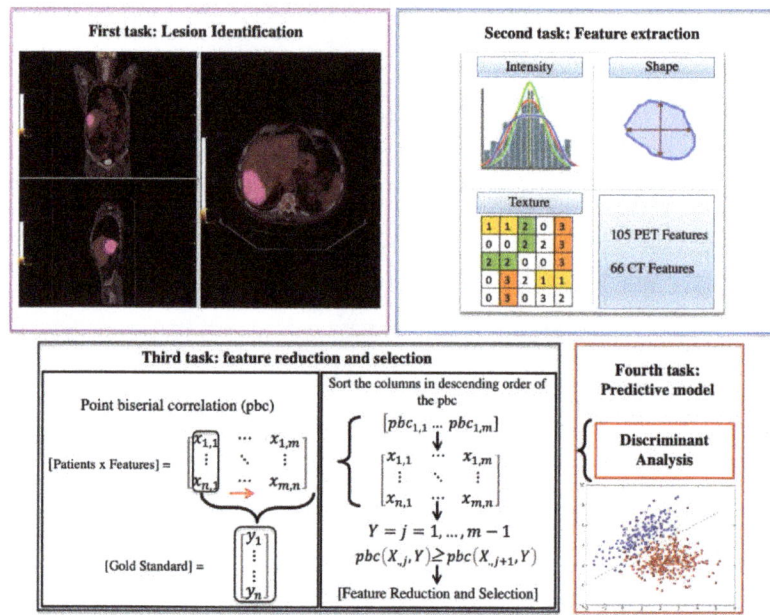

Figure 1. Radiomics flow chart applied in this study.

The results were as follow:

- For lesion analysis, GLRLM-based feature gray-level non-uniformity (GLZLM_GLNU) was selected [15,16] considering the only PET data set obtaining a Sensitivity 90.11%, Specificity 36.78%, Accuracy 66.72%, and AUROC 56.52% for the predictive DA classifier, while three features (GLZLM_ Zone Length Non-Uniformity—GLZLM_ ZLNU, and GLRLM_Short Run High Gray-Level Emphasis—GLRLM_SRHGE—between the CT features and GLZLM_GLNU between the PET features) were selected considering the PET/CT data set with Sensitivity 78.22%, Specificity 51.75%, Accuracy 66.63%, and AUROC 65.22%;
- For patient analysis, three features (GLZLM_ZLNU, GLZLM_High Gray-level Zone -GLZLM_HGZ-, Conventional Radial Intensity Mean Standardized Uptake Value body weight standard deviation squared -CONVENTIONAL_RIM_SUVbwstdev2-) were selected considering the PET-only data set with Sensitivity 32.07%, Specificity 92.11%, Accuracy 73.95% and AUROC 47.97%, and one feature (Conventional Hounsfield Unit Kurtosis -CONVENTIONAL_HUKurtosis-) was selected considering the PET/CT data set with Sensitivity 33.81%, Specificity 83.76%, Accuracy 68.70%, and AUROC 61%.

Figure 2 shows the ROCs for the four implemented models, while Table 2 shows all obtained performances.

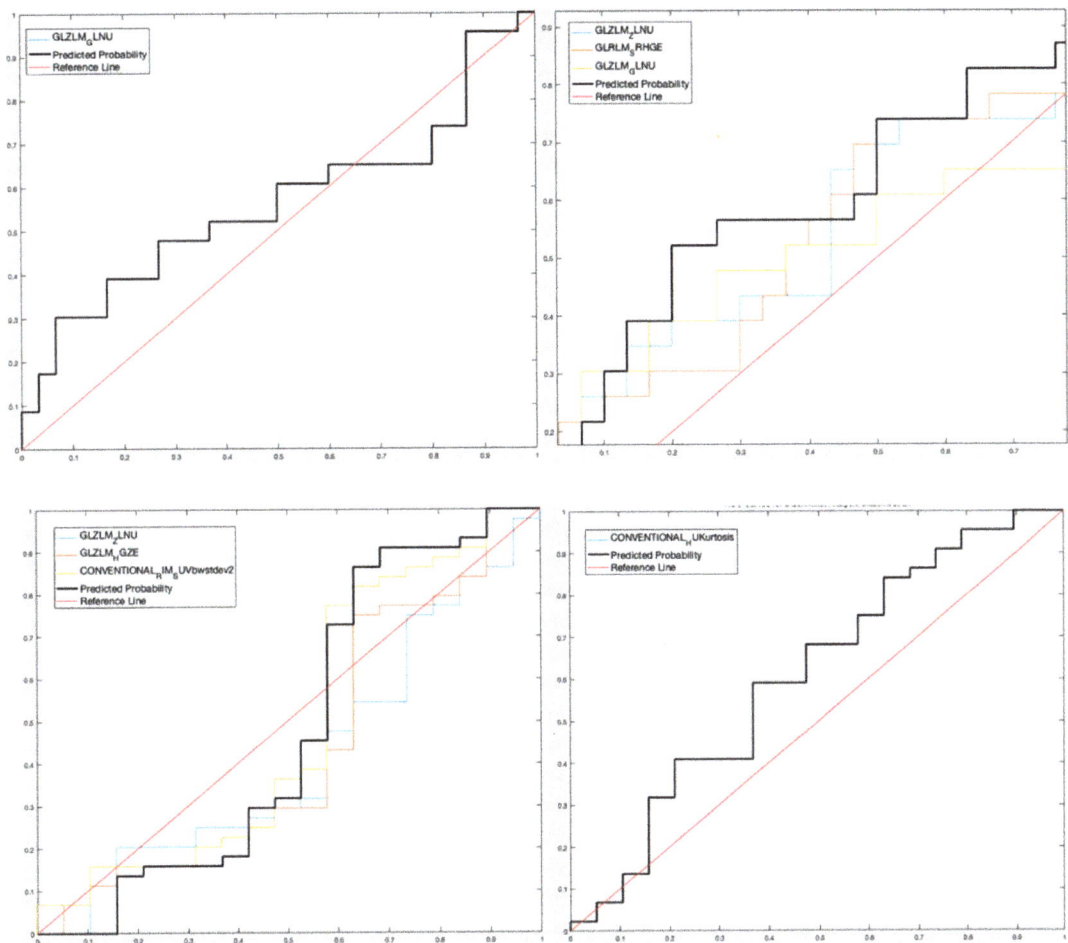

Figure 2. ROCs for the four radiomics models obtained per lesion (first row) and per-patient analyses (second row) for PET-only (first column) and PET/CT images (second column), with an AUROC of 56.52%, 65.22%, 47.97%, and 61%, respectively.

Table 2. Performances of radiomics features in prediction of progression of disease in all lesions, per-patient, and per-lesion analysis.

	Sensitivity	Specificity	Accuracy	AUROC	Features Selected		
PET per-lesion	90.11%	36.78%	66.72%	56.52%	GLZLM_G LNU		
PET/CT per-lesion	78.22%	51.75%	66.63%	65.22%	GLZLM_ZL NU (CT)	GLRLM_ SRHGE (CT)	GLZLM_G LNU (PET)
PET per-patient	32.07%	92.11%	73.95%	47.97%	GLZLM_ZL NU	GLZLM_ HGZ	CONVEN TIONAL_ RIM_SUV bwstdev2
PET/CT per-patient	33.81%	83.76%	68.70%	61.00%	CONVENT IONAL_H UKurtosis		

In addition, the study was similarly repeated, focusing only on liver lesions, for a total of two different radiomics models, with the following results:

- For lesion analysis, one PET feature (GLZLM_GLNU) with Sensitivity 70.15%, Specificity 23.48%, Accuracy 54.21%, and AUROC 39.94%, and three PET/CT features (GLZLM_ZLNU, and GLRLM_SRHGE between the CT features and GLZLM_GLNU between the PET features) with Sensitivity 64.39%, Specificity 76.71%, Accuracy 68.69%, and AUROC 55.26%;
- For patient analysis, three PET features (GLZLM_ZLNU, GLZLM_HGZ, CONVENTIONAL_RIM_SUVbwstdev2) with Sensitivity 44.42%, Specificity 84.37%, Accuracy 59.03%, and AUROC 60.11%, and one PET/CT feature (CONVENTIONAL_HUKurtosis) with Sensitivity 33.12%, Specificity 73.74%, Accuracy 47.88%, and AUROC 43.48%.

Figure 3 shows the ROCs for the four implemented models, while Table 3 shows all obtained performances.

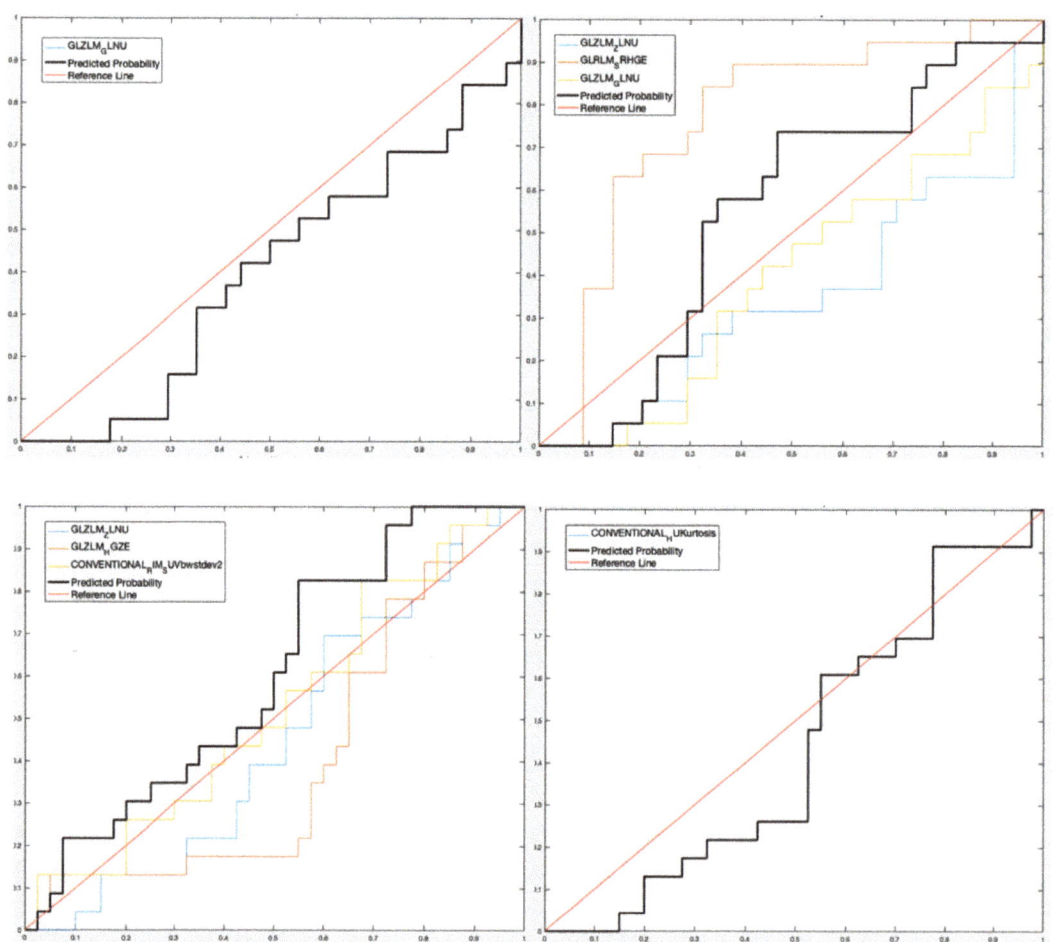

Figure 3. Liver subset: ROCs for the four radiomics models obtained per lesion (first row) and per-patient analyses (second row) for PET (first column) and PET/CT images (second column), with an AUROC of 39.94%, 55.26%, 60.11%, and 43.48%, respectively.

Table 3. Radiomics features performance for liver lesions in prediction of disease progression per-patient and per-lesion analysis.

	Sensitivity	Specificity	Accuracy	AUROC	Features Selected		
PET per-lesion	70.15%	23.48%	54.21%	39.94%	GLZLM_GLNU		
PET/CT per-lesion	64.39%	76.71%	68.69%	55.26%	GLZLM_ZLNU (CT)	GLRLM_SRHGE (CT)	GLZLM_GLNU (PET)
PET per-patient	44.42%	84.37%	59.03%	60.11%	GLZLM_ZLNU	GLZLM_HGZ	CONVENTIONAL_RIM_SUVbwstdev2
PET/CT per-patient	33.12%	73.74%	47.88%	43.48%	CONVENTIONAL_HUKurtosis		

Finally, all lesions were again considered to assess the diagnostic performance of the features in discriminating liver metastasis:

- For PET images, one feature (Discretized SUVbw minimum—DISCRETIZED_SUVbwmin-) was extracted with Sensitivity 73.78%, Specificity 83.02%, Accuracy 76.91%, and AUROC 88.91%;
- For PET/CT images, two features (Discretized histogram energy—DISCRETIZED_HISTO_Energy—between the CT features and DISCRETIZED_SUVbwmin between the PET features) were extracted with Sensitivity 89.46%, Specificity 93.63%, Accuracy 91.02%, and AUROC 95.33%.

Figure 4 shows the ROCs for the two implemented models, while Table 4 shows all obtained performances.

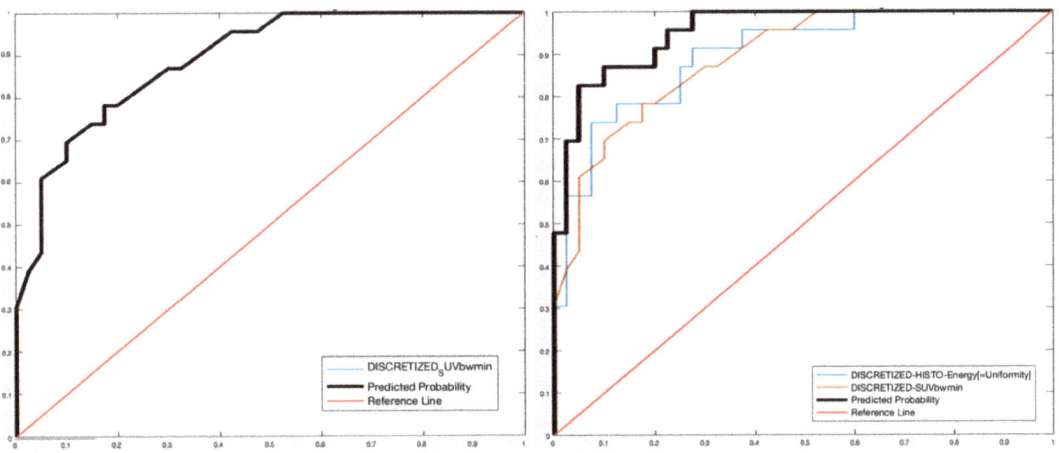

Figure 4. ROCs for the radiomics models implemented for discrimination of liver metastasis using PET and PET/CT images with an AUROC of 88.91% and 95.33%, respectively.

Table 4. Radiomics features performance for liver metastasis discrimination.

	Sensitivity	Specificity	Accuracy	AUROC	Features Selected	
PET liver	73.38%	83.02%	76.91%	88.91%	DISCRETIZED_SUVbwmin	
PET/CT liver	89.46%	93.63%	91.02%	95.33%	DISCRETIZED_HISTO_Energy (CT)	DISCRETIZED_SUVbwmin (PET)

4. Discussion

To the best of our knowledge, the present study is one of the first to explore [^{18}F]FDG PET/CT textural features analysis after first adjuvant therapy to potentially predict disease progression and survival outcome as an indirect predictive parameter of second-line therapy responses in metastatic colon cancer patients, using an innovative mixed descriptive-inferential sequential approach for features reduction and selection, and by using DA as a predictive model [17].

Radiomics literature in CRC is highly heterogeneous, but it holds promise for the prediction of outcomes. Most evidence is available for MRI-based radiomics in rectal cancer [23]. A few studies on textural features derived from [^{18}F]FDG PET images at baseline for locally advanced colorectal cancer and before or after starting any neoadjuvant treatments may enable detailed stratification of prognosis in patients with CRC [24–27].

Our study focused on the potential usefulness to extract PET radiomics features and also low-dose CT radiomic features for a "hybrid" textural PET/CT analysis mimicking the qualitative assessment in the clinical routine evaluation of PET/CT images. The scope of this design study was to confirm the feasibility of our ML methods and to analyze how all the information related to restaging PET/CT imaging after first-line treatments might be able to predict the disease status outcomes after further treatments. Radiomics features were extracted from each lesion (including all the sites of metastasis), divided into three feature subsets: 105 features from PET images, 66 features from CT, and 171 features from both PET and CT. Features were automatically extracted using the well-known IBSI compliant LifeX software to perform a totally objective and reproducible study. Prediction of outcome in patients with CRC is challenging because of the lack of a robust biomarker and heterogeneity between and within tumors to modulate treatment strategies. In this scenario, a study conducted on third-line treatment patients with metastatic colorectal cancer showed that high tumor heterogeneity, volume, and low sphericity on baseline [^{18}F]FDG PET were related to reduced survival [28]. Similarly, textural parameters as the coefficient of variation, kurtosis of the absolute gradient (GrKurtosis), and other features on [^{18}F]FDG PET images have been proposed in other papers as predictive and prognostic factors in the assessment of therapy response and survival outcomes in patients with rectal cancer [29,30].

Our study results, differently from others studies for study design and ML models adopted, demonstrate the potential predictive value of radiomics features derived from an innovative machine learning model adapted by using the disease status at follow-up as the gold standard for the performances analysis. This approach was proposed, as in other studies conducted by our group [31,32], to define the real value of PET/CT as a predictive tool for the stratification of patients with different diseases (prostate and primary brain tumors) that for specific characteristics are more susceptible to have a scarce sensitivity to therapies and a poor disease outcome. For this reason, the apparent sub-optimal results obtained in the present study need to be interpreted with caution because we are not presenting the performance on the identification of disease but the capability of some radiomics features to predict the disease status outcome of the patients with metastatic colon cancer after the standard first adjuvant therapy.

Underlining the results on the PET radiomics analysis in the whole patient group, among per-lesion analysis, the feature selected as the most accurate for the DA classifier was GLZLM_GLNU, while three features (GLZLM_ZLNU and GLRLM_SRHGE between CT features and GLZLM_GLNU between PET features) were selected from PET/CT images obtaining slight enhancement of accuracy when CT analysis was merged with PET performances (AUROC 65.22%).

In per-patient analysis, 3 PET features (GLZLM_ZLNU, GLZLM_HGZ, RIM_SUV bwstdev2), and 1 PET/CT feature (HUKurtosis) were selected by DA classifier (AUROC 61%). Considering these first two analysis groups, three features belonging to the GLZLM class were identified as the most accurate for the DA classifier. The GLZLM, also called gray-level size-zone matrix (GLSZM), is the texture class that provides information on the size of homogeneous zones for each gray-level. Consequently, it is indirectly linked to the heterogeneity of the lesions, which, reflecting biological characteristics, has a potential value in predicting the progression of the disease [9].

In regard to colorectal liver metastasis, the presence of metastasis in this site is widely considered as one of the unfavorable prognosis parameters. However, commonly employed SUV metrics (SUV_{max}, SUV_{peak}, SUV_{mean}) from [^{18}F]FDG PET images perform relatively poorly in outcome prediction tasks (OS, PFS, EFS). In contrast, the use of liver metastasis number and volumetric measurements of MTV and TLG appears to be capable of providing significant performance [33]. Our radiomics model results, similarly, showed sub-optimal performances in the prediction of disease outcome by defining, at per-lesion analysis, one PET feature (GLZLM_GLNU with AUROC 39.94%) and three PET/CT features (GLZLM_ZLNU and GLRLM_SRHGE between CT features and GLZLM_GLNU between PET features with AUROC 55.26%). Similarly, in liver lesions per-patient analysis, we found 3 PET features (GLZLM_ZLNU, GLZLM_HGZ, RIM_SUVbwstdev2 with AUROC 60.11%) and one PET/CT feature (HUKurtosis with AUROC 43.48%).

Furthermore, to quantify the influence of liver metastasis over all PET/CT findings, one only feature considering PET imaging (i.e., DISCRETIZED_SUVbwmin) and two features considering PET/CT imaging (DISCRETIZED_HISTO_Energy between the CT features and DISCRETIZED_SUVbwmin between the PET features) was able to discriminate liver metastasis from the rest of the other lesions (AUROC = 88.91% and 95.33%, respectively). These results, confirmed after further investigations, may be interpreted as crucial in the diagnostic and prognostic impact of liver lesions in patients affected by metastatic colorectal cancer.

Potential limitations of the study must be considered. First, some intrinsic biases as the well-known sub-optimal accuracy of PET in some conditions due to FDG uptake variability, depending on the histology, size, location (particularly relevant for primary lesion in terms of prognosis: right vs. left colorectal cancer), pH, and possible overestimation of metabolic activity due to associate inflammation, could have affected the results. Furthermore, this is a retrospective single-center study, with a relatively small number of patients and a design study limited by data available. All patients who underwent [^{18}F]FDG PET/CT after the first adjuvant therapy were at different disease stages, treated with different chemotherapy combinations following Italian oncological guidelines (5FU or oral capecitabine in combination with either oxaliplatin or irinotecan in various schedules) and a different number of cycles based on patients clinical conditions. All these variables might affect the patient's outcome. In addition, radiomics features were extracted only from the [^{18}F]FDG-positive tumor to construct the model, and the remaining normal tissue in the image may still contain invisible but useful data. To properly analyze the entire images, 3D deep learning methods will be necessary.

Our study results could benefit from validation in a prospective multi-center study. Nevertheless, our preliminary experience suggests that PET texture analysis is feasible and could carefully be used as an independent indicator for the prognosis of patients with a high risk of disease progression and supporting clinicians for a more accurate selection of patients that may benefit from tailored therapies.

As future research direction of our study, radiomics analyses based on wavelet and Laplacian of Gaussian features will also be considered (e.g., using Pyradiomics) [34]. Furthermore, machine learning investigation could be conducted in the staging preoperative scan, aiming to identify patients with an increased risk of liver metastases susceptible to liver-directed therapies, as previously reported in CT textural analysis by Creasy et al. [35].

5. Conclusions

Our machine learning model on restaging [^{18}F]FDG PET/CT demonstrated to be feasible and potentially useful in the predictive evaluation of disease progression in metastatic colon cancer after first-line therapies. New investigations might propose morpho-functional-based radiomics algorithms for risk stratification and impact on treatment management in colorectal cancer.

Author Contributions: Conceptualization, P.A.; methodology, P.A., A.S. (Alessandro Stefano) and A.C.; software, A.C.; validation, A.S. (Alessandro Stefano); formal analysis, F.P., C.L. and R.L. (Riccardo Laudicella); investigation, A.C.; resources, A.S. (Alessandro Spataro), G.F., H.L., F.M., V.B. and L.L.G.; writing—original draft preparation, P.A., A.S. (Alessandro Stefano), A.C. and R.L. (Riccardo Laudicella); writing—review and editing, P.A., A.S. (Alessandro Stefano) and A.C.; visualization, A.C.; supervision, I.A.B., T.V.B., S.B., R.L. (Roberto Lagalla), M.M. and G.R. All authors have read and agreed to the published version of the manuscript.

Funding: This research received no external funding.

Institutional Review Board Statement: The study was conducted according to the Declaration of Helsinki principles and good clinical practice guidelines, and written informed consent was obtained by each patient included in the study. For this type of study, ethical approbation was not required in our institution.

Informed Consent Statement: Informed consent was obtained from all subjects involved in the study.

Data Availability Statement: Data are available for bona fide researchers who request it from the authors.

Conflicts of Interest: The authors of this manuscript declare no relationships with any companies whose products or services may be related to the subject matter of the article.

References

1. Sung, H.; Ferlay, J.; Siegel, R.L.; Laversanne, M.; Soerjomataram, I.; Jemal, A.; Bray, F. Global Cancer Statistics 2020: GLOBOCAN Estimates of Incidence and Mortality Worldwide for 36 Cancers in 185 Countries. *CA Cancer J. Clin.* **2021**, *71*, 209–249. [CrossRef]
2. Li, Y.; Eresen, A.; Lu, Y.; Yang, J.; Shangguan, J.; Velichko, Y.; Yaghmai, V.; Zhang, Z. Radiomics signature for the preoperative assessment of stage in advanced colon cancer. *Am. J. Cancer Res.* **2019**, *9*, 1429–1438. [PubMed]
3. Laudicella, R.; Comelli, A.; Stefano, A.; Szostek, M.; Crocè, L.; Vento, A.; Spataro, A.; Comis, A.D.; La Torre, F.; Gaeta, M.; et al. Artificial Neural Networks in Cardiovascular Diseases and its Potential for Clinical Application in Molecular Imaging. *Curr. Radiopharm.* **2020**, *14*, 209–219. [CrossRef] [PubMed]
4. Cook, G.J.; Azad, G.; Owczarczyk, K.; Siddique, M.; Goh, V. Challenges and Promises of PET Radiomics. *Int. J. Radiat. Oncol. Biol. Phys.* **2018**, *102*, 1083–1089. [CrossRef] [PubMed]
5. Liberini, V.; Laudicella, R.; Capozza, M.; Huellner, M.; Burger, I.; Baldari, S.; Terreno, E.; Deandreis, D. The Future of Cancer Diagnosis, Treatment and Surveillance: A Systemic Review on Immunotherapy and Immuno-PET Radiotracers. *Molecules* **2021**, *26*, 2201. [CrossRef]
6. Mayerhoefer, M.E.; Materka, A.; Langs, G.; Häggström, I.; Szczypiński, P.; Gibbs, P.; Cook, G. Introduction to Radiomics. *J. Nucl. Med.* **2020**, *61*, 488–495. [CrossRef]
7. Alongi, P.; Laudicella, R.; Gentile, R.; Scalisi, S.; Stefano, A.; Russo, G.; Emanuele, G.; Domenico, A.; Giancarlo, P.; Sinagra, E.; et al. Potential clinical value of quantitative fluorine-18-fluorodeoxyglucose-PET/computed tomography using a graph-based method analysis in evaluation of incidental lesions of gastrointestinal tract: Correlation with endoscopic and histopathological findings. *Nucl. Med. Commun.* **2019**, *40*, 1060–1065. [CrossRef]
8. Watanabe, A.; Harimoto, N.; Yokobori, T.; Araki, K.; Kubo, N.; Igarashi, T.; Tsukagoshi, M.; Ishii, N.; Yamanaka, T.; Handa, T.; et al. FDG-PET reflects tumor viability on SUV in colorectal cancer liver metastasis. *Int. J. Clin. Oncol.* **2019**, *25*, 322–329. [CrossRef]
9. Chowdhury, R.; Ganeshan, B.; Irshad, S.; Lawler, K.; Eisenblätter, M.; Milewicz, H.; Rodriguez-Justo, M.; Miles, K.; Ellis, P.; Ng, T.; et al. The use of molecular imaging combined with genomic techniques to understand the heterogeneity in cancer metastasis. *Br. J. Radiol.* **2014**, *87*, 20140065. [CrossRef]
10. Chen, S.-W.; Shen, W.-C.; Chen, W.T.-L.; Hsieh, T.-C.; Yen, K.-Y.; Chang, J.-G.; Kao, C.-H. Metabolic Imaging Phenotype Using Radiomics of [^{18}F]FDG PET/CT Associated with Genetic Alterations of Colorectal Cancer. *Mol. Imaging Biol.* **2019**, *21*, 183–190. [CrossRef]
11. Li, J.; Yang, Z.; Xin, B.; Hao, Y.; Wang, L.; Song, S.; Xu, J.; Wang, X. Quantitative Prediction of Microsatellite Instability in Colorectal Cancer with Preoperative PET/CT-Based Radiomics. *Front. Oncol.* **2021**, *11*, 702055. [CrossRef] [PubMed]
12. Boellaard, R.; Delgado-Bolton, R.; Oyen, W.J.G.; Giammarile, F.; Tatsch, K.; Eschner, W.; Verzijlbergen, F.J.; Barrington, S.F.; Pike, L.C.; Weber, W.A.; et al. FDG PET/CT: EANM procedure guidelines for tumour imaging: Version 2. *Eur. J. Nucl. Med. Mol. Imaging* **2015**, *42*, 328–354. [CrossRef] [PubMed]
13. Nioche, C.; Orlhac, F.; Boughdad, S.; Reuzé, S.; Goya-Outi, J.; Robert, C.; Pellot-Barakat, C.; Soussan, M.; Frouin, F.; Buvat, I. LIFEx: A Freeware for Radiomic Feature Calculation in Multimodality Imaging to Ac-celerate Advances in the Characterization of Tumor Heterogeneity. *Cancer Res.* **2018**, *78*, 4786–4789. [CrossRef] [PubMed]

14. Stefano, A.; Leal, A.; Richiusa, S.; Trang, P.; Comelli, A.; Benfante, V.; Cosentino, S.; Sabini, M.G.; Tuttolomondo, A.; Altieri, R.; et al. Robustness of PET Radiomics Features: Impact of Co-Registration with MRI. *Appl. Sci.* **2021**, *11*, 10170. [CrossRef]
15. Comelli, A.; Stefano, A.; Coronnello, C.; Russo, G.; Vernuccio, F.; Cannella, R.; Salvaggio, G.; Lagalla, R.; Barone, S. Radiomics: A New Biomedical Workflow to Create a Predictive Model. In *Annual Conference on Medical Image Understanding and Analysis*; Communications in Computer and Information Science; Springer: Cham, Switzerland, 2020; pp. 280–293, Volume 1248 CCIS, ISBN 9783030527907. [CrossRef]
16. Barone, S.; Cannella, R.; Comelli, A.; Pellegrino, A.; Salvaggio, G.; Stefano, A.; Vernuccio, F. Hybrid descriptive-inferential method for key feature selection in prostate cancer radiomics. *Appl. Stoch. Model. Bus. Ind.* **2021**, *37*, 961–972. [CrossRef]
17. Stefano, A.; Comelli, A.; Bravatà, V.; Barone, S.; Daskalovski, I.; Savoca, G.; Sabini, M.G.; Ippolito, M.; Russo, G. A preliminary PET ra-diomics study of brain metastases using a fully automatic segmentation method. *BMC Bioinform.* **2020**, *21*, 325. [CrossRef]
18. Russo, G.; Stefano, A.; Alongi, P.; Comelli, A.; Catalfamo, B.; Mantarro, C.; Longo, C.; Altieri, R.; Certo, F.; Cosentino, S.; et al. Feasibility on the Use of Radiomics Features of 11[C]-MET PET/CT in Central Nervous System Tumours: Preliminary Results on Potential Grading Discrimination Using a Machine Learning Model. *Curr. Oncol.* **2021**, *28*, 5318–5331. [CrossRef]
19. Comelli, A.; Stefano, A.; Bignardi, S.; Coronnello, C.; Russo, G.; Sabini, M.G.; Ippolito, M.; Yezzi, A. Tissue Classification to Support Local Active Delineation of Brain Tumors. In *Annual Conference on Medical Image UnderStanding and Analysis*; Communications in Computer and Information Science; Springer: Cham, Switzerland, 2020; pp. 3–14, Volume 1065 CCIS, ISBN 9783030393427. [CrossRef]
20. Cuocolo, R.; Comelli, A.; Stefano, A.; Benfante, V.; Dahiya, N.; Stanzione, A.; Castaldo, A.; De Lucia, D.R.; Yezzi, A.; Imbriaco, M. Deep Learning Whole-Gland and Zonal Prostate Segmentation on a Public MRI Dataset. *J. Magn. Reson. Imaging* **2021**, *54*, 452–459. [CrossRef]
21. Comelli, A.; Coronnello, C.; Dahiya, N.; Benfante, V.; Palmucci, S.; Basile, A.; Vancheri, C.; Russo, G.; Yezzi, A.; Stefano, A. Lung Segmentation on High-Resolution Computerized Tomography Images Using Deep Learning: A Preliminary Step for Radiomics Studies. *J. Imaging* **2020**, *6*, 125. [CrossRef]
22. Stefano, A.; Comelli, A. Customized Efficient Neural Network for COVID-19 Infected Region Identification in CT Images. *J. Imaging* **2021**, *7*, 131. [CrossRef]
23. Staal, F.C.; van der Reijd, D.J.; Taghavi, M.; Lambregts, D.M.; Beets-Tan, R.G.; Maas, M. Radiomics for the Prediction of Treatment Outcome and Survival in Patients with Colorectal Cancer: A Systematic Review. *Clin. Color. Cancer* **2020**, *20*, 52–71. [CrossRef] [PubMed]
24. Kang, J.; Lee, J.H.; Lee, H.S.; Cho, E.S.; Park, E.J.; Baik, S.H.; Lee, K.Y.; Park, C.; Yeu, Y.; Clemenceau, J.R.; et al. Radiomics Features of ^{18}F-Fluorodeoxyglucose Positron-Emission Tomography as a Novel Prog-nostic Signature in Colorectal Cancer. *Cancers* **2021**, *13*, 392. [CrossRef] [PubMed]
25. Shen, W.-C.; Chen, S.-W.; Wu, K.-C.; Lee, P.-Y.; Feng, C.-L.; Hsieh, T.-C.; Yen, K.-Y.; Kao, C.-H. Predicting pathological complete response in rectal cancer after chemoradiotherapy with a random forest using ^{18}F-fluorodeoxyglucose positron emission tomography and computed tomography radiomics. *Ann. Transl. Med.* **2020**, *8*, 207. [CrossRef] [PubMed]
26. Lovinfosse, P.; Polus, M.; Van Daele, D.; Martinive, P.; Daenen, F.; Hatt, M.; Visvikis, D.; Koopmansch, B.; Lambert, F.; Coimbra, C.; et al. FDG PET/CT radiomics for predicting the outcome of locally advanced rectal cancer. *Eur. J. Pediatr.* **2018**, *45*, 365–375. [CrossRef]
27. Giannini, V.; Mazzetti, S.; Bertotto, I.; Chiarenza, C.; Cauda, S.; Delmastro, E.; Bracco, C.; Di Dia, A.; Leone, F.; Medico, E.; et al. Predicting locally advanced rectal cancer response to neoadjuvant therapy with ^{18}F-FDG PET and MRI radiomics features. *Eur. J. Pediatr.* **2019**, *46*, 878–888. [CrossRef]
28. Van Helden, E.J.; Vacher, Y.J.L.; van Wieringen, W.N.; van Velden, F.H.P.; Verheul, H.M.W.; Hoekstra, O.S.; Boellaard, R.; Menke-van der Houven van Oordt, C.W. Radiomics analysis of pre-treatment [^{18}F]FDG PET/CT for patients with metastatic colorectal cancer undergoing palliative systemic treatment. *Eur. J. Nucl. Med. Mol. Imaging.* **2018**, *45*, 2307–2317. [CrossRef]
29. Bundschuh, R.A.; Dinges, J.; Neumann, L.; Seyfried, M.; Zsótér, N.; Papp, L.; Rosenberg, R.; Becker, K.; Astner, S.T.; Essler, M.; et al. Textural Parameters of Tumor Heterogeneity in ^{18}F-FDG PET/CT for Therapy Response Assessment and Prognosis in Patients with Locally Advanced Rectal Cancer. *J. Nucl. Med.* **2014**, *55*, 891–897. [CrossRef]
30. Bang, J.-I.; Ha, S.; Kang, S.-B.; Lee, K.-W.; Lee, H.S.; Kim, J.-S.; Oh, H.-K.; Lee, H.-Y.; Kim, S.E. Prediction of neoadjuvant radiation chemotherapy response and survival using pretreatment [^{18}F]FDG PET/CT scans in locally advanced rectal cancer. *Eur. J. Pediatr.* **2015**, *43*, 422–431. [CrossRef]
31. Alongi, P.; Laudicella, R.; Stefano, A.; Caobelli, F.; Comelli, A.; Vento, A.; Sardina, D.; Ganduscio, G.; Toia, P.; Ceci, F.; et al. Choline PET/CT features to predict survival outcome in high risk prostate cancer restaging: A preliminary machine-learning radiomics study. *Q. J. Nucl. Med. Mol. Imaging* **2020**. [CrossRef] [PubMed]
32. Alongi, P.; Stefano, A.; Comelli, A.; Laudicella, R.; Scalisi, S.; Arnone, G.; Barone, S.; Spada, M.; Purpura, P.; Bartolotta, T.V.; et al. Radiomics analysis of 18F-Choline PET/CT in the prediction of disease outcome in high-risk prostate cancer: An explorative study on machine learning feature classification in 94 patients. *Eur. Radiol.* **2021**, *31*, 4595–4605. [CrossRef]
33. Rahmim, A.; Bak-Fredslund, K.P.; Ashrafinia, S.; Lu, L.; Schmidtlein, C.; Subramaniam, R.M.; Morsing, A.; Keiding, S.; Horsager, J.; Munk, O.L. Prognostic modeling for patients with colorectal liver metastases incorporating FDG PET radiomic features. *Eur. J. Radiol.* **2019**, *113*, 101–109. [CrossRef] [PubMed]

34. Jha, A.K.; Mithun, S.; Jaiswar, V.; Sherkhane, U.B.; Purandare, N.C.; Prabhash, K.; Rangarajan, V.; Dekker, A.; Wee, L.; Traverso, A. Repeatability and reproducibility study of radiomic features on a phantom and human cohort. *Sci. Rep.* **2021**, *11*, 2055. [CrossRef] [PubMed]
35. Creasy, J.M.; Cunanan, K.M.; Chakraborty, J.; McAuliffe, J.C.; Chou, J.; Gonen, M.; Ba, V.S.K.; Weiser, M.R.; Balachandran, V.P.; Drebin, J.A.; et al. Differences in Liver Parenchyma are Measurable with CT Radiomics at Initial Colon Resection in Patients that Develop Hepatic Metastases from Stage II/III Colon Cancer. *Ann. Surg. Oncol.* **2020**, *28*, 1982–1989. [CrossRef] [PubMed]

Article

Pathologic Complete Response Prediction after Neoadjuvant Chemoradiation Therapy for Rectal Cancer Using Radiomics and Deep Embedding Network of MRI

Seunghyun Lee [1], Joonseok Lim [2], Jaeseung Shin [2], Sungwon Kim [2,*] and Heasoo Hwang [1,*]

1. Department of Computer Science and Engineering, University of Seoul, Seoul 02504, Korea; easter3163@naver.com
2. Department of Radiology, Severance Hospital, College of Medicine, Yonsei University, Seoul 03722, Korea; jslim1@yuhs.ac (J.L.); drshinjs@yuhs.ac (J.S.)
* Correspondence: dinbe@yuhs.ac (S.K.); hwang@uos.ac.kr (H.H.); Tel.: +82-2-6490-2454 (H.H.)

Citation: Lee, S.; Lim, J.; Shin, J.; Kim, S.; Hwang, H. Pathologic Complete Response Prediction after Neoadjuvant Chemoradiation Therapy for Rectal Cancer Using Radiomics and Deep Embedding Network of MRI. *Appl. Sci.* **2021**, *11*, 9494. https://doi.org/10.3390/app11209494

Academic Editor: Alessandro Stefano

Received: 6 September 2021
Accepted: 8 October 2021
Published: 13 October 2021

Publisher's Note: MDPI stays neutral with regard to jurisdictional claims in published maps and institutional affiliations.

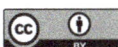

Copyright: © 2021 by the authors. Licensee MDPI, Basel, Switzerland. This article is an open access article distributed under the terms and conditions of the Creative Commons Attribution (CC BY) license (https://creativecommons.org/licenses/by/4.0/).

Abstract: Assessment of magnetic resonance imaging (MRI) after neoadjuvant chemoradiation therapy (nCRT) is essential in rectal cancer staging and treatment planning. However, when predicting the pathologic complete response (pCR) after nCRT for rectal cancer, existing works either rely on simple quantitative evaluation based on radiomics features or partially analyze multi-parametric MRI. We propose an effective pCR prediction method based on novel multi-parametric MRI embedding. We first seek to extract volumetric features of tumors that can be found only by analyzing multiple MRI sequences jointly. Specifically, we encapsulate multiple MRI sequences into multi-sequence fusion images (MSFI) and generate MSFI embedding. We merge radiomics features, which capture important characteristics of tumors, with MSFI embedding to generate multi-parametric MRI embedding and then use it to predict pCR using a random forest classifier. Our extensive experiments demonstrate that using all given MRI sequences is the most effective regardless of the dimension reduction method. The proposed method outperformed any variants with different combinations of feature vectors and dimension reduction methods or different classification models. Comparative experiments demonstrate that it outperformed four competing baselines in terms of the AUC and F1-score. We use MRI sequences from 912 patients with rectal cancer, a much larger sample than in any existing work.

Keywords: convolutional neural network (CNN); magnetic resonance imaging (MRI); neoadjuvant chemoradiation therapy (nCRT); pathologic complete response (pCR); radiomics; rectal cancer

1. Introduction

Rectal cancer is a carcinoma with a high incidence, accounting for 11.4% of the total cancer incidence, with 25,330 new cases in Korea in 2019, according to the Korea Central Cancer Registry [1]. Magnetic resonance imaging (MRI) is considered one of the most effective tools for staging rectal cancer by evaluating the local progression of tumors and lymph node metastasis.

Recently, for locally advanced rectal cancer, neoadjuvant chemoradiation therapy (nCRT) has been suggested to perform chemoradiation therapy before surgery [2]. If a patient is highly likely to have a pathologic complete response (pCR) after nCRT, they can avoid or postpone surgery while monitoring recurrence. Therefore, if we can predict pCR after nCRT accurately through MRI assessment, surgery could be avoided in the case of some patients, thereby greatly improving their quality of life by preserving their organs, which surgery might otherwise damage [3]. However, treatments, such as nCRT, may cause fibrosis, desmoplastic reaction, or colloid formation; therefore, MRI analysis becomes increasingly challenging.

To predict the pCR of rectal cancer, radiologists have used various MRI sequences, such as T2-weighted images (T2), diffusion-weighted imaging (DWI) [4,5], and contrast-enhanced imaging (CE) [6]. While T2 is considered as an essential MRI sequence, radiologists can achieve higher accuracy by using DWI along with T2 than using T2 alone [7]. This can be improved further by replacing T2 and DTW with T2/Gabor (T2 after applying the Gabor filter) and DWI/ADC (apparent diffusion coefficient of DWI) [8,9].

To quantitatively evaluate MRI for the pCR prediction of rectal cancer, many prior studies [8,10–12] have focused on radiomics features that can quantify the texture and non-texture characteristics of tumors. For example, a random forest classifier on T2/Gabor radiomics features outperformed qualitative analysis of T2 and DWI by radiologists [8]. By merging the radiomics features of multi-parametric MRI [10] and additional information, such as tumor length [11], simple classifiers based on multi-layer perceptron (MLP), and logistic regression, have shown high pCR prediction accuracy.

Recently, convolutional neural network (CNN) architectures have been widely used to extract new features of tumors in medical images, such as MRI and CT/PET [13–18]. Using 2D-CNN pre-trained on non-medical images, 2D features of the tumor are extracted from CE MRI and used for an effective logistic regression classifier [13,14]. To improve the pCR prediction accuracy, 2D-features from multi-parametric MRI [15] and radiomics features [16] can be combined. Some approaches have used pre-trained 3D-CNN to extract 3D features of tumor volume [17,18]. However, they neither analyze multi-parametric MRI nor consider radiomics features; they analyze 3D CT/PET images [18] or the DWI/ADC MRI sequence [17] only.

In this study, given pre-operative MRI sequences, {T2, DWI/ADC, and CE}, we predict the pCR of rectal cancer after nCRT by using multi-parametric MRI embedding. Specifically, we focus on extracting 3D features of tumor volume and radiomics features and fusing them to generate novel and diverse features of multi-parametric MRI. To this end, we encapsulate multiple MRI sequences into a multi-sequence fusion image (MSFI) and extract features directly from it, instead of simply merging the features extracted from each MRI sequence.

We generate MSFI embedding using a 3D-CNN, which is known to capture non-linear correlations of volumetric features extracted by 3D convolutional filters. As the number of 3D filters to tune for a deep 3D-CNN is very large, training randomly initialized filters will be more likely to overfit as the size of training set becomes smaller. For better generalization ability, we use transfer learning [19] with a 3D-CNN pre-trained on a large collection of videos.

Finally, we generate multi-parametric MRI embedding by concatenating MSFI embedding and radiomics features and performing dimension reduction for pCR prediction. This enables us to consider both diverse structural features of the tumor volume present in each MRI sequence and novel volumetric features that can only be found by analyzing multiple MRI sequences jointly.

We utilize the annotated MRI sequences of 912 rectal cancer patients, a sample size that is significantly larger than those used in previous works. We construct our pCR prediction model and existing models using MRI sequences of 592 patients after enlarging the number of MRI sequences using image augmentation techniques. For the model evaluation, we use the MRI sequences of 320 patients.

Our main contributions are as follows.

- We propose a method for encapsulating multiple MRI sequences into an MSFI and generating MSFI embedding using 3D-CNN to extract novel volumetric features of tumors.
- We introduce multi-parametric MRI embedding that contains diverse discriminative features of tumors by incorporating MSFI embedding and radiomics.
- We show the superiority of the proposed method through extensive experiments using the pre-operative MRI sequences of 912 rectal cancer patients.

2. Related Works

2.1. Qualitative Evaluation of Rectal Cancer Using MRI

Various types of MRI sequences, such as T2, DWI, and CE, have been used by radiologists for the qualitative evaluation of rectal cancer. In particular, radiologists can assess rectal cancer more accurately by simultaneously examining multiple MRI sequences at the same time. T2 has been considered as the best MRI sequence for evaluating rectal cancer, while DWI can help predict pCR after nCRT because it shows rectal cancer in a scar more clearly [4,5,20]. Recently, it has been shown that by using both T2 and DWI, radiologists can predict pCR more accurately than using T2 alone, since DWI enables them to interpret qualitative characteristics of rectal cancer that are invisible in T2 [21]. CE is helpful in assessing rectal cancer by providing the perfusion properties of tumors [6,22].

2.2. Quantitative Evaluation of Rectal Cancer using Radiomics Features

Radiomics features are quantities that can be automatically extracted from medical images and used to assist clinical decision-making [23]. Given a sequence of medical images and tumor masks, 2D/3D radiomics features pertaining to the tumor shape, voxel intensity histogram, and texture of tumor areas (such as the gray-level co-occurrence matrix and gray-level size-zone matrix), can be extracted [24]. Since radiomics features effectively quantify both texture and non-texture characteristics of tumors, many prior studies have used them for pCR prediction.

Recently, in diagnosing pCR after nCRT, a random forest classifier on T2/Gabor radiomics features has shown higher performance (AUC = 0.93) than qualitative assessment of T2 and DWI by radiologists, based on a cohort of 114 rectal cancer patients [8]. Given the computerized tomography (CT) radiomics features of 222 patients, an MLP classifier (AUC = 0.72) was shown to outperform a logistic regression classifier (AUC = 0.59) and support vector machine (SVM) classifier (AUC = 0.62), because it can capture non-linear correlations between CT radiomics features and the pCR of rectal cancer [25].

Radiomics features obtained from multi-parametric MRI have been used to predict the pCR of rectal cancer. Multi-parametric MRI provides more comprehensive information on rectal tumor areas than a particular MRI sequence does. Given the radiomics features of multi-parametric MRI, {T2, DWI/ADC, and CE}, of 48 patients, a three-layer MLP classifier (AUC = 0.79) was shown to outperform conventional voxelized heterogeneity analysis by radiologists (AUC = 0.71) [10]. By fusing T2 and DWI radiomics features before and after the CRT of 152 patients and additional information, such as tumor length, one logistic regression classifier showed an AUC of 0.9756 in a validation cohort of 70 patients [11]. Using the radiomics features of T2, DWI, and CE obtained before and after nCRT of 186 patients, another logistic regression classifier achieved an AUC of 0.948 [12].

2.3. Quantitative Evaluation of Rectal Cancer using Deep Learning

While radiomics features capture the essential characteristics of rectal tumor areas, we can extract new discriminative features using various CNN architectures. Using features of CE MRI extracted by 2D-CNN pre-trained on non-medical images, logistic regression classifiers can effectively predict the pCR of breast cancer (AUC = 0.85 [13] AUC = 0.77 [14]). With the features of multi-parametric MRI, T2, and CE, extracted by pre-trained 2D-CNN, an SVM classifier can accurately predict the pCR of breast cancer (AUC = 0.87) [15]. Given the multi-parametric MRI of DWI/ADC and CE, an MLP classifier has been shown to achieve higher accuracy and robustness by exploiting both 2D-CNN embedding and radiomics features of MRI [16].

However, 2D-CNN cannot capture features of tumor volumes, because it analyzes each slice of MRI sequences separately. 3D-CNN can capture volumetric features by applying 3D filters across consecutive slices of an MRI sequence. Given 3D rectal CT/PET images of tumors, 3D-CNN has been used to extract volumetric features for pCR prediction [18]. This end-to-end deep learning method shows a 0.64 c-index score, which is higher than the Cox proportional hazards model (0.62) [26] and random survival forests (0.60) [27], based on a cohort of 84 patients. Given DWI/ADC MRI sequences obtained before nCRT, a logistic regression model on 3D-CNN embedding (AUC = 0.73) was shown to outperform a logistic regression model on its radiomics features (AUC = 0.64), based on a cohort of 43 rectal cancer patients [17].

Our method differs from these works in three aspects. First, we focus on extracting the discriminative volumetric features of rectal cancer by applying 3D-CNN to multi-parametric MRI. Next, we exploit both our novel volumetric features and radiomics features of multi-parametric MRI to generate multi-parametric MRI embedding for pCR prediction of rectal cancer. Lastly, our experimental evaluation is based on a large collection of multi-parametric MRI scans of 912 rectal cancer patients. To the best of our knowledge, very few studies have used a cohort of more than 200 rectal cancer patients.

3. Method

3.1. Data Preprocessing

In this study, we use pre-operative MRI sequences of 912 patients with rectal cancer after nCRT. To split the samples into train and test sets, we partition them into two disjoint cohorts based on surgery date. In this way, we want to predict the prognosis of future patients by using the data of past patients before a specific point in time. This data partitioning scheme is frequently used in medical research because it naturally reflects the actual disease incidence and prevents random selection bias.

The training set consists of MRI sequences of 592 patients, 114 pCR patients, and 478 non-pCR patients, and the test set contains the MRI sequences of 320 patients, of which 78 are pCR, and 242 are non-pCR patients. We excluded the MRI sequences of 13 patients because it was impossible to evaluate their MRI reliably due to metal artifacts caused by metal stents for rectal obstruction. The disease stage information is summarized in Table 1. During the MRI examination, we followed the MRI protocol described in Appendix A.

Table 1. Disease stages of rectal cancer patients (total = 912).

	Train (n = 592)	Validation (n = 320)
Age (mean ± SD years)	58.8 ± 12.1	59.5 ± 11.8
Male (n (%))/Female (n (%))	388 (65.5)/204 (34.5)	199 (62.2)/121 (37.8)
pCR (n (%))	114 (19.3)	78 (24.4)
ypT stage (n (%))		
T0	114 (19.3)	78 (24.4)
Tis	6 (1.0)	8 (2.5)
T1	36 (6.1)	14 (4.4)
T2	145 (24.5)	60 (18.8)
T3	285 (48.1)	156 (48.8)
T4	6 (1.0)	4 (1.3)
ypN stage (n (%))		
N0	409 (69.1)	231 (72.2)
N1	139 (23.5)	76 (23.8)
N2	44 (7.4)	13 (4.1)

A board-certified abdominal radiologist with 6 years of experience registered multi-parametric MRI sequences. Fully automated co-registration was performed, and then the radiologist validated the co-registered MRI sequences. Automated co-registration of rectal MRI is known to be effective because rectum is in the pelvic cavity and, thus, moves much less during respiration. No manual correction was performed. Then, the radiologist drew the volume of interest (VOI) to include the whole tumor volume on T2 images semi-automatically using a 3D Slicer tool [28]. All VOIs were confirmed by a senior abdominal radiologist with 19 years of experience to ensure the quality of tumor annotations.

Disagreements on annotations were resolved by consensus-based discussion. The radiologists were blinded to the clinical and histopathologic data, except for information on the diagnosis of rectal cancer. During training, we oversampled pCR MRI images in the training set to alleviate the class imbalance between pCR and non-pCR [29].

Figure 1 shows snapshots of MRI sequences, {T2, DWI/ADC, and CE}, of a pCR patient (upper) and those of a non-pCR patient (lower). Yellow masks depict rectal tumor areas segmented and validated by radiologists. As the resolution or the number of slices may differ across MRI sequences, we executed MRI alignment and z-normalization as preprocessing steps.

To equalize the resolution of different MRI sequences, images were resampled to an isovoxel size of 1 mm^3 using the B-Spline method [30]. Then, the signal intensities of the images were converted to values in the range $(-3, 3)$ using z-score normalization. These values were multiplied by 100 and converted to a value between $(-300, 300)$. Radiomic features were extracted by assigning a bin size of 5 for grayscale discretization. Due to the lack of a standardized signal intensity scale of MRI, signal intensity normalization is recommended before comparing MRI images [31].

Grayscale normalization improves the robustness of radiomics features [32,33]. As with T2, we applied z-score normalization to the post contrast enhanced MRI during the preprocessing stage. All processes, including voxel resampling and signal intensity normalization, were performed using the functions implemented in pyradiomics. As the width and height of the interpolated MRI slices ranged from 224 to 230 after voxel size resampling, we cropped larger ones slightly to obtain slices of equal resolution. After data preprocessing, each MRI sequence has 30 slices of resolution (224 × 224).

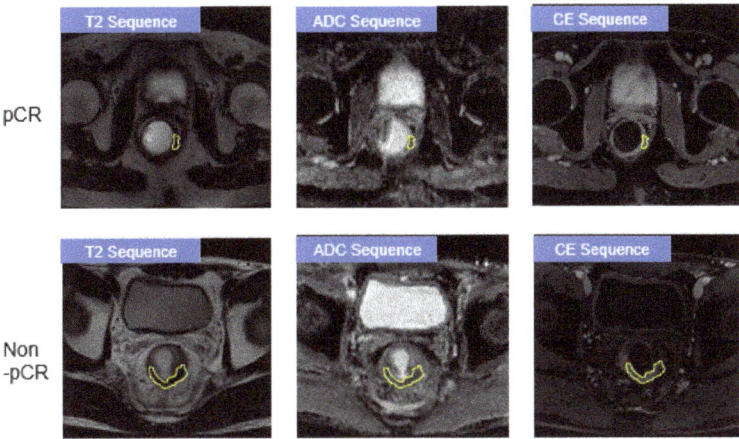

Figure 1. Three types of MRI images {T2, DWI/ADC, and CE} of a pCR patient (**upper**) and a non-pCR one (**lower**). Yellow masks are rectal tumor areas segmented and validated by radiologists.

3.2. Suggested Method

3.2.1. Representing Multiple MRI Sequences as MSFI Embedding

Figure 2 depicts our pCR prediction process used to transform given multi-parametric MRI sequences into embedding. To extract features of tumor volumes, we highlight tumor areas in each MRI image and select the MRI images related to the major tumor volume as follows. First, we highlight the tumor area in each MRI image by filling the region outside its tumor mask with zeros. Then, to select contiguous slices capturing tumor volume, we find the slice with the largest tumor area and pick five and six slices above and below the slice, respectively, in each MRI sequence.

If the tumor size exceeded 12 slices, a total of 12 slices were used above and below the central section with the largest tumor area. The reason is that after nCRT, the viable portion of the tumor is mainly found in the central region of the tumor, and the border region of the tumor has a very small volume or is observed as a streak-like fibrosis, making it difficult to represent the characteristics of the entire tumor volume.

In our study, the number of patients whose tumor size exceeded 12 slices is relatively small (22/592 in the training set and 17/320 in the test set). Lastly, since the input resolution of the 3D-CNN used for transfer learning is 112×112, we center-cropped each slice around the tumor area accordingly.

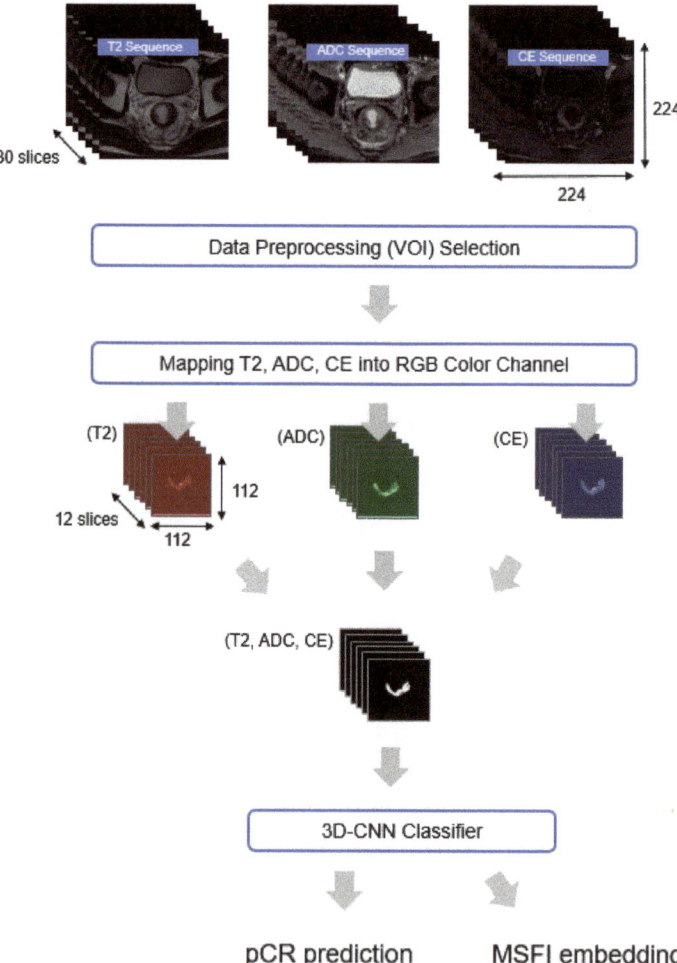

Figure 2. The pCR prediction process using the 3D-CNN classifier from which we extract MSFI embedding, given {T2, DWI/ADC, and CE} MRI sequences.

To alleviate data scarcity and avoid overfitting, we apply data augmentation techniques and transfer learning. We use data augmentation techniques, such as 3D-rotation and 3D-shift [34] during the training stage to increase the size and variety of the training set. We exclude some image augmentation techniques, such as adding Gaussian noise and applying a median filter, because they often distort the texture of tumor areas, which is an essential characteristic of tumors for pCR prediction [35].

In addition to extracting the diverse features from each MRI sequence, we aim to examine novel features that can be found only by considering multiple MRI sequences jointly. For this, we transform the given three MRI sequences, {T2, DWI/ADC, and CE}, into an MSFI. The MSFI is a sequence of slices containing 3D values (v_1, v_2, v_3), where v_1, v_2, and v_3 are from T2, DWI/ADC, and CE, respectively. After encapsulating three MRI sequences into the MSFI, we use it as an input for deep learning to represent it as MSFI embedding.

To extract the volumetric features of tumors, we use a 3D-CNN model that is known for its high classification performance on video data. Unlike 2D-CNN, 3D convolutional filters can identify patterns that appear across multiple image slices. As there are many 3D convolutional filters to tune in a deep 3D-CNN model, we perform transfer learning to improve generalization ability [36,37], instead of training randomly initialized 3D filters.

For this, we used 3D-ResNet [38] pre-trained on Kinetic [39], a large-scale, high-quality video dataset that contains 400 classes with at least 400 videos per class and is considered as a de facto standard for the research on 3D image processing. 3D-ResNet is known to distinguish 3D instances very effectively by reducing the gradient-vanishing effect through gradient flow. This means that its pre-trained 3D filters can already extract useful volumetric features from 3D instances. Therefore, by fine-tuning the pre-trained filters in 3D-ResNet, we can construct more effective 3D filters for MSFI embedding extraction. Figure 3 shows the architecture of 3D-ResNet, the 3D-CNN that we use for MSFI embedding extraction. We obtain MSFI embedding from the fully connected layer of the trained 3D-ResNet.

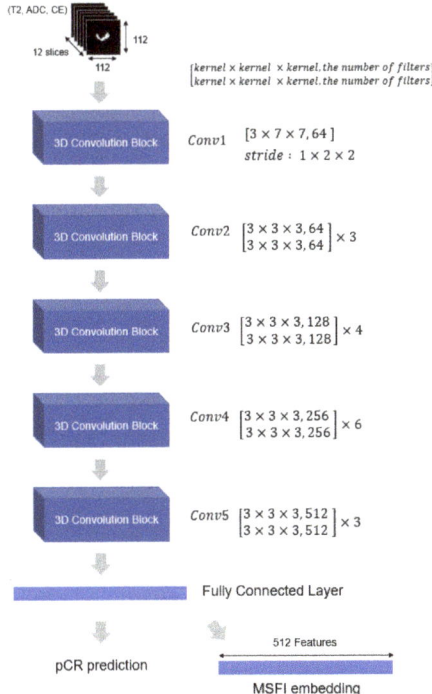

Figure 3. Architecture of the 3D-CNN classifier for MSFI embedding extraction.

3.2.2. Extracting Radiomics Features

Given multi-parametric MRI, we seek to extract another set of features that can capture different aspects of tumor characteristics than MSFI embedding. Radiomics features have already demonstrated a high correlation with pCR after nCRT for rectal cancer. Thus, we merge radiomics features with MSFI embedding to further improve pCR prediction performance. Using the pyradiomics package [40], we extract radiomics features from tumor areas in multiple MRI sequences, {T2, DWI/ADC, and CE}.

Figure 4 shows 3740 radiomics features that were extracted from multiple MRI sequences, {T2, DWI/ADC, and CE}. From each MRI sequence, we extracted 2D/3D radiomics features on the tumor shape, voxel intensity histogram, texture of tumor areas, such as the gray-level co-occurrence matrix (GLCM), gray-level run-length matrix (GLRLM), gray-level size-zone matrix (GLSZM), and gray-level dependence matrix (GLDM). In addition, we applied filters, such as log and wavelet transform, to each MRI sequence to extract higher-order statistical features on rectal tumor areas [41]. To extract more diverse textual features from T2, we applied a Gabor filter with four angles, $\{0°, 45°, 90°, \text{and } 135°\}$.

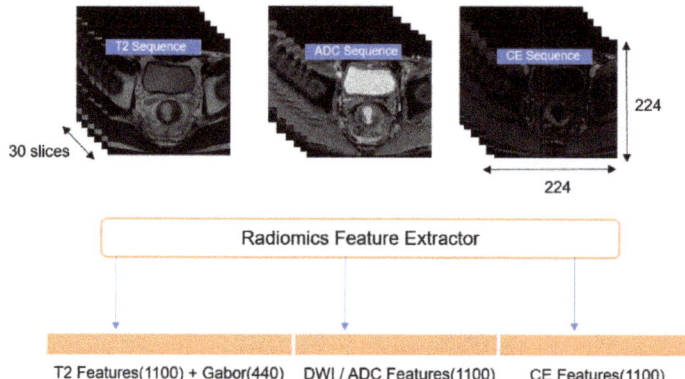

Figure 4. Radiomics feature extraction.

3.2.3. Predicting pCR using Both MSFI Embedding and Radiomics Features

For effective pCR prediction, we seek to use diverse characteristics of tumor areas by considering both MSFI embedding and radiomics features. Radiomics features are extracted through mathematical analysis of each MRI sequence and mainly capture shapes, voxel intensity histograms, and the texture of tumor areas. MSFI embedding is generated through deep learning of multi-parametric MRI and consists of novel volumetric features highly related to pCR prediction.

Figure 5 presents an overview of our pCR prediction method. Given three MRI sequences, {T2, DWI/ADC, and CE}, we extracted 512-dimensional MSFI embedding and 3740 radiomics features, as shown in Figures 2 and 4. Then, we obtained a novel multi-parametric MRI embedding, a compact and effective representation of multi-parametric MRI, by combining MSFI embedding and radiomics features and compressing them into 150 features using kernel principal component analysis (PCA) [42].

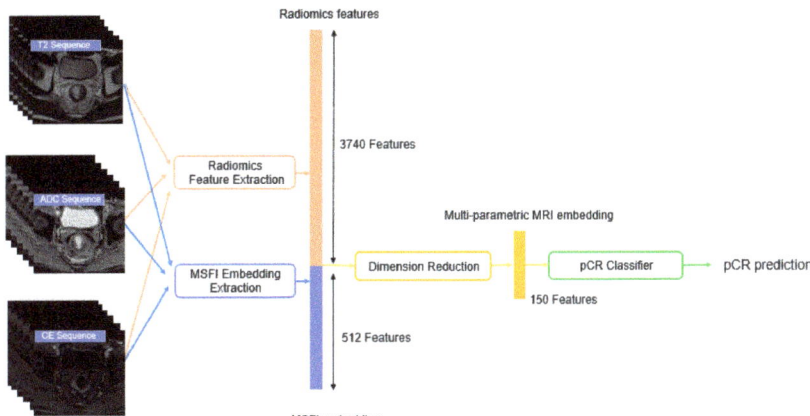

Figure 5. The overall pCR prediction method using both radiomics features and MSFI embedding, given three MRI sequences.

Kernel PCA is a dimension reduction method that modifies linear PCA [43] by replacing the linear kernel with a Gaussian kernel. Thus, non-linear transformation is performed so that feature vectors can be represented in a linearly separable feature space. We use this multi-parametric MRI embedding as input to a random forest classifier for pCR prediction [44]. We build our pCR classifier based on the random forest model, because random forest classifiers on radiomics features have shown high performance in predicting pCR after nCRT for rectal cancer—sometimes higher than qualitative MRI assessment by radiologists [8,45].

Note that a deep neural network classifier is likely to overfit when trained with multi-parametric MRI embeddings, because they are no longer images; thus, data augmentation or transfer learning cannot be applied.

4. Experiments

We evaluate the pCR prediction performance of the proposed method through the experiments listed as follows. Specifically, we investigate the impact of input MRI sequences, analyze the pCR prediction performance of the proposed method and compare it with existing methods.

1. Comparison of five types of input MRI sequences:
   (a) {T2}
   (b) {DWI/ADC}
   (c) {CE}
   (d) {T2, DWI/ADC} and
   (e) {T2, DWI/ADC, and CE} (ours).

2. Comparison of the proposed method with its variants that differ in two factors, MRI feature vector extraction and pCR classification:
   - Three MRI feature vectors: radiomics features, MSFI embedding, and multi-parametric MRI embedding (ours).
   - Six classification models: logistic regression, xgboost, lightgbm, random forest (ours), MLP, and ensemble of the five classifiers.

3. Comparative evaluation of the proposed method with four competing baselines:
   (a) SVM classifier on radiomics features [46],
   (b) RF classifier on radiomics features [8],
   (c) MLP classifier on radiomics features [25], and
   (d) 3D-CNN classifier on MRI images [18].

To evaluate the overall pCR prediction performance, we use AUC (Area Under the ROC Curve), because it reflects the sensitivity and specificity of a classifier at the same time.

$$AUC(f) = \frac{\sum_{t_0 \in \mathcal{D}_0} \sum_{t_1 \in \mathcal{D}_1} \mathbb{1}[f(t_0) < f(t_1)]}{|\mathcal{D}_0| \cdot |\mathcal{D}_1|}. \quad (1)$$

For a classifier f, we estimate its AUC based on the Wilcoxon–Mann–Whitney statistic [47], as shown in Equation (1). $\mathcal{D}_0$ and $\mathcal{D}_1$ are the set of non-pCR patients and the set of pCR patients, respectively, and $\mathbb{1}[f(t_0) < f(t_1)]$ is an indicator function. We use an independent test cohort to measure the AUC of each classifier.

4.1. Experimental Setup

To generate MSFI embedding, we set the hyperparameters of 3D-ResNet as follows. The batch size was 2, and the number of training epochs was set to 100. We used the Radam optimizer [48] to alleviate the local minima convergence problem that may occur when an adaptive learning rate is used. Initial learning rate was 10^{-3}, and warmup-proportion was 0.1. We used 512 as the dimension of MSFI embedding throughout the experiments.

The hyperparameters of existing pCR classifiers were set as follows. For tree-based classifiers, such as xgboost, lightgbm, and random forest, the number of decision trees was set to 1000 to obtain stable pCR prediction results. For a logistic regression classifier, we selected features with L2 regularization. For an MLP-based classifier, a two-layer MLP was used with ReLU as an activation function. We trained it using the Adam optimizer [49]. An ensemble classifier performs soft voting by averaging the pCR probabilities predicted by five classifiers: logistic regression, xgboost, lightgbm, random forest, and MLP.

We examine three different dimension reduction methods in {No dimension reduction, PCA, and Kernel PCA} and compare the AUC of an ensemble classifier.

4.2. Impact of Input MRI Sequences

To demonstrate the impact of the input MRI sequences on the pCR prediction performance, we compare the pCR prediction performance of five types of input MRI sequences in Table 2: {T2}, {DWI/ADC}, {CE}, {T2, DWI/ADC}, {T2, DWI/ADC, and CE}. Note that pCR prediction performance is affected not only by the input MRI sequences but also by the feature vector extraction method and the pCR classification model. For a fair comparison, we use both radiomics features and MSFI embedding extracted by the same architecture, 3D-ResNet, and apply different dimension reduction methods, as in {no dimension reduction, PCA, and Kernel PCA}. We report the AUC of an ensemble classifier because it corresponds to the average performance of five different pCR classification models.

Table 2. Comparison of pCR prediction performance of five types of input MRI sequences. For a fair comparison, we extract both MSFI embedding and radiomics features from input MRI sequences, apply three different dimension reduction methods in {No dimension reduction, PCA, and Kernel PCA} and report the AUC of an ensemble classifier.

Input MRI Sequences	No Dimension Reduction	PCA	Kernel PCA
{T2}	0.765	0.791	0.787
{DWI/ADC}	0.721	0.801	0.791
{CE}	0.716	0.800	0.801
{T2, DWI/ADC}	0.764	0.793	0.800
{T2, DWI/ADC, and CE}	0.811	0.804	0.819

Table 2 shows that the AUC of pCR prediction using three MRI sequences, {T2, DWI/ADC, and CE}, as the input is higher than that using one of these MRI sequences separately, regardless of the dimension reduction method. In particular, while T2 is widely known to be the most effective in evaluating rectal cancer, pCR prediction performance can be further improved when DWI/ADC and CE are used simultaneously. When comparing {T2, DWI/ADC} and {T2, DWI/ADC, and CE}, we observe that pCR prediction using three input MRI sequences, {T2, DWI/ADC, and CE}, outperforms {T2, DWI/ADC}.

Among the three possible pairs of MRI sequences from {T2, DWI/ADC, and CE}, we include only {T2, DWI/ADC} in Table 2, because using T2 and DWI together is already known to be highly effective in evaluating rectal cancer. Radiologists achieve higher pCR prediction accuracy by using both T2 and DWI than by using T2 alone [21] and simple classification methods, such as logistic regression and random forest on radiomics features from T2 and DWI, outperform MRI assessment by radiologists [8].

4.3. Analysis of Our pCR Prediction Model

We evaluated the effectiveness of the proposed pCR prediction method by examining two major factors: MRI feature vector extraction and pCR classification. Recall that for effective pCR classification, we suggest using multi-parametric MRI embedding as an input to a random forest classifier.

In the proposed pCR prediction method, we generate multi-parametric MRI embedding by concatenating MSFI embedding and radiomics features extracted from given MRI sequences, {T2, DWI/ADC, and CE}, and applying kernel PCA. To check the impact of multi-parametric MRI embedding, we apply nine different input vectors to a random forest classifier by combining a feature vector of {radiomics features, MSFI embedding, concatenation of both} and a dimension reduction method of {No dimension reduction, PCA, and Kernel PCA}.

Table 3 presents the pCR prediction performance of random forest classifiers using nine input vectors. We observe, among various input vectors, that with the input vector obtained by concatenating MSFI embedding and radiomics features and then applying kernel PCA, that is, our multi-parametric MRI embedding, random forest classifier achieved the highest AUC of 0.837.

Table 3. Comparison of pCR prediction performance of various combinations of feature vectors and dimension reduction methods. Three types of feature vectors, {radiomics features, MSFI embedding, concatenation of both}, and three dimension reduction methods, {No dimension reduction, PCA, and Kernel PCA}, are considered. The pCR classification model is fixed to a random forest.

Feature Vector	No Dimension Reduction	PCA	Kernel PCA
MSFI embedding	0.776	0.739	0.732
Radiomics features	0.811	0.754	0.819
Concatenation of both	0.796	0.746	0.837

From this, we observe that MSFI embedding extracts novel volumetric features that cannot be found in the pool of radiomics features. At the same time, radiomics features explain some essential characteristics of rectal cancer that MSFI embedding cannot represent. Thus, multi-parametric MRI embedding succeeds in capturing more diverse features from the given MRI sequences. We also observe that kernel PCA can extract discriminative features for pCR prediction from MSFI embedding and radiomics features.

Then, we compare the effectiveness of MSFI embedding and radiomics features. In Table 3, MSFI embedding shows a lower AUC than the radiomics features when used as the input to the random forest classifier. However, while we use 3D-ResNet only for MSFI embedding extraction, it should be noted that its pCR classification performance has already reached 0.807 just as (B4) in Section 4.4. Recall that the random forest classifier on radiomics features is known to be highly effective in pCR prediction for rectal cancer [8].

Given three MRI sequences, {T2, DWI/ADC, and CE}, we can obtain multi-parametric MRI embedding by concatenating MSFI embedding and radiomics features and performing kernel PCA. Through this novel embedding, we aim to show the effectiveness of our random forest classifier by comparing it with various classification models.

Table 4 presents the AUC of six pCR classifiers built on multi-parametric MRI embedding: logistic regression, xgboost, lightgbm, random forest, MLP, and an ensemble of all the classifiers. The random forest classifier outperforms all the other classifiers, including the ensemble, demonstrating an AUC of 0.837.

Table 4. Comparison of pCR prediction performance of various classifiers built on multi-parametric MRI embedding.

Classifier	Logistic Regression	Xgboost	Lightgbm	Random Forest	MLP	Ensemble
AUC	0.804	0.783	0.792	**0.837**	0.798	0.819

4.4. Comparison with Existing pCR Prediction Methods

To demonstrate the superiority of our method in predicting pCR after nCRT for rectal cancer, we compared it with four competing baselines: (B1) SVM classifier on radiomics features [46]; (B2) random forest classifier on radiomics features [8]; (B3) MLP classifier on radiomics features [25]; and (B4) 3D-CNN classifier on MRI images [18].

For a fair comparison, we re-implemented all the baselines to re-train them with our large training set containing three MRI sequences, {T2, DWI/ADC, and CE}, of 592 rectal cancer patients. As input to the three baselines, (B1)–(B3), we used 3740 radiomics features extracted as shown in Figure 4. We also re-implemented the 3D-CNN classifier [18], (B4), so that it could accept three MRI sequences, instead of CT/PET images, of rectal cancer as the input.

We compared the proposed method with four baselines by evaluating the overall pCR prediction performance using four measures: AUC, F1-score, specificity, and sensitivity. Specificity and sensitivity correspond to the true negative rate and true positive rate, respectively, and the F1-score is their harmonic mean.

In Table 5, we observe that the proposed method outperformed all competing baselines in terms of the AUC and F1-score. (B2) performed the best among (B1)–(B3) built on radiomics features. However, while the sensitivity of the proposed method was slightly lower, the overall performance of the proposed method was better than that of (B2). This implies that MSFI embedding successfully represents novel features of tumors that radiomics features cannot capture. Compared with (B4), all four measures of the proposed method were higher, which indicates that radiomics features contribute to the improved performance of the proposed method.

Table 5. Comparison of pCR prediction performance with competing baselines.

pCR Prediction Method	AUC	F1-Score	Specificity	Sensitivity
(B1) SVM classifier (input = radiomics features) [46]	0.799	0.53	0.45	0.67
(B2) RF classifier (input = radiomics features) [8]	0.811	0.63	0.56	0.74
(B3) MLP classifier (input = radiomics features) [25]	0.763	0.54	0.49	0.62
(B4) 3D-CNN classifier (input = MRI images) [18]	0.807	0.63	0.59	0.68
Proposed Method	0.837	0.65	0.60	0.72

5. Discussion

This is the first study that fully exploits both radiomics features and a deep embedding network of multi-parametric MRI to predict pCR after nCRT in patients with locally advanced rectal cancer. We demonstrated the superiority of the proposed method by analyzing its pCR prediction performance and comparing it with competing baselines based on a large cohort of 912 rectal cancer patients.

Before analyzing the pCR prediction performance of our method, we showed that the average pCR prediction performance was the highest (AUC = 0.819) when using various features from the entire multi-parametric MRI (Table 2). Given multi-parametric MRI, we generated radiomics features and MSFI embedding and merged them through kernel PCA to obtain multi-parametric MRI embedding. The multi-parametric MRI embedding exhibited higher pCR prediction performance than radiomics features or MSFI embedding (Table 3).

This means that some tumor characteristics that are highly relevant to pCR prediction are captured by either radiomics features or MSFI embedding but not both. It also indicates that MSFI embedding can represent novel volumetric features of tumors in multi-parametric MRI. Given multi-parametric MRI embedding, we demonstrated that a random forest classifier was the most effective pCR prediction model (Table 4), as suggested in our method. Then, we confirmed that our method outperformed four competing baselines in terms of overall prediction performance (AUC = 0.837 and F1-score = 0.65) for pCR after nCRT for locally advanced rectal cancer (Table 5).

The 3740 radiomics features and 512 features in MSFI embedding are not equally important to the pCR prediction. Using kernel PCA, we performed non-linear dimensionality reduction over the vector of 4252 features to obtain a low-dimensional embedding that maximizes the variance. In our experiments, we selected 150 as the optimal number of components through hyperparameter tuning. Instead of tuning the output dimension manually, advanced feature selection techniques [50] that automatically determine the optimal number of features can be used. To explore non-linear combinations of features, we can also consider performing kernel PCA by fixing the variance threshold instead of specifying the number of components.

Our MRI data is heterogeneous as it was acquired from different patients using MRI scanners of various vendors, as stated in Appendix A. Due to the lack of a standardized signal intensity scale, heterogeneous MRI images are not directly comparable [31]. To deal with such heterogeneity, we used pyradiomics, the most widely used tool for reliable radiomics feature extraction. During preprocessing, we applied voxel size resampling and signal intensity normalization implemented in pyradiomics because these two techniques have been known to improve the robustness of radiomics features [32,33]. We used the preprocessed MRI data as an input to 3D-CNN for MSFI embedding to improve the robustness of MSFI embedding. We expect that we can further improve the pCR prediction performance by applying semi-supervised training techniques for heterogeneous medical image data [51].

Segmentation variability also affects the pCR prediction performance of the proposed method. As we performed semi-automatic VOI segmentation using 3D Slicer tool that requires manual adjustment, inter- and intra-observer variability still needs to be resolved. The proposed method uses features extracted from segmented VOI of multi-parametric MRI, and thus the pCR prediction performance will gradually drop as segmentation variability increases. While there is a lack of reliable and validated fully automatic VOI segmentation tools for MRI [52], there have been efforts to develop automated VOI segmentation tools based on deep learning [53–55]. By using automatic VOI segmentation, we can fully automate the proposed method and perform more reliable and consistent pCR prediction.

This study has clinical significance in that it increases the applicability of a new treatment method, such as "wait-and-see" without surgery [56,57] by achieving a higher prediction performance of pCR after nCRT based on a large number of patients. For the past decade, the two-step process of performing nCRT followed by surgery has been considered as the standard treatment. pCR is often achieved after nCRT only, although the surgery was unavoidable even in the case of pCR. This is because we can determine the presence or absence of pCR only after performing surgery.

Rectal cancer surgery often causes anal function loss and sexual dysfunction. Although these are not directly related to survival, they severely reduce the quality of life. If we can predict pCR after nCRT before surgery with higher accuracy than existing methods as shown in Table 5, this means that more patients can avoid surgery in the case of pCR. Therefore, it is important to predict pCR more accurately and reliably before surgery.

As the wait-and-see method is not included in the internationally standardized medical guidelines, it is currently being conducted only as a clinical study by some professors at our hospital and is not a routine process. Therefore, it is not mandatory for radiologists to provide information on the prediction of pCR. More studies on reliable pre-operative pCR prediction are necessary to establish clinical guidelines for pre-operative pCR prediction, and this study will contribute to it. The inability to compare the results of this study with clinical practice is a limitation of this study, and further research is needed.

6. Conclusions

Given pre-operative multiple MRI sequences, {T2, DWI/ADC, and CE}, of rectal cancer after nCRT, we proposed an effective pCR prediction method by building a random forest classifier through novel multi-parametric MRI embedding. We obtained multi-parametric MRI embedding by MSFI embedding and incorporating it with radiomics features. We extracted MSFI embedding using 3D-ResNet to capture novel volumetric features of tumors by considering multiple MRI sequences jointly.

Through extensive experiments, we demonstrated the superiority of the proposed method by demonstrating the effectiveness of (1) multiple input MRI sequences, (2) multi-parametric MRI embedding, and (3) the random forest pCR classifier. Then, we compared the proposed method with four competing baselines and showed that our method achieved the highest overall pCR prediction performance. Our experimental results are robust in that we used a large dataset of 912 patients' MRI sequences, which is much larger than that of any existing work.

Author Contributions: Conceptualization, S.K.; methodology, S.K. and S.L.; software, S.K. and S.L.; validation, S.L., S.K. and H.H.; formal analysis, S.L.; investigation, S.L., S.K. and H.H.; resources, J.S., J.L. and S.K.; data curation, J.S., J.L. and S.K.; writing—original draft preparation, S.L., S.K. and H.H.; writing—review and editing, S.L., S.K. and H.H.; visualization, S.L.; supervision, H.H.; project administration, S.K.; funding acquisition, S.K. and H.H. All authors have read and agreed to the published version of the manuscript.

Funding: This study was supported by the National Research Foundation of Korea (NRF) grant funded by the Korea government (MSIT) (NRF-2019R1A2C1008743) and a Basic Science Research Program through the National Research Foundation of Korea (NRF) funded by the Ministry of Education (NRF-2018R1D1A1B07048179).

Institutional Review Board Statement: This study was approved by the Institutional Review Board of Severance Hospital, Yonsei University, College of Medicine, Seoul, Republic of Korea.

Informed Consent Statement: Informed consent was waived due to the retrospective nature of the study.

Data Availability Statement: Data sharing is not applicable.

Conflicts of Interest: The authors declare no conflict of interest.

Appendix A. MRI Protocol

MRI examinations [58] were performed with a 1.5-T scanner (Achieva, Philips Healthcare) or a 3.0-T MR scanner (Magnetom Tim Tio, Siemens Healthineers, Germany; or Ingenia, Philips Medical Systems, the Netherlands). For bowel preparation, 20 mg of scopolamine butylbromide (Buscopan; Boehringer Ingelheim) was injected intramuscularly, and sonography transmission gel (50–100 mL) was administered in the rectal lumen for the mass at the lower or middle rectum before MRI scanning.

The MRI sequences included high-resolution T2-weighted images using a respiratory-triggered fast spin echo (axial, sagittal, and oblique axial and coronal orientations), axial T1-weighted images, axial diffusion-weighted images using single-shot echo-planar imaging (the highest b-values 1000 s/mm^2), as well as gadolinium contrast enhanced T1 weighted images using a three-dimensional gradient-echo sequence. The oblique T2-weighted image sequence was obtained orthogonal or parallel to the long axis of the tumor. An intravenous bolus of gadobutrol (Gadovist; Bayer AG, Berlin, German: 0.1 mL/kg of body weight) or gadopentetate dimeglumine (Magnevist; Bayer Healthcare, Berlin, Germany: 0.2 mL/kg of body weight) was injected at a rate of 2.0 mL/s. The details on MRI sequences are summarized in Table A1.

The effectiveness of T2 and ADC in staging/restaging rectal cancer has been widely accepted. Regarding DCE, however, a consensus meeting of 14 abdominal imaging experts from the European Society of Gastrointestinal and Abdominal Radiology (ESGAR) recommended that, although some promising data are available, it should currently be considered as a research tool and not be adopted routinely [59]. Therefore, we acquired contrast enhanced T1 weighted gradient echo images but not DCE.

Table A1. The MRI parameters.

	1.5 T			3.0 T		
	Fast Spin-Echo T2-Weighted Image (T2)	Diffusion-Weighted Image (DWI)	3D T1-Weighted Gradient Echo (CE)	Fast Spin-Echo T2-Weighted Image (T2)	Diffusion-Weighted Image (DWI)	3D T1-Weighted Gradient Echo (CE)
Plane	Axial, Sagittal, Oblique axial, Oblique coronal	Axial	Axial	Axial, Sagittal, Oblique axial, Oblique coronal	Axial	Axial
Repetition time(ms)	2740–4200	6900–9100	3.51	3800–5500	9500–12,000	3.51
Echo time(ms)	80	64–90	1.44	80–120	62–95	1.44
Flip angle(degrees)	137	90		90–150	90	
B factor(s/mm^2)		0, 300, 1000			0, 300, 1000	
Field of view(mm)	180 or 240	220	240	180 or 240	220	240
Matrix without interpolation	304	128 or 150	240	320–448	126 or 153	240
Slice thickness (mm)	3	3	3	3	3	3
Slice gap (mm)	0	0		0	0	
Echo train length	16			17 or 35		

References

1. Jung, K.W.; Won, Y.J.; Kong, H.J.; Lee, E.S. Prediction of cancer incidence and mortality in Korea, 2019. *Cancer Res. Treat. Off. J. Korean Cancer Assoc.* **2019**, *51*, 431. [CrossRef] [PubMed]
2. Renehan, A.G.; Malcomson, L.; Emsley, R.; Gollins, S.; Maw, A.; Myint, A.S.; Rooney, P.S.; Susnerwala, S.; Blower, A.; Saunders, M.P.; et al. Watch-and-wait approach versus surgical resection after chemoradiotherapy for patients with rectal cancer (the OnCoRe project): A propensity-score matched cohort analysis. *Lancet Oncol.* **2016**, *17*, 174–183. [CrossRef]
3. Maas, M.; Lambregts, D.M.; Nelemans, P.J.; Heijnen, L.A.; Martens, M.H.; Leijtens, J.W.; Sosef, M.; Hulsewé, K.W.; Hoff, C.; Breukink, S.O.; et al. Assessment of clinical complete response after chemoradiation for rectal cancer with digital rectal examination, endoscopy, and MRI: selection for organ-saving treatment. *Ann. Surg. Oncol.* **2015**, *22*, 3873–3880. [CrossRef] [PubMed]
4. Patel, U.B.; Brown, G.; Rutten, H.; West, N.; Sebag-Montefiore, D.; Glynne-Jones, R.; Rullier, E.; Peeters, M.; Van Cutsem, E.; Ricci, S.; et al. Comparison of magnetic resonance imaging and histopathological response to chemoradiotherapy in locally advanced rectal cancer. *Ann. Surg. Oncol.* **2012**, *19*, 2842–2852. [CrossRef] [PubMed]
5. Dzik-Jurasz, A.; Domenig, C.; George, M.; Wolber, J.; Padhani, A.; Brown, G.; Doran, S. Diffusion MRI for prediction of response of rectal cancer to chemoradiation. *Lancet* **2002**, *360*, 307–308. [CrossRef]
6. Villers, A.; Puech, P.; Mouton, D.; Leroy, X.; Ballereau, C.; Lemaitre, L. Dynamic contrast enhanced, pelvic phased array magnetic resonance imaging of localized prostate cancer for predicting tumor volume: correlation with radical prostatectomy findings. *J. Urol.* **2006**, *176*, 2432–2437. [CrossRef] [PubMed]
7. Weiser, M.R.; Gollub, M.J.; Saltz, L.B. Assessment of clinical complete response after chemoradiation for rectal cancer with digital rectal examination, endoscopy, and MRI. *Ann. Surg. Oncol.* **2015**, *22*, 3769–3771. [CrossRef]
8. Horvat, N.; Veeraraghavan, H.; Khan, M.; Blazic, I.; Zheng, J.; Capanu, M.; Sala, E.; Garcia-Aguilar, J.; Gollub, M.J.; Petkovska, I. MR imaging of rectal cancer: radiomics analysis to assess treatment response after neoadjuvant therapy. *Radiology* **2018**, *287*, 833–843. [CrossRef]

9. Lambregts, D.M.; Maas, M.; Riedl, R.G.; Bakers, F.C.; Verwoerd, J.L.; Kessels, A.G.; Lammering, G.; Boetes, C.; Beets, G.L.; Beets-Tan, R.G. Value of ADC measurements for nodal staging after chemoradiation in locally advanced rectal cancer—A per lesion validation study. *Eur. Radiol.* **2011**, *21*, 265–273. [CrossRef]
10. Nie, K.; Shi, L.; Chen, Q.; Hu, X.; Jabbour, S.K.; Yue, N.; Niu, T.; Sun, X. Rectal cancer: Assessment of neoadjuvant chemoradiation outcome based on radiomics of multiparametric MRI. *Clin. Cancer Res.* **2016**, *22*, 5256–5264. [CrossRef]
11. Liu, Z.; Zhang, X.Y.; Shi, Y.J.; Wang, L.; Zhu, H.T.; Tang, Z.; Wang, S.; Li, X.T.; Tian, J.; Sun, Y.S. Radiomics analysis for evaluation of pathological complete response to neoadjuvant chemoradiotherapy in locally advanced rectal cancer. *Clin. Cancer Res.* **2017**, *23*, 7253–7262. [CrossRef]
12. Cui, Y.; Yang, X.; Shi, Z.; Yang, Z.; Du, X.; Zhao, Z.; Cheng, X. Radiomics analysis of multiparametric MRI for prediction of pathological complete response to neoadjuvant chemoradiotherapy in locally advanced rectal cancer. *Eur. Radiol.* **2019**, *29*, 1211–1220. [CrossRef]
13. Huynh, B.Q.; Antropova, N.; Giger, M.L. Comparison of breast DCE-MRI contrast time points for predicting response to neoadjuvant chemotherapy using deep convolutional neural network features with transfer learning. In Proceedings of the Medical imaging 2017: Computer-Aided Diagnosis. International Society for Optics and Photonics, Orlando, FL, USA, 11–16 February 2017; Volume 10134, p. 101340U.
14. Ravichandran, K.; Braman, N.; Janowczyk, A.; Madabhushi, A. A deep learning classifier for prediction of pathological complete response to neoadjuvant chemotherapy from baseline breast DCE-MRI. In Proceedings of the Medical Imaging 2018: Computer-Aided Diagnosis, International Society for Optics and Photonics, Houston, TX, USA, 10–15 February 2018; Volume 10575, p. 105750C.
15. Hu, Q.; Whitney, H.M.; Giger, M.L. A deep learning methodology for improved breast cancer diagnosis using multiparametric MRI. *Sci. Rep.* **2020**, *10*, 1–11. [CrossRef]
16. Yun, J.; Park, J.E.; Lee, H.; Ham, S.; Kim, N.; Kim, H.S. Radiomic features and multilayer perceptron network classifier: A robust MRI classification strategy for distinguishing glioblastoma from primary central nervous system lymphoma. *Sci. Rep.* **2019**, *9*, 1–10. [CrossRef]
17. Fu, J.; Zhong, X.; Li, N.; Van Dams, R.; Lewis, J.; Sung, K.; Raldow, A.C.; Jin, J.; Qi, X.S. Deep learning-based radiomic features for improving neoadjuvant chemoradiation response prediction in locally advanced rectal cancer. *Phys. Med. Biol.* **2020**, *65*, 075001. [CrossRef]
18. Li, H.; Boimel, P.; Janopaul-Naylor, J.; Zhong, H.; Xiao, Y.; Ben-Josef, E.; Fan, Y. Deep convolutional neural networks for imaging data based survival analysis of rectal cancer. In Proceedings of the 2019 IEEE 16th International Symposium on Biomedical Imaging (ISBI 2019), Venice, Italy, 8–11 April 2019; pp. 846–849.
19. Kornblith, S.; Shlens, J.; Le, Q.V. Do better imagenet models transfer better? In Proceedings of the IEEE Conference on Computer Vision and Pattern Recognition, Long Beach, CA, USA, 15–20 June 2019; pp. 2661–2671.
20. Lubner, M.G.; Stabo, N.; Abel, E.J.; del Rio, A.M.; Pickhardt, P.J. CT textural analysis of large primary renal cell carcinomas: pretreatment tumor heterogeneity correlates with histologic findings and clinical outcomes. *Am. J. Roentgenol.* **2016**, *207*, 96–105. [CrossRef]
21. Park, J.H.; Seo, N.; Lim, J.S.; Hahm, J.; Kim, M.J. Feasibility of Simultaneous Multislice Acceleration Technique in Diffusion-Weighted Magnetic Resonance Imaging of the Rectum. *Korean J. Radiol.* **2020**, *21*, 77–87. [CrossRef]
22. Gollub, M.; Gultekin, D.; Akin, O.; Do, R.; Fuqua, J.; Gonen, M.; Kuk, D.; Weiser, M.; Saltz, L.; Schrag, D.; et al. Dynamic contrast enhanced-MRI for the detection of pathological complete response to neoadjuvant chemotherapy for locally advanced rectal cancer. *Eur. Radiol.* **2012**, *22*, 821–831. [CrossRef]
23. Gillies, R.J.; Kinahan, P.E.; Hricak, H. Radiomics: images are more than pictures, they are data. *Radiology* **2016**, *278*, 563–577. [CrossRef]
24. Lambin, P.; Rios-Velazquez, E.; Leijenaar, R.; Carvalho, S.; Van Stiphout, R.G.; Granton, P.; Zegers, C.M.; Gillies, R.; Boellard, R.; Dekker, A.; et al. Radiomics: extracting more information from medical images using advanced feature analysis. *Eur. J. Cancer* **2012**, *48*, 441–446. [CrossRef]
25. Bibault, J.E.; Giraud, P.; Housset, M.; Durdux, C.; Taieb, J.; Berger, A.; Coriat, R.; Chaussade, S.; Dousset, B.; Nordlinger, B.; et al. Deep Learning and Radiomics predict complete response after neo-adjuvant chemoradiation for locally advanced rectal cancer. *Sci. Rep.* **2018**, *8*, 1–8.
26. Cox, D.R. Regression models and life-tables. *J. R. Stat. Soc. Ser. (Methodol.)* **1972**, *34*, 187–202. [CrossRef]
27. Ishwaran, H.; Kogalur, U.B.; Blackstone, E.H.; Lauer, M.S. Random survival forests. *Ann. Appl. Stat.* **2008**, *2*, 841–860. [CrossRef]
28. Pieper, S.; Halle, M.; Kikinis, R. 3D Slicer. In Proceedings of the 2004 2nd IEEE International Symposium on Biomedical Imaging: Nano to Macro (IEEE Cat No. 04EX821), Arlington, VA, USA, 15–18 April 2004; pp. 632–635.
29. Gosain, A.; Sardana, S. Handling class imbalance problem using oversampling techniques: A review. In Proceedings of the 2017 International Conference on Advances in Computing, Communications and Informatics (ICACCI), Udupi, India, 13–16 September 2017; pp. 79–85.
30. Unser, M.; Aldroubi, A.; Eden, M. B-spline signal processing. I. Theory. *IEEE Trans. Signal Process.* **1993**, *41*, 821–833. [CrossRef]
31. Schwier, M.; van Griethuysen, J.; Vangel, M.G.; Pieper, S.; Peled, S.; Tempany, C.; Aerts, H.J.; Kikinis, R.; Fennessy, F.M.; Fedorov, A. Repeatability of multiparametric prostate MRI radiomics features. *Sci. Rep.* **2019**, *9*, 1–16. [CrossRef] [PubMed]

32. Park, S.H.; Lim, H.; Bae, B.K.; Hahm, M.H.; Chong, G.O.; Jeong, S.Y.; Kim, J.C. Robustness of magnetic resonance radiomic features to pixel size resampling and interpolation in patients with cervical cancer. *Cancer Imaging* **2021**, *21*, 1–11. [CrossRef] [PubMed]
33. Duron, L.; Balvay, D.; Vande Perre, S.; Bouchouicha, A.; Savatovsky, J.; Sadik, J.C.; Thomassin-Naggara, I.; Fournier, L.; Lecler, A. Gray-level discretization impacts reproducible MRI radiomics texture features. *PLoS ONE* **2019**, *14*, e0213459. [CrossRef] [PubMed]
34. Hussain, Z.; Gimenez, F.; Yi, D.; Rubin, D. Differential data augmentation techniques for medical imaging classification tasks. In Proceedings of the AMIA Annual Symposium Proceedings, American Medical Informatics Association, Washington, DC, USA, 6–8 November 2017; Volume 2017, p. 979.
35. Perez, F.; Vasconcelos, C.; Avila, S.; Valle, E. Data augmentation for skin lesion analysis. In *OR 2.0 Context-Aware Operating Theaters, Computer Assisted Robotic Endoscopy, Clinical Image-Based Procedures, and Skin Image Analysis*; Springer: Berlin, Germany, 2018; pp. 303–311.
36. Shin, H.C.; Roth, H.R.; Gao, M.; Lu, L.; Xu, Z.; Nogues, I.; Yao, J.; Mollura, D.; Summers, R.M. Deep convolutional neural networks for computer-aided detection: CNN architectures, dataset characteristics and transfer learning. *IEEE Trans. Med. Imaging* **2016**, *35*, 1285–1298. [CrossRef]
37. Almourish, M.H.; Saif, A.A.; Radman, B.M.; Saeed, A.Y. Covid-19 Diagnosis Based on CT Images Using Pre-Trained Models. In Proceedings of the 2021 International Conference of Technology, Science and Administration (ICTSA), Taiz, Yemen, 22–24 March 2021; pp. 1–5.
38. Tran, D.; Wang, H.; Torresani, L.; Ray, J.; LeCun, Y.; Paluri, M. A closer look at spatiotemporal convolutions for action recognition. In Proceedings of the IEEE conference on Computer Vision and Pattern Recognition, Salt Lake City, UT, USA, 18–23 June 2018; pp. 6450–6459.
39. Kay, W.; Carreira, J.; Simonyan, K.; Zhang, B.; Hillier, C.; Vijayanarasimhan, S.; Viola, F.; Green, T.; Back, T.; Natsev, P.; et al. The kinetics human action video dataset. *arXiv* **2017**, arXiv:1705.06950.
40. Van Griethuysen, J.J.; Fedorov, A.; Parmar, C.; Hosny, A.; Aucoin, N.; Narayan, V.; Beets-Tan, R.G.; Fillion-Robin, J.C.; Pieper, S.; Aerts, H.J. Computational radiomics system to decode the radiographic phenotype. *Cancer Res.* **2017**, *77*, e104–e107. [CrossRef]
41. Rizzo, S.; Botta, F.; Raimondi, S.; Origgi, D.; Fanciullo, C.; Morganti, A.G.; Bellomi, M. Radiomics: the facts and the challenges of image analysis. *Eur. Radiol. Exp.* **2018**, *2*, 1–8. [CrossRef]
42. Sarveniazi, A. An actual survey of dimensionality reduction. *Am. J. Comput. Math.* **2014**, *4*, 55–72.. [CrossRef]
43. Schölkopf, B.; Smola, A.; Müller, K.R. Kernel principal component analysis. In *International Conference on Artificial Neural Networks*; Springer: Berlin, Germany, 1997; pp. 583–588.
44. Breiman, L. Random forests. *Machine Learn.* **2001**, *45*, 5–32. [CrossRef]
45. Ospina, J.D.; Zhu, J.; Chira, C.; Bossi, A.; Delobel, J.B.; Beckendorf, V.; Dubray, B.; Lagrange, J.L.; Correa, J.C.; Simon, A.; et al. Random forests to predict rectal toxicity following prostate cancer radiation therapy. *Int. J. Radiat. Oncol. Biol. Phys.* **2014**, *89*, 1024–1031. [CrossRef]
46. Petkovska, I.; Tixier, F.; Ortiz, E.J.; Pernicka, J.S.G.; Paroder, V.; Bates, D.D.; Horvat, N.; Fuqua, J.; Schilsky, J.; Gollub, M.J.; et al. Clinical utility of radiomics at baseline rectal MRI to predict complete response of rectal cancer after chemoradiation therapy. *Abdom. Radiol.* **2020**, *45*, 3608–3617. [CrossRef]
47. Calders, T.; Jaroszewicz, S. Efficient AUC optimization for classification. In *European Conference on Principles of Data Mining and Knowledge Discovery*; Springer: Berlin, Germany, 2007; pp. 42–53.
48. Liu, L.; Jiang, H.; He, P.; Chen, W.; Liu, X.; Gao, J.; Han, J. On the variance of the adaptive learning rate and beyond. *arXiv* **2019**, arXiv:1908.03265.
49. Kingma, D.P.; Ba, J. Adam: A method for stochastic optimization. *arXiv* **2014**, arXiv:1412.6980.
50. Comelli, A.; Stefano, A.; Coronnello, C.; Russo, G.; Vernuccio, F.; Cannella, R.; Salvaggio, G.; Lagalla, R.; Barone, S. Radiomics: A new biomedical workflow to create a predictive model. In *Annual Conference on Medical Image Understanding and Analysis*; Springer: Berlin, Germany, 2020; pp. 280–293.
51. Marini, N.; Otálora, S.; Müller, H.; Atzori, M. Semi-supervised training of deep convolutional neural networks with heterogeneous data and few local annotations: An experiment on prostate histopathology image classification. *Med. Image Anal.* **2021**, *73*, 102165. [CrossRef]
52. Granzier, R.; Verbakel, N.; Ibrahim, A.; van Timmeren, J.; van Nijnatten, T.; Leijenaar, R.; Lobbes, M.; Smidt, M.; Woodruff, H. MRI-based radiomics in breast cancer: feature robustness with respect to inter-observer segmentation variability. *Sci. Rep.* **2020**, *10*, 1–11. [CrossRef]
53. Ronneberger, O.; Fischer, P.; Brox, T. U-net: Convolutional networks for biomedical image segmentation. In *International Conference on Medical Image Computing and Computer-Assisted Intervention*; Springer: Berlin, Germany, 2015; pp. 234–241.
54. He, K.; Gkioxari, G.; Dollár, P.; Girshick, R. Mask r-cnn. In Proceedings of the IEEE International Conference on Computer Vision, Venice, Italy, 22–29 October 2017; pp. 2961–2969.
55. Comelli, A.; Dahiya, N.; Stefano, A.; Vernuccio, F.; Portoghese, M.; Cutaia, G.; Bruno, A.; Salvaggio, G.; Yezzi, A. Deep Learning-Based Methods for Prostate Segmentation in Magnetic Resonance Imaging. *Appl. Sci.* **2021**, *11*, 782. [CrossRef]

56. Habr-Gama, A.; Perez, R.O.; Nadalin, W.; Sabbaga, J.; Ribeiro Jr, U.; e Sousa Jr, A.H.S.; Campos, F.G.; Kiss, D.R.; Gama-Rodrigues, J. Operative versus nonoperative treatment for stage 0 distal rectal cancer following chemoradiation therapy: long-term results. *Ann. Surg.* **2004**, *240*, 711. [CrossRef]
57. Habr-Gama, A.; Perez, R.O.; Proscurshim, I.; Campos, F.G.; Nadalin, W.; Kiss, D.; Gama-Rodrigues, J. Patterns of failure and survival for nonoperative treatment of stage c0 distal rectal cancer following neoadjuvant chemoradiation therapy. *J. Gastrointest. Surg.* **2006**, *10*, 1319–1329. [CrossRef]
58. Horvat, N.; Carlos Tavares Rocha, C.; Clemente Oliveira, B.; Petkovska, I.; Gollub, M.J. MRI of rectal cancer: tumor staging, imaging techniques, and management. *Radiographics* **2019**, *39*, 367–387. [CrossRef]
59. Beets-Tan, R.G.; Lambregts, D.M.; Maas, M.; Bipat, S.; Barbaro, B.; Curvo-Semedo, L.; Fenlon, H.M.; Gollub, M.J.; Gourtsoyianni, S.; Halligan, S.; et al. Magnetic resonance imaging for clinical management of rectal cancer: Updated recommendations from the 2016 European Society of Gastrointestinal and Abdominal Radiology (ESGAR) consensus meeting. *Eur. Radiol.* **2018**, *28*, 1465–1475. [CrossRef]

Article

Robustness of PET Radiomics Features: Impact of Co-Registration with MRI

Alessandro Stefano [1], Antonio Leal [2], Selene Richiusa [1,3], Phan Trang [3], Albert Comelli [4,*], Viviana Benfante [1,4,5], Sebastiano Cosentino [6], Maria G. Sabini [6], Antonino Tuttolomondo [5], Roberto Altieri [7,8], Francesco Certo [7,8], Giuseppe Maria Vincenzo Barbagallo [7,8], Massimo Ippolito [6] and Giorgio Russo [1,3,6]

[1] Institute of Molecular Bioimaging and Physiology, National Research Council (IBFM-CNR), 90015 Cefalù, Italy; alessandro.stefano@ibfm.cnr.it (A.S.); selene.richiusa@ibfm.cnr.it (S.R.); viviana.benfante@unipa.it (V.B.); giorgio.russo@ibfm.cnr.it (G.R.)
[2] Departamento de Fisiología Médica y Biofísica, University de Seville/Instituto de Biomedicina de Sevilla (IBiS), 41013 Seville, Spain; alplaza@us.es
[3] Department of Physics and Astronomy "E. Majorana", University of Catania, 95124 Catania, Italy; trangphan046@gmail.com
[4] Ri.Med Foundation, Via Bandiera 11, 90133 Palermo, Italy
[5] Department of Health Promotion, Mother and Child Care, Internal Medicine and Medical Specialties, Molecular and Clinical Medicine, University of Palermo, 90127 Palermo, Italy; bruno.tuttolomondo@unipa.it
[6] Nuclear Medicine Department, Cannizzaro Hospital, 95126 Catania, Italy; sebastiano.cosentino@aoec.it (S.C.); mgabsabini@gmail.com (M.G.S.); centro_pet@ospedale-cannizzaro.it (M.I.)
[7] Neurosurgical Unit, AOU Policlinico "G. Rodolico-San Marco", University of Catania, 95123 Catania, Italy; roberto.altieri.87@gmail.com (R.A.); cicciocerto@yahoo.com (F.C.); gbarbagallo@unict.it (G.M.V.B.)
[8] Interdisciplinary Research Center on Diagnosis and Management of Brain Tumors, University of Catania, 95123 Catania, Italy
* Correspondence: acomelli@fondazionerimed.com; Tel.: +39-09-2192-0149

Featured Application: The study proposes an analysis of the robustness of Positron Emission Tomography (PET) radiomics features after PET image co-registration with two different Magnetic Resonance Imaging sequences, namely T1 and FLAIR.

Abstract: Radiomics holds great promise in the field of cancer management. However, the clinical application of radiomics has been hampered by uncertainty about the robustness of the features extracted from the images. Previous studies have reported that radiomics features are sensitive to changes in voxel size resampling and interpolation, image perturbation, or slice thickness. This study aims to observe the variability of positron emission tomography (PET) radiomics features under the impact of co-registration with magnetic resonance imaging (MRI) using the difference percentage coefficient, and the Spearman's correlation coefficient for three groups of images: (i) original PET, (ii) PET after co-registration with T1-weighted MRI and (iii) PET after co-registration with FLAIR MRI. Specifically, seventeen patients with brain cancers undergoing [11C]-Methionine PET were considered. Successively, PET images were co-registered with MRI sequences and 107 features were extracted for each mentioned group of images. The variability analysis revealed that shape features, first-order features and two subgroups of higher-order features possessed a good robustness, unlike the remaining groups of features, which showed large differences in the difference percentage coefficient. Furthermore, using the Spearman's correlation coefficient, approximately 40% of the selected features differed from the three mentioned groups of images. This is an important consideration for users conducting radiomics studies with image co-registration constraints to avoid errors in cancer diagnosis, prognosis, and clinical outcome prediction.

Keywords: radiomics feature robustness; imaging quantification; [11C]-methionine positron emission tomography; PET/MRI co-registration

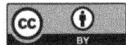

1. Introduction

Cancer is one of the leading causes of mortality, and anatomical and functional imaging is of vital importance for diagnosis, treatment planning, and treatment response, which has become standard in clinical protocols for many different oncological disease types. However, qualitative analyses are not always sufficient to reveal disease characteristics and to make a treatment decision or final diagnosis with the utmost confidence. To date, interest has emerged in characterizing tumor heterogeneity and phenotypes based on innovative image-based biomarkers related to the pathological, genomic, proteomic, and clinical data. Recent advances in computational power and the use of automated algorithms have generated a new area of research termed radiomics [1,2] that can be applied on imaging data sets such as computed tomography (CT) [3,4], positron emission tomography (PET) [5,6], and magnetic resonance imaging (MRI) [7,8]. It is based on the extraction of a large variety of biomarkers from images in order to improve diagnosis and treatment response prediction, and thus potentially allow for the personalization of cancer treatments. The fundamental hypothesis of radiomics is that much more information is presented in medical images than what visual assessment can understand, and therefore, the pathophysiological information of tumors can be captured using image biomarkers. In computer vision and image processing, a biomarker is an information about the content of an image and can be renamed as feature. Specifically, these features express properties regarding the shape, histogram, and texture of the images. Shape features are based on the surface reconstruction whereas first-order metrics are obtained from the histogram that describes the distribution of voxel intensities in the image. Information about inter-voxel relationships within the image can be interpreted using higher-order statistics based on texture analysis. As a result, quantitative analysis based on these features is considered one of the key findings in clinical studies for cancer detection, diagnosis and therapy assessment, resulting in improved decision support systems. Nevertheless, their clinical application may be challenging. A major obstacle is that the "robustness" of the extracted radiomics features is unclear. Robustness is understood as the level of variability of features as a result of perturbations, such as image co-registration. In other words, an essential ingredient to establish novel quantitative imaging biomarkers in clinical practice is to quantify and ascertain the consistency of radiomics features.

Recently, many researchers have focused on gaining a deeper understanding of feature robustness. However, most studies used phantoms, and consequently, it is difficult to ensure that their results could be applied to imaging studies of real patients [9]. Furthermore, standardizing the parameters during image acquisition in clinical settings is a challenge. To date, there are various studies on the robustness of radiomics features due to various factors, such as the impact of voxel size resampling and interpolation, image perturbation, different slice thickness, etc. [10–12], and many works have discussed the potential uncertainty of feature extraction, i.e., [13].

In PET imaging, some standardized semi-quantitative measurements are usually extracted and used in clinical practice, such as the standardized uptake value (SUV), and the metabolically active tumor volume (MTV) [14]. Tixier et al. [15] investigated the reproducibility of SUV, intensity histogram features, intensity-size zone features, and co-occurrence matrices features. The results showed that these features were insensitive to the discretization range. Hatt et al. [16] investigated the robustness of PET based heterogeneity textural features with respect to the delineation of volumes and partial volume effects correction. These features were significantly affected by the differences in the volume delineation. The authors further reported that local features, e.g., entropy and heterogeneity, were more robust when compared to regional features, e.g., intensity variability and size-zone variability. To the best of our knowledge, no studies have analyzed the robustness of PET radiomics features in a real patients' dataset after the co-registration with MRI.

We hypothesize that image co-registration can change the voxel intensity relationships between neighboring voxels which in turn changes the feature values. Furthermore, the volume shape is likely to differ from the original one, changing the shape based feature values, such as the sphericity, compactness, convexity, etc. [17]. In practice, we expected that the image co-registration would introduce further uncertainty to radiomics studies. Specifically, we consider PET images, and we assess the variation in PET radiomics features after the co-registration with T1-weighted MRI, and FLAIR MR images obtained using the same acquisition protocols and the same scanners. MRI is generally used for standard clinical care of patients with brain tumors (i.e., diagnoses, monitor tumor progression, and treatment response assessment) but the clinical role of PET in the management of these patients has evolved considerably in recent years. Consequently, MRI and PET are applied to diagnose and classify brain tumors before surgery, to plan and manage intraoperative phase, to monitor and evaluate response to treatment, and to understand the effects of treatment on the patient's brain.

A recent radiomics study [18] suggests that [18F]-Fluorodeoxiglucose (FDG) PET-based radiomics is a reliable non-invasive method to distinguish lymphoma and glioblastoma. Specifically, thirteen features were selected for the differential diagnosis of lymphoma and glioblastoma. The same research group [19] affirms that the radiomics signature based on FDG-PET is a promising method for the non-invasive measurement of glioma proliferative activity and facilitates the prediction of patient prognoses. Nevertheless, although FDG is considered the best oncology radio-tracer in PET, it shows a high-glucose metabolism in normal brain tissue, which hinders the identification of a low- or intermediate-grade tumor with similar or less activity. For this reason, an alternative radio-tracer, [11C]- Methionine (MET), is studied since it provides a high detection rate of focal lesions in the central nervous system [20]. Particularly, [11C]-MET reflects amino acid transport in tumor which demonstrates a higher efficiency compared to [18F]-FDG in delineating the tumor extent, especially in the low-grade gliomas. The uptake of amino acid in a normal brain is relatively low as compared to those with gliomas since cancers need to consume more methionine for extensive proliferation and survival, while normal cells do not [21]. For this reason, it is important to incorporate MET-PET imaging in addition to MRI to provide specific information for defining the target volume for the radio-surgical treatment in patients with recurrent brain tumors to optimize target identification for infiltrating or ill-defined brain lesions.

Considering MET-PET radiomics studies, Stefano, et al. [5] were able to select a sub-panel of three features (namely asphericity, low-intensity run emphasis, and complexity) with valuable association with patient outcome (sensitivity, 81.23%; specificity, 73.97%; accuracy, 78.27%). Hotta et al. [22] developed a radiomics model to differentiate recurrent brain tumor from radiation necrosis based on MET-PET in a mixed cohort of 41 patients with brain metastasis or glioma. A random forest classifier was trained to separate radiation necrosis from recurrent brain tumor. The implemented radiomics model obtained an area under the receiver operating characteristic curve (AUC) of 0.98 (specificity, 94%; sensitivity, 90%). Papp at al. [23] considered machine-learning-driven survival models for glioma built on in vivo MET-PET characteristics, ex vivo characteristics, and patient characteristics with an AUC of 0.9. However, many technical challenges still remain, including image co-registration, such that PET radiomics can effectively contribute to personalized medicine [24].

For this reason, seventeen glioblastoma patients who underwent both MET-PET and MRI between a time range of three years (2016–2019) were used for our analysis by extracting radiomics features grouped into shape, first- and higher-order features. Usually, the feature extraction task is one of the five fundamental tasks of a radiomics workflow [25] together with image acquisition, target segmentation, feature selection, and implementation of the classification model to predict the clinical outcome. Nevertheless, our study will omit the final task focusing on the first four steps by newly adding the PET/MRI co-registration prior to the feature extraction process to evaluate its impact in a radiomics study.

2. Materials and Methods

To analyze the stability of PET radiomics features after co-registration with MRI, the PET volume of interest was delineated before and after co-registration using a semi-automatic threshold segmentation approach, followed by the extraction of radiomics features. Afterward, a robustness analysis was performed considering the different feature groups and, since not all radiomics features are useful in predicting a particular outcome of an event, the most representative features were identified from the large number of extracted features through an appropriate selection algorithm. An overview of our workflow is shown in Figure 1. Each step is detailed in the following sections.

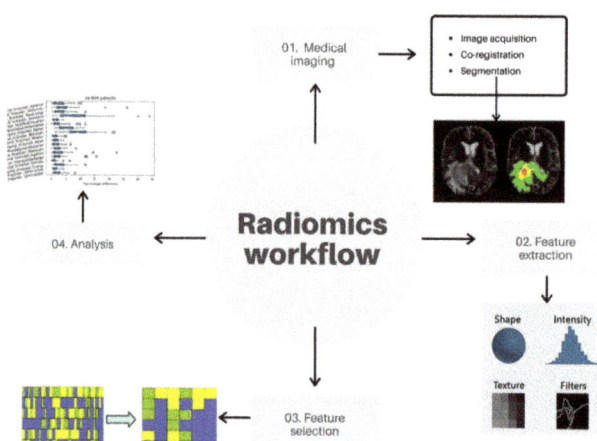

Figure 1. An overview of the study workflow.

2.1. Medical Imaging

While MRI images are anatomical imaging with high spatial resolutions but a limited physiological information, PET images provide metabolic details on the target but with poor spatial resolution leading to low-valued anatomical information. As a consequence, it would be advantageous to integrate useful data from those two images into a single one with complementary anatomical and functional information yielding more accurate disease information that will significantly aid in the early detection of tumors and enhance the efficiency of diagnosis. Compared with PET/CT, hybrid PET/MRI is capable of providing superior anatomical detail while reducing the cost of significant radiation exposure. The adoption of hybrid PET/MRI, however, is still limited. Consequently, while PET/CT is an image acquired with a single device in almost all hospital centers, PET/MRI performed in a single scanning session is not yet a widely used technology. For this reason, PET/MRI image co-registration, which is a process of overlaying images from different modalities taken at different time points of the same organ, plays an increasingly important role in the part of medical imaging analysis. Therefore, seventeen glioblastoma patients undergoing [11C]-MET PET (Biograph Horizon, Siemens Healthcare, Erlangen, Germany) and MRI (T1-weighted and FLAIR sequences, Achieva, Philips Healthcare, Best, The Netherlands) examinations were considered. An interval of no more than 15 days between PET and MRI examinations was considered. Specifically, the mean interval was of 6.6 days (range 2–15 days). PET images were reconstructed using the Ordered Subset Expectation Maximization (OSEM) with 4 iterations with a 512×512 image matrix and a voxel size of 0.4821 mm $\times$ 0.4821 mm $\times$ 3 mm. T1-weithted sequences had a matrix resolution of 288×288 with a voxel size of 0.8888 mm $\times$ 0.8888 mm $\times$ 2 mm, while FLAIR sequences had a matrix resolution 240×240 image matrix with a voxel size of 1 mm $\times$ 1 mm $\times$ 2 mm. PET/MRI co-registrations were obtained using the automatic registration MIM software (MIM v.7.0.5 software; Cleveland, OH, USA). Rigid Assisted Alignment is MIM's default method for aligning images by maximization of mutual information. An optimization routine adjusts the translation and rotation between the two series in order to maximize a mutual information metric. The mutual information metric is based on the intensities of the overlapping voxels between the two images that are being aligned and is partially based on joint entropy calculations between the volumes. The theory is that the ratio of intensity levels should vary little in regions of similar structures contained in the series. Therefore, the variability of this ratio should be minimized, and mutual information maximized, when the images are aligned correctly. The advantage of this technique is that it is general in nature and can be used to align series of the same modality or different modalities. In our study, this function produces a link between PET and MRI series that allows you to localize and scroll on both series simultaneously, transfer contours, and more.

The following steps were performed for all patient studies such that there were no differences in the co-registration algorithm while avoiding other sources of bias:

1. In an open session, click the "Create Fusion" tool;
2. Select the main series;
3. Select the secondary series;
4. The co-registered image is created and appears on the current page.

The primary series is the series that remains unaltered when co-registration is performed (MRI in our study). The secondary series (PET) is rotated and translated to be alignment with the main series which aligns images by maximization of mutual information. An optimization routine adjusts translation and rotation between the two series in order to maximize a mutual information metric. After that, the segmentation task was performed on the original and co-registered PET images. This process is challenging because many tumors show unclear borders [26]. Radiologists can flexibly delineate targets manually resulting in highly accurate segmentations. Nevertheless, manual segmentation is labor-intensive, time-consuming, and not always feasible for radiomics analysis requiring huge datasets. Additionally, manual segmentation is subject to inter- and intra-observer variability [27]. Hence, many semi-automatic delineation algorithms, such as region growing or thresholding, are used in the clinical environment although less precise than manual segmentation. Conversely, they reduce the operator interaction in the segmentation process, improving time efficiency, and reproducibility. Consequently, the stand-alone and freely available Local Image Feature Extraction (LifeX, IMIV/CEA, Orsay, France) platform [28] was used. Specifically, the threshold method was applied in the regions including the target roughly determined by the user. With this approach, the region is identified by the user, but no accurate drawing is required. Once the inclusion of the anomalous region was chosen, the algorithm performed all the subsequent processes automatically leading in the delineation of the volume of interest (VOI). According to [29], the threshold value was set at 40% of the maximum SUV (SUV_{max}). This operation was performed for each PET study, before and after image co-registration.

2.2. Feature Extraction

After VOI identification, the extraction of radiomics features was performed for each patient in the data set. One of the main points in radiomics is to increase the reproducibility of the extracted features. For this, the image biomarker standardization initiative (IBSI) [30], which is an independent international collaborative study towards the standardization of radiomics features for the purpose of high-throughput quantitative image analyses, has been introduced. For this reason, we used a comprehensive open source IBSI-compliant platform called PyRadiomics (Harvard Medical School, Boston, MA, USA) [31], which enables processing and extraction of radiomics features from medical image data using a large panel of engineered hard-coded feature algorithms, and currently is one of the most commonly used software for radiomics studies. PyRadiomics is implemented in Python, a language that has established itself as a popular open-source language for scientific computing, and which can be installed on any system. PyRadiomics provides a flexible analysis platform with a back-end interface allowing automation in data processing, feature definition, and batch handling. The Pyradiomics platform calculates different feature classes, namely first-order statistics, shape descriptors, and five texture classes: gray level cooccurrence matrix (GLCM), gray level run-length matrix (GLRLM), gray level dependence matrix (GLDM), gray level size-zone matrix (GLSZM) and neighboring gray level dependence matrix (NGLDM).

Shape-based features are based on the VOI voxel representation and are independent of the distribution of gray level intensity in the image. They are used to describe the three-dimensional shape, size of the lesion and other geometric aspects such as volume, maximum diameter along different orthogonal directions, surface, tumor compactness, and sphericity (a measure of roundness). Specifically, compactness and sphericity describe how the VOI shape differs from that of a circle (for 2D analyses) or a sphere (for 3D analyses). Additionally, the surface area is calculated by triangulation (a process that produces a net of triangles that completely cover the tumor surface) and serves as a base for calculation of the surface-volume ratio: spiculated tumors show higher values than those of a round tumor of similar volume. Furthermore, flatness describes whether the surface of the object is flat or has raised areas or indentations. In short, these radiomics features provide physical measurements and significantly contribute to clinical outcome.

First-order statistical features describe the frequency distribution of voxels within a VOI. This information can be obtained from the histogram of gray-level intensity values; for this, they are referred as "histogram-based" features. Sophisticated features include skewness and kurtosis, which describe the shape of the intensity distribution of data: skewness reflects the asymmetry of the data distribution curve to lower or higher values than the mean one (negative skew and positive skew, respectively), whereas kurtosis reflects the tail of a data distribution with respect to a gaussian distribution due to outliers. Other features include histogram entropy and uniformity (also called energy).

Texture analysis is a key concept in radiomics. It refers to wide variety of quantitative methods that are used to assess the relative voxel positions within the image to derive texture features. As a result, the texture features provide information on the spatial organization of color or intensities in an image or a selected region of an image. The texture is a linked set of voxels fulfilling a given gray level property that occurs repeatedly in an image region thus creating a textured region. Due to the fact that the texture is characterized by the spatial distribution of gray levels in a neighborhood, it cannot be defined for a point. Texture features are sub-categorized according to particular matrices from which they are obtained. These matrices are calculated to describe the spatial voxel differences by considering the spatial correlation properties of gray scales and therefore are the most capable of expressing the correlation between different parts of the tumor. In particular, GLCM is used to quantify the incidence of voxels with same intensities at a predetermined distance along a fixed direction while GLRLM quantifies consecutive voxels with the same intensity along fixed directions and GLDM is created by counting the number of voxel segments having the same intensity in a given direction. In addition, GLSZM is defined as number of connected voxels that have equal gray level intensity. Finally, NGTDM valuates the spatial interrelationships between 3 or more voxels. These features provide a complete information of the tumor; therefore, it is believed to match and resemble the visual experience of a human.

To evaluate the difference percentage (DP) coefficient between the feature values extracted from the original PET images and the co-registered PET ones, we used the following formula:

$$\mathrm{DP} = 100 \times \mathrm{ABS}\left(\frac{\text{Feature Value}_{\text{original PET}} - \text{Feature Value}_{\text{co-registered PET}}}{\text{Feature Value}_{\text{original PET}}}\right) \qquad (1)$$

2.3. Feature Selection and Analysis

The process of identifying small sets of features useful for diagnostic purposes, namely the selection feature process, is a challenging task in radiomics studies. The aim is to obtain the smallest possible set of features, considered as optimal set for achieving a good predictive performance, thus leading to exclusion of non-reproducible, redundant, and irrelevant features from the dataset. In this study, we want to investigate whether the same optimal set of radiomic features is obtained from three sets of images, namely original PET, PET co-registered with T1-weighted MRI, and PET co-registered with FLAIR MRI. In that way, the robustness of radiomics features can be evaluated after co-registration. Spearman's rank correlation coefficient, which belongs to the filter method group [25], is used to assess whether there is any association between two observed features and to estimate the strength of this relationship. In this way, it is possible to eliminate all features whose level of correlation is above a user-specified threshold. For two sets of variables x and y, each raw score x_i and y_i is converted to ranks X_i and Y_i. The Spearman's correlation coefficient is then used on the ranked variables which can be expressed mathematically by the following formula:

$$\rho = 1 - \frac{6 \sum d_i^2}{n(n^2 - 1)} \quad (2)$$

where $d_i = X_i - Y_i$ is the difference between ranks and n is the number of paired observations. The coefficient ranges from -1 to $+1$, where negative values indicate that y decreases with x and positive values indicate that y increases with x. In other words, a correlation of 1.0 indicates a perfect positive correlation, and a correlation of -1.0 indicates a perfect negative correlation. Particularly, the strength of association between the two variables is considered very strong if the coefficient ranges from 0.8 to 1, moderate from 0.6 to 0.7, weak from 0.3 to 0.5, and very weak when less than 0.2. When the correlation coefficient is equal to 0, the two variables are independent from one another [32] (see Table 1).

Table 1. The Spearman's rank correlation coefficient ranges from -1 to 1 indicating various degrees of association between radiomics features.

Correlation Coefficient	Degree of Association
±1	Perfect
±0.9	Very Strong
±0.8	Very Strong
±0.7	Moderate
±0.6	Moderate
±0.5	Fair
±0.4	Fair
±0.3	Fair
±0.2	Poor
±0.1	Poor
0	None

In our study, a threshold of 0.8 was selected such that a number of high correlated features will be extracted. Consequently, a list of features that are not correlated, i.e., have the correlation coefficient lower than the chosen threshold, is obtained. After applying this correlation-based method, observation of different radiomic features from three different sets of images is obtained to evaluate the robustness of radiomics features following co-registration interference.

3. Results and Discussions

A total of 107 features (14 shape features, 18 first-order statistical features, and 65 texture features) were extracted from each PET study before and after co-registration with T1-weighted (for 15 patients because two T1 images were unavailable), and FLAIR (for all 17 patients) MRI sequences, for a total of three feature datasets for each lesion.

Starting from an exploratory analysis of the difference percentage between the feature values obtained from original PET images and co-registered PET ones, the shape-based feature group showed a mean less than 5% for all features indicating that this group has significantly robust features (see Figure 2). This is because a similar VOI is used before and after co-registration, and as a result, the shape characteristics are not supposed to change significantly from each other after the co-registration process. Even the first-order statistical GLCM and NGTDM features showed a median of less than 20% (<10% for first-order statistical features); thus, they are quite robust (see Figure 3).

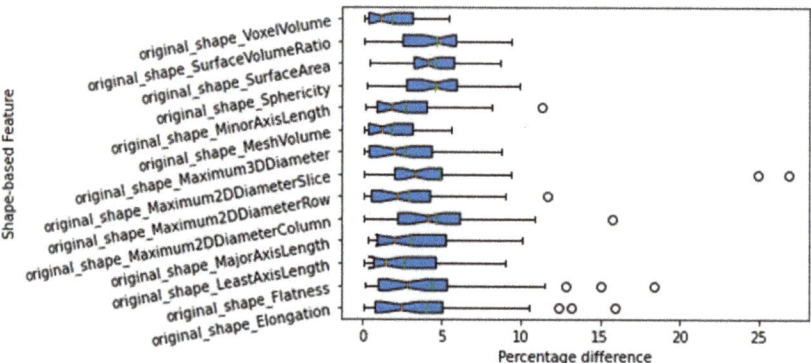

Figure 2. Difference percentage between non-co-registered and co-registered PET with T1-weighted and FLAIR MRI (the median is indicated in orange, while mean in green) for shape-based features.

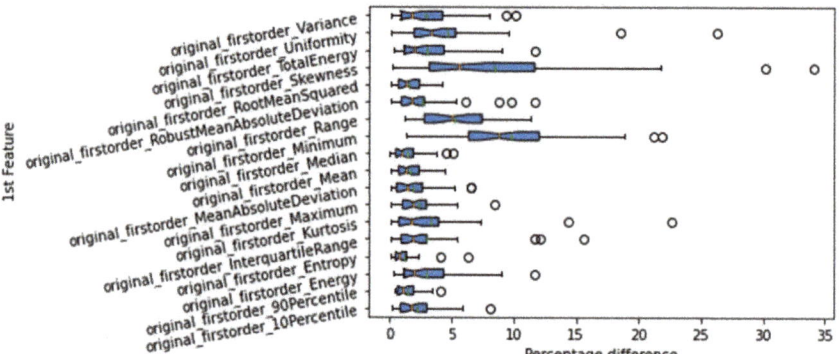

Figure 3. *Cont.*

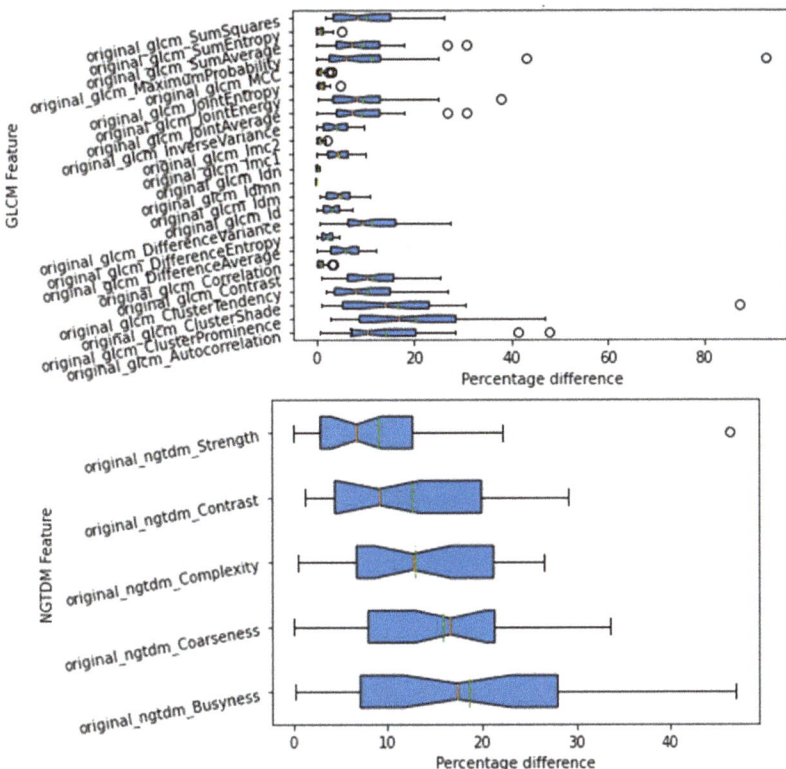

Figure 3. Difference percentage between non-co-registered and co-registered PET with T1-weighted and FLAIR MRI (the median is indicated in orange, while mean in green) for first-order, and GLCM, and NGTDM features, respectively.

Vice versa, significant differences were found for the remaining texture matrices with mean values above 40% (Figure 4). In the case of the GLSZM Large Area High Gray Level Emphasis feature, the main exceeded 70%. These results are consistent with previous results published in [33]. In addition, in GLSZM group, a peculiarly high difference percentage was obtained for one patient (DP = 546% for the Large Area Low Gray Level Emphasis feature). Once again, this result shows a similarity with Meijer's findings [33], where the GLSZM class is the one with the highest variation. Specifically, a difference of 106.58% was reported for the Large Area Low Gray Level Emphasis feature. This value refers to the variability analysis of the PET features when image acquisition is repeated five times. Conversely, in our study, the comparison is not between PET phantom studies obtained at different times but between PET and co-registered PET studies. Consequently, we can expect that this difference increases in our study where image co-registration is considered. In other studies dealing with other types of images, i.e., CT imaging [17] where deformable image registration was applied, the shape-based features were 100% robust, while GLSZM and NGTDM were the most unstable feature groups. Furthermore, features from the categories of intensity and GLCM were considered as stable. This is in good agreement with our results. In a MRI study, Joonsang Lee's [34] found that the variation of radiomics features were intermediate or high for Skewness, glcm-Autocorrelation, glcm-ClusterShade, glcm-Imc1, glrlm-LongRunLow (or High) GrayLevelEmphasis, firstorder-90Percentile, glcm-ClusterTendency, glcm-Correlation, and ngtdm-Complexity. This also matches with our study.

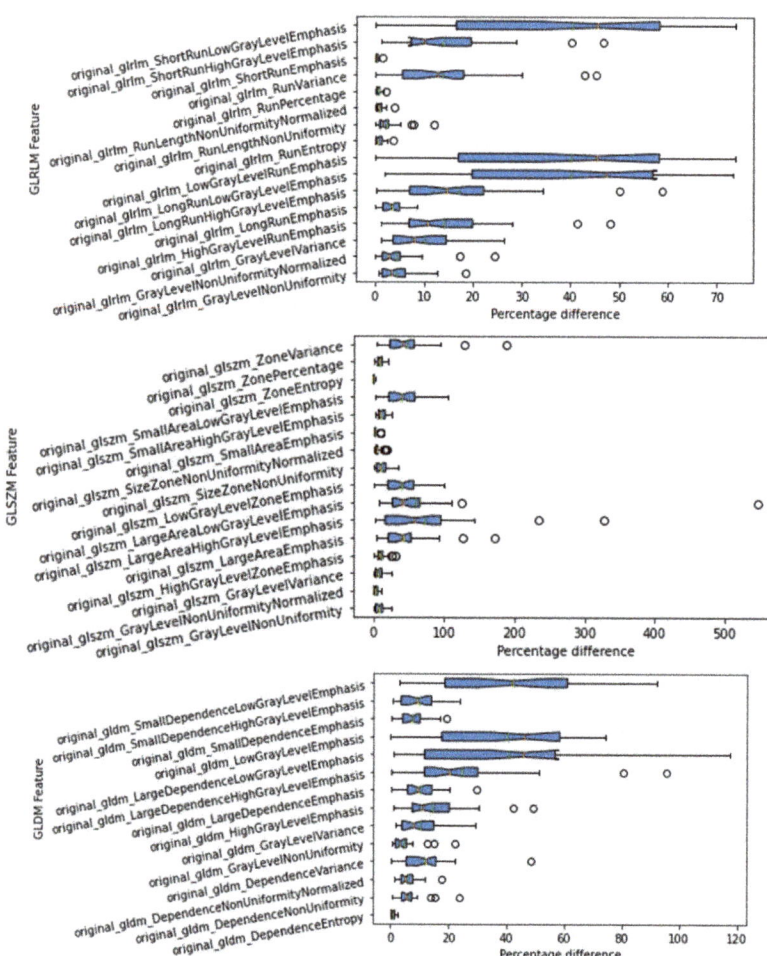

Figure 4. Difference percentage between non-co-registered and co-registered PET with T1-weighted and FLAIR MRI (the median is indicated in orange, while mean in green) for GLRLM, GLSZM, and GLDM features.

The next step was to verify if the same optimal set of radiomics features was obtained in the three groups of images after the selection process based on the Spearman rank correlation coefficient. This approach was replicated for all patient studies producing a matrix that showed the correlation coefficient for all extracted features (see Figure 5).

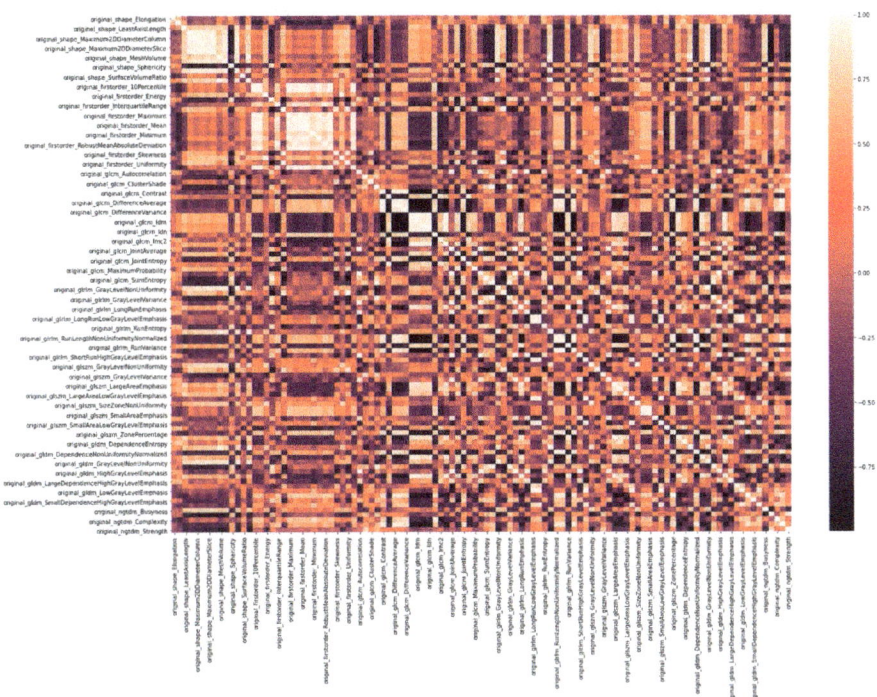

Figure 5. Correlation matrix for the 107 radiomics features.

A threshold of 0.8 (see Table 1) was chosen to reduce the amount of radiomics features that are highly correlated. In this way, only uncorrelated features were considered. Specifically, 21 features were identified both for PET, and PET co-registered with FLAIR while 19 for PET co-registered with T1. Although the number of uncorrelated features is similar (in the case of PET and PET/T1 is identical), the same features were not selected. In particular, nine features were different between PET and PET co-registered with FLAIR, while eight were different between PET and PET co-registered with T1. Approximately 40% of the uncorrelated features were different within the three image datasets. The different features from each other group are detailed in Tables 2 and 3.

Table 2. The different features selected in PET and PET co-registered with FLAIR datasets.

PET	PET FLAIR Co-Registration
shape-MinorAxisLength	firstorder-90Percentile
shape-Sphericity	glcm-Autocorrelation
firstorder-10Percentile	glcm-ClusterShade
firstorder-InterquartileRange	glcm-ClusterTendency
firstorder-Skewness	glcm-Correlation
glrlm-LongRunHighGrayLevelEmphasis	glrlm-LowGrayLevelRunEmphasis
glszm-GrayLevelNonUniformity	glrlm-RunVariance
glszm-GrayLevelNonUniformityNormalized	glszm-SmallAreaEmphasis
gldm-SmallDependenceLowGrayLevelEmphasis	glszm-SmallAreaEmphasis

Table 3. The different features selected in PET and PET co-registered with T1 datasets.

PET	PET T1 Co-Registration
shape-MinorAxisLength	shape-Maximum2DDiameterSlice
shape-Sphericity	glcm-ClusterShade
firstorder-Skewness	glcm-Imc1
glrlm-LongRunHighGrayLevelEmphasis	glrlm-LongRunLowGrayLevelEmphasis
glszm-GrayLevelNonUniformity	glrlm-RunVariance
glszm-GrayLevelNonUniformityNormalized	glszm-SizeZoneNonUniformity
gldm-LargeDependenceLowGrayLevelEmphasis	
gldm-SmallDependenceLowGrayLevelEmphasis	

These results show that the co-registration process not only modifies the value of the features, as shown in the previous analysis based on the difference percentage value, but that the changes are severe enough that the selection process identifies about 40% of different features in the three image datasets. Arguably, resizing voxels can be the parameter with the greatest impact on feature robustness when co-registration is performed. However, we cannot say for sure which parameter harmed the process the most. In general, it can be argued that feature robustness can be improved if an effort is made to harmonize image acquisition and processing as defined by EARL accreditations [35]. Further analyses will be needed to provide more detailed information on this issue.

4. Conclusions

Radiomics involves the extraction of a huge number of quantitative features from medical images to predict patient outcomes and to support clinical decision-making systems. However, the clinical application of radiomics is limited due to uncertainty about the robustness of the extracted features. To analyze this aspect in the context of PET/MRI co-registration, we applied a semi-automatic segmentation based on the thresholding method combined with an automatic PET feature extraction process using Pyradiomics. In this way, the difference in percentage coefficients was evaluated between features extracted from: i) original PET, ii) PET after co-registration with T1-weighted MRI and iii) PET after co-registration with FLAIR MRI. In addition, feature selection using Spearman's correlation method was proposed to reduce the high dimension of extracted features and verify if the selected radiomics features are consistent after co-registration of PET images on MRI ones. The results showed that the shape features, first-order statistical features, NGTDM and GLCM features are robust, as the percentage difference is less than 20%. Conversely, GLSZM, GLRLM and GLDM showed very weak robustness due to co-registration. In addition, approximately 40% of different features were identified in the three image datasets after eliminating all highly correlated features in each dataset. In conclusion, co-registration compromises the robustness of radiomics features; thus, authors need to be careful when radiomics studies are performed on co-registered images. Any results found using PET images are not transferable to the co-registered images. Understanding the robustness of radiomics features after image co-registration can aid future radiomics research to enhance the clinical outcome prediction and improve diagnosis and prognosis of cancer.

Author Contributions: Conceptualization, A.S. and G.R.; Data curation, A.S., S.R. and P.T.; Formal analysis, A.S. and P.T.; Funding acquisition, A.S. and A.C.; Investigation; A.S. and P.T.; Methodology, A.S.; Project administration, A.S.; Resources, S.R., A.C., V.B., S.C., M.G.S., A.T., R.A., F.C., G.M.V.B. and M.I.; Software, P.T.; Supervision, A.S., A.L., and G.R.; Validation, A.S.; Visualization, A.S. and P.T.; Writing—original draft, A.S. and P.T.; Writing—review and editing, A.L. All authors have read and agreed to the published version of the manuscript.

Funding: This research received no external funding.

Institutional Review Board Statement: The proposed research has no implication on patient treatment. Review board approval was not sought: the proposed image analysis was performed offline and thus did not change the current treatment protocol.

Informed Consent Statement: Informed consent was obtained from all subjects involved in the study.

Data Availability Statement: Data sharing not applicable.

Conflicts of Interest: The authors declare no conflict of interest. The funders had no role in the design of the study; in the collection, analyses, or interpretation of data; in the writing of the manuscript; or in the decision to publish the results.

References

1. Hatt, M.; Tixier, F.; Visvikis, D.; Cheze Le Rest, C. Radiomics in PET/CT: More Than Meets the Eye? *J. Nucl. Med.* **2017**, *58*, 365–366. [CrossRef]
2. Castiglioni, I.; Gilardi, M.C. Radiomics: Is it time to compose the puzzle? *Clin. Transl. Imaging* **2018**, *6*, 411–413. [CrossRef]
3. Fang, M.; He, B.; Li, L.; Dong, D.; Yang, X.; Li, C.; Meng, L.; Zhong, L.; Li, H.; Li, H.; et al. CT radiomics can help screen the Coronavirus disease 2019 (COVID-19): A preliminary study. *Sci. China Inf. Sci.* **2020**, *63*, 1–8. [CrossRef]
4. Stefano, A.; Gioè, M.; Russo, G.; Palmucci, S.; Torrisi, S.E.; Bignardi, S.; Basile, A.; Comelli, A.; Benfante, V.; Sambataro, G.; et al. Performance of radiomics features in the quantification of idiopathic pulmonary fibrosis from HRCT. *Diagnostics* **2020**, *10*, 306. [CrossRef]
5. Stefano, A.; Comelli, A.; Bravatà, V.; Barone, S.; Daskalovski, I.; Savoca, G.; Sabini, M.G.; Ippolito, M.; Russo, G. A preliminary PET radiomics study of brain metastases using a fully automatic segmentation method. *BMC Bioinform.* **2020**, *21*, 325. [CrossRef] [PubMed]
6. Alongi, P.; Laudicella, R.; Stefano, A.; Caobelli, F.; Comelli, A.; Vento, A.; Sardina, D.; Ganduscio, G.; Toia, P.; Ceci, F.; et al. Choline PET/CT features to predict survival outcome in high risk prostate cancer restaging: A preliminary machine-learning radiomics study. *Q. J. Nucl. Med. Mol. Imaging* **2020**. Online ahead of print. [CrossRef]
7. Comelli, A.; Stefano, A.; Coronnello, C.; Russo, G.; Vernuccio, F.; Cannella, R.; Salvaggio, G.; Lagalla, R.; Barone, S. Radiomics: A New Biomedical Workflow to Create a Predictive Model. In *Annual Conference on Medical Image Understanding and Analysis*; Springer: Cham, Switzerland, 2020; pp. 280–293.
8. Cuocolo, R.; Cipullo, M.B.; Stanzione, A.; Ugga, L.; Romeo, V.; Radice, L.; Brunetti, A.; Imbriaco, M. Machine learning applications in prostate cancer magnetic resonance imaging. *Eur. Radiol. Exp.* **2019**, *3*, 35. [CrossRef] [PubMed]
9. Cattell, R.; Chen, S.; Huang, C. Robustness of radiomic features in magnetic resonance imaging: Review and a phantom study. *Vis. Comput. Ind. Biomed. Art* **2019**, *2*, 1–16. [CrossRef]
10. Moradmand, H.; Aghamiri, S.M.R.; Ghaderi, R. Impact of image preprocessing methods on reproducibility of radiomic features in multimodal magnetic resonance imaging in glioblastoma. *J. Appl. Clin. Med. Phys.* **2020**, *21*, 179–190. [CrossRef]
11. Chaddad, A.; Kucharczyk, M.J.; Daniel, P.; Sabri, S.; Jean-Claude, B.J.; Niazi, T.; Abdulkarim, B. Radiomics in Glioblastoma: Current Status and Challenges Facing Clinical Implementation. *Front. Oncol.* **2019**, *9*, 374. [CrossRef]
12. Castiglioni, I.; Gallivanone, F.; Soda, P.; Avanzo, M.; Stancanello, J.; Aiello, M.; Interlenghi, M.; Salvatore, M. AI-based applications in hybrid imaging: How to build smart and truly multi-parametric decision models for radiomics. *Eur. J. Nucl. Med. Mol. Imaging* **2019**, *46*, 2673–2699. [CrossRef]
13. Ibrahim, A.; Primakov, S.; Beuque, M.; Woodruff, H.C.; Halilaj, I.; Wu, G.; Refaee, T.; Granzier, R.; Widaatalla, Y.; Hustinx, R.; et al. Radiomics for precision medicine: Current challenges, future prospects, and the proposal of a new framework. *Methods* **2021**, *188*, 20–29. [CrossRef]
14. Banna, G.L.; Anile, G.; Russo, G.; Vigneri, P.; Castaing, M.; Nicolosi, M.; Strano, S.; Gieri, S.; Spina, R.; Patanè, D.; et al. Predictive and Prognostic Value of Early Disease Progression by PET Evaluation in Advanced Non-Small Cell Lung Cancer. *Oncology* **2017**, *92*, 39–47. [CrossRef]
15. Tixier, F.; Hatt, M.; Le Rest, C.C.; Le Pogam, A.; Corcos, L.; Visvikis, D. Reproducibility of Tumor Uptake Heterogeneity Characterization Through Textural Feature Analysis in 18 F-FDG PET. *J. Nucl Med.* **2012**, *53*, 693–700. [CrossRef]
16. Hatt, M.; Tixier, F.; Cheze Le Rest, C.; Pradier, O.; Visvikis, D. Robustness of intratumour 18F-FDG PET uptake heterogeneity quantification for therapy response prediction in oesophageal carcinoma. *Eur. J. Nucl. Med. Mol. Imaging* **2013**, *40*, 1662–1671. [CrossRef] [PubMed]
17. Chou, K.-T.; Latifi, K.; Moros, E.G.; Feygelman, V.; Huang, T.-C.; Dilling, T.J.; Perez, B.; Zhang, G.G. Evaluation of Radiomic Features Stability When Deformable Image Registration Is Applied. In Proceedings of the International Joint Conference on Biomedical Engineering Systems and Technologies, Funchal, Portugal, 19–21 January 2018.
18. Kong, Z.; Jiang, C.; Zhu, R.; Feng, S.; Wang, Y.; Li, J.; Chen, W.; Liu, P.; Zhao, D.; Ma, W.; et al. 18F-FDG-PET-based radiomics features to distinguish primary central nervous system lymphoma from glioblastoma. *NeuroImage Clin.* **2019**, *23*, 101912. [CrossRef] [PubMed]
19. Kong, Z.; Li, J.; Liu, Z.; Liu, Z.; Zhao, D.; Cheng, X.; Li, L.; Lin, Y.; Wang, Y.; Tian, J.; et al. Radiomics signature based on FDG-PET predicts proliferative activity in primary glioma. *Clin. Radiol.* **2019**, *74*, e15–e815. [CrossRef]

20. Comelli, A.; Stefano, A.; Bignardi, S.; Coronnello, C.; Russo, G.; Sabini, M.G.; Ippolito, M.; Yezzi, A. Tissue Classification to Support Local Active Delineation of Brain Tumors. In *Proceedings of the Communications in Computer and Information Science*; Springer: Cham, Switzerland, 2020; Volume 1065, pp. 3–14.
21. Stefano, A.; Vitabile, S.; Russo, G.; Ippolito, M.; Sardina, D.; Sabini, M.G.; Gallivanone, F.; Castiglioni, I.; Gilardi, M.C. A Graph-Based Method for PET Image Segmentation in Radiotherapy Planning: A Pilot Study. In *International Conference on Image Analysis and Processing*; Springer: Berlin/Heidelberg, Germany, 2013; Volume 8157, pp. 711–720, ISBN 9783642411830.
22. Hotta, M.; Minamimoto, R.; Miwa, K. 11C-methionine-PET for differentiating recurrent brain tumor from radiation necrosis: Radiomics approach with random forest classifier. *Sci. Rep.* **2019**, *9*, 1–7. [CrossRef] [PubMed]
23. Papp, L.; Pötsch, N.; Grahovac, M.; Schmidbauer, V.; Woehrer, A.; Preusser, M.; Mitterhauser, M.; Kiesel, B.; Wadsak, W.; Beyer, T.; et al. Glioma Survival Prediction with Combined Analysis of In Vivo 11C-MET PET Features, Ex Vivo Features, and Patient Features by Supervised Machine Learning. *J. Nucl. Med.* **2018**, *59*, 892–899. [CrossRef] [PubMed]
24. Cook, G.J.R.; Azad, G.; Owczarczyk, K.; Siddique, M.; Goh, V. Challenges and Promises of PET Radiomics. *Int. J. Radiat. Oncol. Biol. Phys.* **2018**, *102*, 1083–1089. [CrossRef]
25. Barone, S.; Cannella, R.; Comelli, A.; Pellegrino, A.; Salvaggio, G.; Stefano, A.; Vernuccio, F. Hybrid descriptive-inferential method for key feature selection in prostate cancer radiomics. *Appl. Stoch. Model. Bus. Ind.* **2021**, *37*, 961–972. [CrossRef]
26. Comelli, A.; Stefano, A. A Fully Automated Segmentation System of Positron Emission Tomography Studies. In *Proceedings of the Communications in Computer and Information Science*; Zheng, Y., Williams, B.M., Chen, K., Eds.; Springer International Publishing: Cham, Switzerland, 2020; Volume 1065, pp. 353–363.
27. Alongi, P.; Stefano, A.; Comelli, A.; Laudicella, R.; Scalisi, S.; Arnone, G.; Barone, S.; Spada, M.; Purpura, P.; Bartolotta, T.V.; et al. Radiomics analysis of 18F-Choline PET/CT in the prediction of disease outcome in high-risk prostate cancer: An explorative study on machine learning feature classification in 94 patients. *Eur. Radiol.* **2021**, *31*, 4595–4605. [CrossRef] [PubMed]
28. Nioche, C.; Orlhac, F.; Boughdad, S.; Reuze, S.; Goya-Outi, J.; Robert, C.; Pellot-Barakat, C.; Soussan, M.; Frouin, F.; Buvat, I. Lifex: A freeware for radiomic feature calculation in multimodality imaging to accelerate advances in the characterization of tumor heterogeneity. *Cancer Res.* **2018**, *78*, 4786–4789. [CrossRef] [PubMed]
29. Stefano, A.; Vitabile, S.; Russo, G.; Ippolito, M.; Marletta, F.; D'Arrigo, C.; D'Urso, D.; Gambino, O.; Pirrone, R.; Ardizzone, E.; et al. A fully automatic method for biological target volume segmentation of brain metastases. *Int. J. Imaging Syst. Technol.* **2016**, *26*, 29–37. [CrossRef]
30. Fornacon-Wood, I.; Mistry, H.; Ackermann, C.J.; Blackhall, F.; McPartlin, A.; Faivre-Finn, C.; Price, G.J.; O'Connor, J.P.B. Reliability and prognostic value of radiomic features are highly dependent on choice of feature extraction platform. *Eur. Radiol.* **2020**, *30*, 6241–6250. [CrossRef] [PubMed]
31. Van Griethuysen, J.J.M.; Fedorov, A.; Parmar, C.; Hosny, A.; Aucoin, N.; Narayan, V.; Beets-Tan, R.G.H.; Fillion-Robin, J.C.; Pieper, S.; Aerts, H.J.W.L. Computational radiomics system to decode the radiographic phenotype. *Cancer Res.* **2017**, *77*, e104–e107. [CrossRef]
32. Akoglu, H. User's guide to correlation coefficients. *Turkish J. Emerg. Med.* **2018**, *18*, 91–93. [CrossRef]
33. Meijer, K.M. Accuracy and Stability of Radiomic Features for Characterising Tumour Heterogeneity Using Multimodality Imaging: A Phantom Study. Master's Thesis, University of Twente, Enschede, The Netherlands, 2019; pp. 1–48.
34. Lee, J.; Steinmann, A.; Ding, Y.; Lee, H.; Owens, C.; Wang, J.; Yang, J.; Followill, D.; Ger, R.; MacKin, D.; et al. Radiomics feature robustness as measured using an MRI phantom. *Sci. Rep.* **2021**, *11*, 1–14.
35. Kaalep, A.; Sera, T.; Oyen, W.; Krause, B.J.; Chiti, A.; Liu, Y.; Boellaard, R. EANM/EARL FDG-PET/CT accreditation-summary results from the first 200 accredited imaging systems. *Eur. J. Nucl. Med. Mol. Imaging* **2018**, *45*, 412. [CrossRef]

Article
Early Monitoring Response to Therapy in Patients with Brain Lesions Using the Cumulative SUV Histogram

Alessandro Stefano [1], Pietro Pisciotta [1,2,3], Marco Pometti [4,5], Albert Comelli [1,6,*], Sebastiano Cosentino [5], Francesco Marletta [5], Salvatore Cicero [5], Maria G. Sabini [2,5], Massimo Ippolito [5] and Giorgio Russo [1,2,5]

1. Institute of Molecular Bioimaging and Physiology, National Research Council (IBFM-CNR), 90015 Cefalù, Italy; alessandro.stefano@ibfm.cnr.it (A.S.); pietro.pisciotta@ibfm.cnr.it (P.P.); giorgio.russo@ibfm.cnr.it (G.R.)
2. Laboratori Nazionali del Sud, Istituto Nazionale di Fisica Nucleare, 95125 Catania, Italy; mgabsabini@gmail.com
3. University Medical Center Groningen, Department of Radiotherapy, University of Groningen, 9713 GZ Groningen, The Netherlands
4. FORA S.p.A., Via Alfred Bernhard Nobel 11/A, 43122 Parma, Italy; marco.pometti@gmail.com
5. Nuclear Medicine and NeuroRadiosurgery Departments, Cannizzaro Hospital, 95126 Catania, Italy; sebastiano.cosentino@aoec.it (S.C.); francescomarletta1@gmail.com (F.M.); cicerosalvatore@yahoo.it (S.C.); centro_pet@ospedale-cannizzaro.it (M.I.)
6. Ri.MED Foundation, Via Bandiera 11, 90133 Palermo, Italy
* Correspondence: acomelli@fondazionerimed.com; Tel.: +39-092-192-0149

Featured Application: The study proposes a methodology to evaluate the response of patients with brain lesions to Gamma Knife treatments through the use of Positron Emission Tomography imaging.

Citation: Stefano, A.; Pisciotta, P.; Pometti, M.; Comelli, A.; Cosentino, S.; Marletta, F.; Cicero, S.; Sabini, M.G.; Ippolito, M.; Russo, G. Early Monitoring Response to Therapy in Patients with Brain Lesions Using the Cumulative SUV Histogram. *Appl. Sci.* **2021**, *11*, 2999. https://doi.org/10.3390/app11072999

Academic Editor: Qi-Huang Zheng

Received: 19 February 2021
Accepted: 23 March 2021
Published: 27 March 2021

Publisher's Note: MDPI stays neutral with regard to jurisdictional claims in published maps and institutional affiliations.

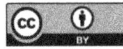

Copyright: © 2021 by the authors. Licensee MDPI, Basel, Switzerland. This article is an open access article distributed under the terms and conditions of the Creative Commons Attribution (CC BY) license (https://creativecommons.org/licenses/by/4.0/).

Abstract: Gamma Knife treatment is an alternative to traditional brain surgery and whole-brain radiation therapy for treating cancers that are inaccessible via conventional treatments. To assess the effectiveness of Gamma Knife treatments, functional imaging can play a crucial role. The aim of this study is to evaluate new prognostic indices to perform an early assessment of treatment response to therapy using positron emission tomography imaging. The parameters currently used in nuclear medicine assessments can be affected by statistical fluctuation errors and/or cannot provide information on tumor extension and heterogeneity. To overcome these limitations, the Cumulative standardized uptake value (SUV) Histogram (CSH) and Area Under the Curve (AUC) indices were evaluated to obtain additional information on treatment response. For this purpose, the absolute level of [11C]-Methionine (MET) uptake was measured and its heterogeneity distribution within lesions was evaluated by calculating the CSH and AUC indices. CSH and AUC parameters show good agreement with patient outcomes after Gamma Knife treatments. Furthermore, no relevant correlations were found between CSH and AUC indices and those usually used in the nuclear medicine environment. CSH and AUC indices could be a useful tool for assessing patient responses to therapy.

Keywords: gamma knife; imaging quantification; [11C]-methionine positron emission tomography; cancer

1. Introduction

The Leksell Gamma Knife (GK) is a stereotactic radio surgical device capable of treating brain tumors inaccessible to conventional surgery by allowing accurate target irradiation. It is a minimally invasive instrument that does not involve a scalpel or incision [1,2]. Tumor delineation is the crucial step when planning GK treatment because metastatic lesions can show infiltrative natures. Magnetic resonance (MR) is usually used to perform accurate delineation of the target volume. MR provides high-quality images with excellent soft-tissue contrast [3–6]. With the aim of adding another layer of sophistication during radiosurgery, the integration of positron emission tomography (PET) images in the treatment planning phase was evaluated [7–9]. Functional information improves lesion knowledge, as demonstrated by Gempt et al. [10]. The biological tumor volume (BTV) identified by PET can be used to treat the cancer region more precisely [11]. Furthermore, PET imaging has become a standard component of diagnosis and staging in oncology [12–16]. Functional changes are often faster and more indicative of the effects caused by therapy than anatomical imaging, providing a faster method of detecting the treatment response [17,18]. Levivier et al. [19] found that PET conveys complementary information to information derived from computerized tomography (CT) or MR imaging in brain disorders. Historically, the first parameter introduced for the evaluation of PET studies is the maximum standardized uptake value (SUV_{max}), which provides punctual information of the voxel showing the highest uptake value within the tumor. Nevertheless, this parameter can be affected by statistical fluctuation errors and cannot provide information on the extent of the tumor [20]. For this reason, other quantitative indices have been introduced, such as metabolic tumor volume (MTV) and total lesion glycolysis (TLG) [21]. These parameters provide information on the extent of the tumor but no information on the uptake heterogeneity.

To overcome these limitations and considering that the dose distribution is not uniform in GK treatments, sixteen patients underwent [^{11}C]-Methionine (MET) PET scans and GK treatments were considered in this study to calculate new PET indices, such as the Cumulative SUV Histogram (CSH) and Area Under the Curve (AUC), in order to obtain additional PET information, such as the functional heterogeneity [22]. In other words, we focus on the [^{11}C]-MET uptake heterogeneity in pre- and post-treatment PET examinations by calculating CSH and AUC for each patient. Methionine is an amino acid that exhibits increased transport within active cancer cells. It has been reported that the extent of tumor cell invasion can be more clearly detected by [^{11}C]-MET PET than by CT or MR [23]. The correlation between CSH and AUC results with medical reports evaluated by three physicians was also considered in our study. The proposed methodology could represent a useful tool for assessing patient response to GK treatments.

2. Materials and Methods

2.1. Patients

We retrospectively analyzed patients with metastatic brain cancers who underwent restaging PET/CT after GK between March 2014 and December 2015. The inclusion criteria were as follows: (i) [^{11}C]-MET PET/CT performed one week before stereotactic neuro-radiosurgery, (ii) [^{11}C]-MET PET/CT performed two months after stereotactic neuro-radiosurgery for the early treatment assessment, and (iii) MR performed one year after stereotactic neuro-radiosurgery to assess the treatment response. In this way, sixteen patients (8 males, 8 females; mean age ± standard deviation: 60 ± 9.80 years; median age: 57 years; age range: 48 ÷ 78 years) with metastatic brain cancers originating from melanoma ($n = 2$), breast ($n = 2$), kidney ($n = 2$), lung ($n = 9$), and urothelium ($n = 1$) primary cancers were considered.

All subjects were treated with Leksell Gamma Knife® model C, a mini-invasive technique for the treatment of cerebral lesions inaccessible to conventional surgery [24,25]. The dose released during treatment in a single fraction ranged from 16 to 18 Gy at 50% isodose. The qualitative evaluation of the treatment response was carried out by a team of three physicians (S.C., Sebastiano Cosentino, F.M., and S.C., Salvatore Cicero). The clinical staff jointly analyzed brain tumors without any information of the quantitative evaluation performed in this study. Comparing their perspectives, physicians were able to provide a careful assessment for each case.

This study was not a clinical trial but a retrospective study that did not influence management of patients. Image analyses were performed offline. In any case, the informed consent to the processing of personal data was obtained from all the subjects involved in the study.

2.2. [^{11}C]-Methionine PET (MET)

Methionine is the most popular amino acid tracer used in PET imaging. It has a potential role in providing additional information in brain studies, although MR remains the gold-standard for diagnosis and follow-up evaluations after radiotherapy [26,27]. Cell proliferation in brain tumors is associated with protein synthesis and since the amino acids are protein constituents, avid uptake of these precursors indicates a rapidly proliferating cell. As a consequence, an increase in amino acid transport and protein synthesis, compared to normal tissue, indicates the presence of tumor proliferation. For this reason, MET-PET is able to distinguish between malign and benign tissue with great sensitivity and specificity. The MET-PET specificity for cancer delineation and differentiation between relapse and radiation necrosis is higher than MR [28].

Since C-11 isotope has a short half-life (20.3 min) [29], on-site production of MET is essential to perform diagnostic scans. An IBA cyclotron 18 MeV was used to produce C-11. To ensure compatibility with in vivo administration, the final product was subjected to quality control according to European Pharmacopoeia. Radiochemical and enantiomeric purity, higher than 95% and 90%, respectively, were assessed by radio-HPLC-UV, while residual solvents were evaluated by gas chromatography.

2.3. PET/CT

PET brain acquisitions were performed using the PET/CT Discovery 690 with time of flight (TOF) by General Electric Medical Systems (Milwaukee, WI, USA). Patients fasted for 4 hours before PET examination and were injected intravenously with MET. The PET protocol started 10 minutes after injection. PET images consisted of a matrix of 256×256 voxels of $1.1719 \times 1.1719 \times 3.27$ mm^3 voxel size. Imaging data were encoded in the 16-bit Digital Imaging and Communications in Medicine (DICOM) format. The activity of MET administered to patients was 550 MBq.

2.4. PET Feature-Based Measures

Similar to the dose–volume histogram (DVH), which is the radiation dose histogram for tumor treatment [30], the CSH uses the SUV derived from PET imaging instead of the dose value derived from CT imaging. Specifically, the SUV is the widely used PET semiquantitative parameter calculated as the ratio of the tissue radioactivity concentration (RC) in kBq/mL and the MET injected dose (ID) in MBq at the time of injection divided by the body weight in kilograms [31]:

$$SUV = \frac{RC}{ID} \times M_p \qquad (1)$$

where RC is calculated as the ratio between the image intensity and the image scale factor. ID is the product between actual activity and dose calibration factor. Therefore, in the case of PET imaging, the image intensity values were normalized in SUVs. While the SUV$_{mean}$ is the mean intensity value in the region of interest (ROI), the SUV$_{max}$ is defined as the voxel with the highest SUV within a specified ROI. It is the most common PET parameter because it is both a ROI and user independent [32]. A disadvantage is that it represents a small portion of the tumor that may not be a statistically reliable representation of the whole-tumor biology. It does not take into account the SUV distribution within the tumor. Starting from these considerations, the CSH is the representation of the percentage of the tumor volume with a certain SUV [22,33]. The CSH summarizes the 3D functional imaging intensity information in a single curve for the structure of interest, which will be used to derive intensity-volume metrics, such as the area under the CSH (AUC) to take into account the tumor uptake heterogeneity [22] (see Figure 1 for an example of CSH and AUC). In this way, it is possible to analyze changes in the uptake distribution within the tumor due to nonuniform dose distribution during GK treatments. Finally, in addition to the aforementioned PET feature-based measures, MTV and TLG were also calculated [21]. These parameters provide information on the tumor extension but no information on the uptake heterogeneity. MTV is the active volume of oncological lesions obtained using a segmentation algorithm, e.g., [34,35], while TLG was calculated to acquire a simultaneous estimate of volumetric and metabolic information:

$$TLG = MTV \times SUV_{mean} \tag{2}$$

Consequently, TLG is also a segmentation-dependent parameter.

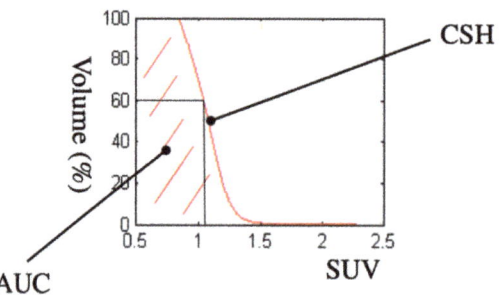

Figure 1. An example of Cumulative standardized uptake value (SUV) Histogram (CSH) and Area Under the Curve (AUC). CSH shows the percentage of the tumor volume with a certain SUV. For example, the 60% of the tumor has a SUV > 1.

2.5. Data Analysis

For the purpose of treatment response monitoring, the quantitative assessment of PET studies before and after treatment can become the standard. In general, however, the uptake of PET radiotracers is not homogeneously distributed across the tumor due to necrosis, cell proliferation, blood flow, microvessel density, and hypoxia [22]. For this reason, it is interesting to quantify heterogeneity in tumor uptake to provide useful information for planning radiation therapy treatment. The area under the CSH can be a quantitative parameter capable of providing additional information on the tumor response and its heterogeneity. Lower values correspond to greater heterogeneity.

To evaluate this innovative PET parameter in the evaluation of the treatment response, we analyzed PET images using a semiautomatic MATLAB tool [36] to reduce intra- and interoperator result variability. As a matter of fact, semiautomatic algorithms provide greater accuracy and consistency in defining PET volumes and they are important to quantify the response to therapy. In our tool, the operator dependence is minimal because it is limited to the change in the size of the bounding area containing the cancer region—no parameter setup is required.

In the following, a brief explanation of the processing steps is presented. The user draws a line on the coronal PET image along the lesion, and the axial slice with SUV_{max} is automatically identified and showed to the user. To manage ambiguous situations, physicians can make corrections to the volume of interest (VOI), including the tumor region, obtained as described in [36]. After a square bounding region enclosing the tumor is shown, the user can reduce the region size to discard any external area with high uptake to target. This approach allows the proper inclusion of cancer, excluding false positives. Furthermore, the number of PET slices containing the tumor in basal examinations is recorded to process the same slice volume in post-GK treatment examinations. In this way, the proposed tool is designed ad hoc to appropriately compare cumulative histograms between follow-up scans. According to the literature [19], the SUV threshold was set at 50% of SUV_{max} and the area under the CSH curve was considered as a quantitative index of the MET uptake heterogeneity within the lesion volume. Figure 2 outlines the overall flow diagram of the proposed approach.

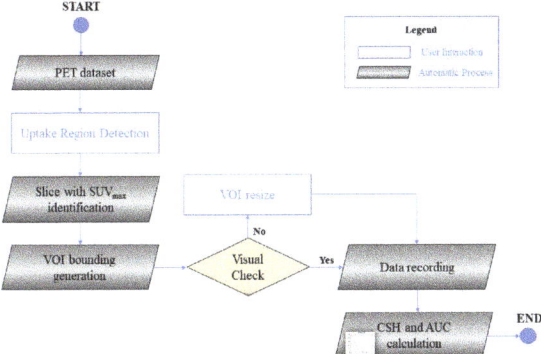

Figure 2. Flow diagram of the proposed semiautomatic approach to calculate CSH and AUC parameters. Adopted graphical and color notations are explained in the legend box.

In order to evaluate the ablation effect, the percentage change of AUC between pre- and post-treatment periods was obtained as follows:

$$\Delta AUC = \frac{AUC_{post} - AUC_{pre}}{AUC_{pre}} \quad (3)$$

AUC variation was analyzed and its correlation with the patients' outcomes was studied. Three outcome classes, based on variation of AUC and on shifting of CSH curve, were identified: positive response, stable response, and negative response. Figure 3 shows the workflow of the proposed study used to compare PET studies before and after GK treatment.

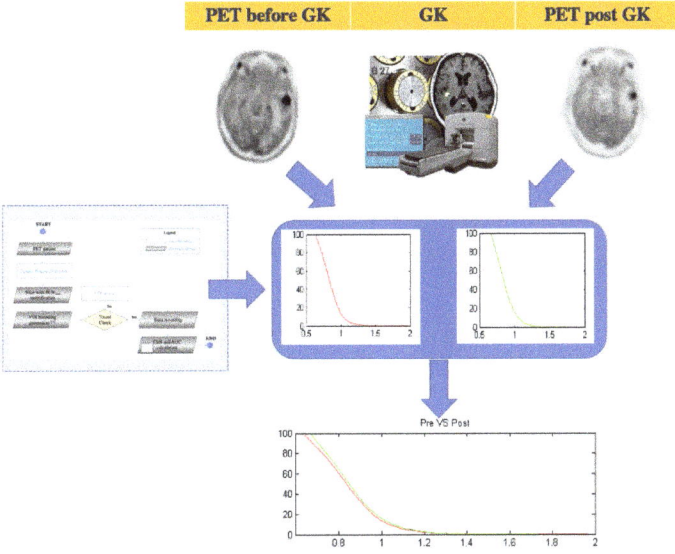

Figure 3. The workflow of the proposed study.

2.6. Statistical Analysis

Statistical analyses were performed to assess whether ΔAUC provides additional information compared to the other PET parameters (ΔMTV, ΔSUV$_{max}$, ΔSUV$_{mean}$ and ΔTLG). For this reason, the Pearson correlation coefficient (r) between ΔAUC and the aforementioned prognostic indices was computed as:

$$r = \frac{COV(X,Y)}{\sigma X \sigma Y} \quad (4)$$

where COV is covariance, σX is the standard deviation of X and σY is the standard deviation of Y. The Pearson correlation coefficient ranged between +1 and −1, where +1 and −1 show total correlation (no difference between ΔAUC and the aforementioned prognostic indices), 0 is no correlation (total difference between ΔAUC and the aforementioned prognostic indices). Consequently, the determination coefficient (R^2) was calculated as:

$$R^2 = r^2 \quad (5)$$

In this way, R^2 ranges from 0 to 1. $R^2 = 0$ means that the dependent variable cannot be predicted by the independent variable. Finally, the paired *t*-test was used to determine whether a result is statistically significant. Particularly, the *t*-test was used to determine whether the correlation coefficient is significantly equal to zero, hence there is no evidence of an association between ΔAUC and the aforementioned indices.

3. Results

A total of 16 patients were involved in this study. All subjects were treated with the Leksell Gamma Knife Model C and they underwent PET/CT Discovery 690 with TOF (GE Medical Systems) before and after the treatment. For basal studies, tumor size ranged from 0.25 to 10.56 cm^3 (mean ± standard deviation: 2.83 ± 2.41 cm^3) with a SUV$_{max}$ between 1.6 and 6.84 (mean ± standard deviation: 3.91 ± 1.57). In follow-up studies, tumor size ranged from 0 (complete response) to 12.02 cm^3 (mean ± standard deviation: 2.40 ± 2.96 cm^3) with a SUV$_{max}$ between 0 (complete response) and 4.6 (mean ± standard deviation: 2.81 ± 1.17). Changes (Δ) in AUC, SUV$_{max}$, SUV$_{mean}$, MTV and TLG between baseline and follow-up scans and medical reports performed by the three nuclear medicine physicians are shown in Table 1 for each patient.

Table 1. Positron emission tomography (PET) parameter variations (%) between pre- and post-Gamma Knife (GK) treatment.

Patient N.	ΔAUC	ΔMTV	ΔSUV$_{max}$	ΔSUV$_{mean}$	ΔTLG	Physician Report
#1	2.33	13.87	−12.63	−12.18	0.05	Stable
#2	−38.62	18.80	−32.72	−25.73	−11.77	Improvement
#3	−59.05	0.12	−47.66	−33.56	−33.48	Improvement
#4	−17.43	−62.72	−20.23	−5.91	−64.93	Improvement
#5	−57.59	−81.16	−41.83	−14.34	−83.86	Improvement
#6	−36.42	24.85	−44.36	−40.85	−26.15	Improvement
#7	8.62	−16.90	9.47	10.10	−8.50	Worsening
#8	16	−100	−100	−100	−100	Complete Response
#9	−11.22	7.73	−2.29	−5.56	1.73	Stable
#10	−4.61	−13.27	−11.28	3.08	−10.60	Stable
#11	−30.37	−31.53	−26.21	−17.96	−43.83	Improvement

Table 1. Cont.

Patient N.	ΔAUC	ΔMTV	ΔSUV$_{max}$	ΔSUV$_{mean}$	ΔTLG	Physician Report
#12	−13.07	14.14	−22.74	−17.40	−5.72	Improvement
#13	−23.03	−94.29	−34.64	−10.65	−94.90	Improvement
#14	−25.48	−62.20	−30.11	−11.82	−66.67	Improvement
#15	1.88	−61.12	−1.00	4.34	−59.43	Stable
#16	−6.11	−5.06	−33.55	−13.41	−17.80	Stable

Starting from an exploratory analysis of PET parameters to understand if ΔAUC could actually provide further information to other PET parameters, Pearson correlation coefficients (r) between ΔAUC and the aforementioned prognostic indices were computed. ΔMTV, ΔSUV$_{max}$, ΔSUV$_{mean}$, and ΔTLG were not highly correlated with ΔAUC (see Figure 4). The determination coefficients (R^2) were low, demonstrating a low correlation between considered measures. As a result, it can be affirmed that ΔAUC provides additional information than other PET parameters. The paired t-test showed a p-value greater than 0.05 in all cases, so there is no evidence of an association between ΔAUC and the aforementioned indices. Finally, three outcome classes were identified based on the variation of AUC and on the shifting of the CSH curve: positive response, stable response, and negative response, as shown in Figure 5.

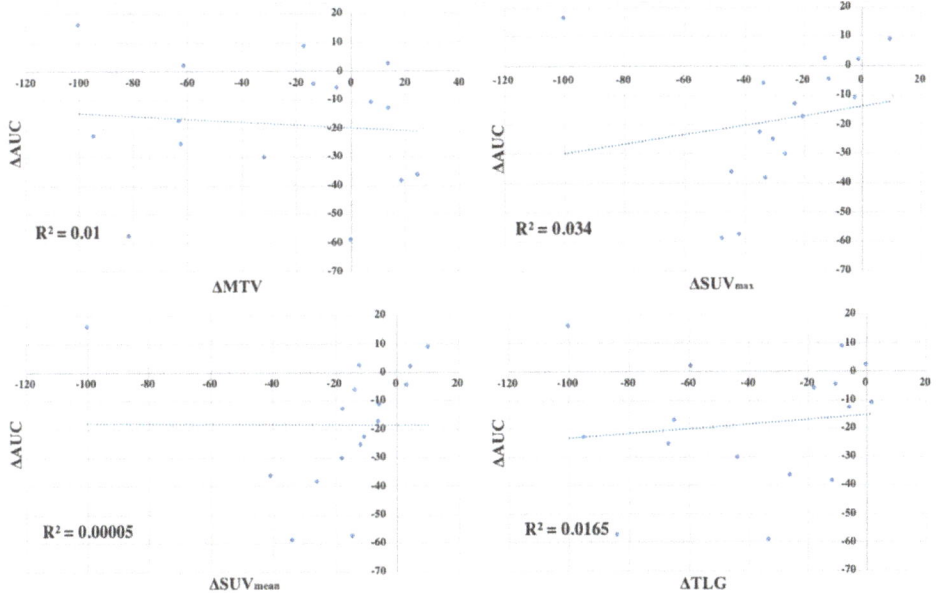

Figure 4. Correlation between ΔAUC and Δmetabolic tumor volume (ΔMTV), ΔSUV$_{max}$, ΔSUV$_{mean}$, and Δtotal lesion glycolysis (ΔTLG).

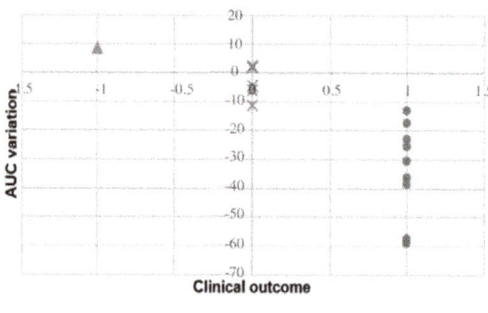

Figure 5. AUC variation correlated to patients' outcomes.

3.1. Positive Response

Nine patients who showed positive responses to treatment show a reduction in the AUC greater than about 10% and a shifting of the CSH to the left, as is possible to see in Figure 6 (patient #3). Patients included in this category show a marked response to the therapy. In particular, all cases show a reduction in the MET uptake (as can be seen in Table 1, where ΔSUV_{mean} is always negative), indicating a probable formation of necrotic areas.

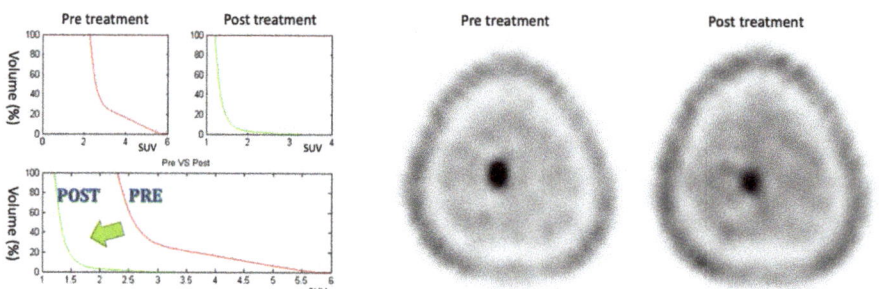

Figure 6. On the left: CSH pretreatment (top left); CSH post-treatment (top right); comparison between pre- and post-treatment (bottom) in positive response case: $\Delta AUC = -59.05\%$. On the right: PET images of pre- and post-treatment. (For interpretation of the references in colour in this figure legend, the reader is referred to the web version of this article.)

3.2. Stable Response

The five patients included in this class show a AUC reduction of less than 10% and no modification of the CSH between the PET pretreatment and the PET post-treatment, as it is possible to see in Figure 7 (patient #1). Patients included in this category show a moderate response to the therapy.

3.3. Negative Response

The patient included in this class shows an increasing AUC and a right shifting of CSH, as it is possible to see in Figure 8 (patient #7). The patient included in this category worsened following therapy.

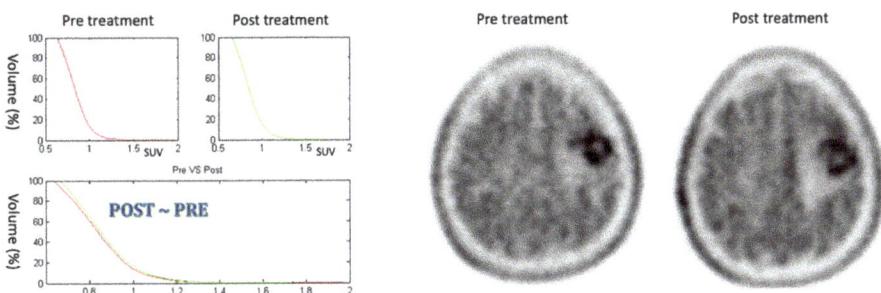

Figure 7. On the left: CSH pretreatment (top left); CSH post-treatment (top right); comparison between pre- and post-treatment (bottom) in stable response case: ΔAUC = 2.33%. On the right: PET images of pre- and post-treatment. (For interpretation of the references in this figure legend in colour, the reader is referred to the web version of this article.)

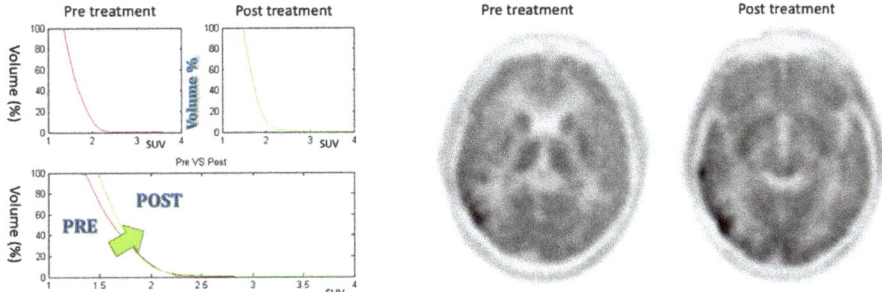

Figure 8. On the left: CSH pretreatment (top left); CSH post-treatment (top right); comparison between pre- and post-treatment (bottom) in negative response case: ΔAUC = 8.62%. On the right: PET images of pre- and post-treatment. (For interpretation of the references to colour in this figure legend, the reader is referred to the web version of this article.)

4. Discussion

The conventional parameters used in the nuclear medicine environment, such as the SUV_{max}, can be affected by statistical fluctuation errors and cannot provide information on the tumor extension and heterogeneity. The other parameters introduced to resolve these limitations have some limitations related to partial volume effect [32] and to the segmentation method chosen to identify the tumor area [37]. TLG is the first parameter that can provide both anatomical and metabolic information. It is calculated by performing a multiplication of SUV_{mean} with the MTV value. Nevertheless, TLG does not take into account the SUV distribution within the VOI.

New parameters were proposed, such as CSH and AUC, in order to provide information about the absolute uptake, the radiotracer distribution, and the lesion dimension [22,33,38,39]. The histograms are similar to DVH used in radiotherapy [30]. The CSH is a cumulative histogram that shows the percentage of the lesion volume with the same SUV. It takes into account the distribution of SUV within the tumor volume. The AUC consists of the value of the area under the histogram curve and can be a quantitative index of tracer uptake heterogeneity or homogeneity tumor response [22].

The aim of this work was to assess these new prognostic indices in order to perform an early assessment of the treatment response to therapy using MET-PET images. The strength of these new parameters is that they can potentially take into account the SUV distribution within the tumor area voxel by voxel and not only a single one, as is the case when using SUV_{max} or a single mean value, i.e., the SUV_{mean}, which does not take into account the tumor heterogeneity. No relevant correlation was found between AUC and other parameters usually used in the nuclear medicine environment. Furthermore, the CSH and AUC parameters showed a good agreement with the patient follow-up after GK treatments. Changes in AUC between baseline and follow-up scans could indicate an increase in necrotic tissue tumour after treatment [22]. In our study, the proposed classification (positive, stable, and negative response) found a good agreement with the patient outcome evaluated by three physicians. In particular, nine patients with a positive response to the treatment showed a reduction in AUC—lower AUC values correspond to greater heterogeneity, which can be associated with an increase in the necrotic tissue, as well as the corresponding MET uptake reduction in the follow-up scans.

Conversely, an increase in heterogeneity (positive ΔAUC) can indicate a negative response to therapy. As a result, AUC represents a potential clinical index for an early assessment of the treatment response. In fact, functional changes are faster to identify the therapy response than anatomical imaging (CT or MRI). However, the current clinical methodology in nuclear medicine departments is limited to visual assessment or uptake value measurements, such as SUV_{max}. Our preliminary results suggest that the proposed parameters could provide better discriminating power for the use of PET imaging in radiotherapy or chemotherapy. These parameters may be incorporated into the planning process to modify patient management. For example, this could be carried out by intensifying chemotherapy treatment after radiotherapy for high-risk patients showing negative responses or providing less toxic regimens for patients at lower risk; in the age of radiomics [40,41], it is mandatory to find the most relevant quantitative features in monitoring or predicting the patient's response to cancer therapy. Further studies are needed to evaluate the proposed PET parameters in depth and enlarge the number of patients involved, as well as improve statistics to validate the patient outcome classes identified in our work.

5. Conclusions

CSH and AUC could be new functional parameters useful for evaluating treatment response considering the heterogeneity information provided by PET studies. An innovative method to monitor the patient's treatment response could be developed to alter patient management in the early stages to maximize results of therapy from the perspective of personalized medicine.

Author Contributions: Conceptualization, A.S.; Data curation, A.S., S.C. (Sebastiano Cosentino), F.M., and S.C. (Salvatore Cicero); Formal analysis, A.S. and P.P.; Funding acquisition, A.S. and A.C.; Investigation; A.S.; Methodology, A.S.; Project administration, A.S.; Resources, P.P. and M.G.S.; Software, A.S.; Supervision, G.R. and M.I.; Validation, P.P.; Visualization, A.S., A.C., and M.P.; Writing—original draft, A.S. and P.P.; Writing—review and editing, A.S., A.C., and M.P. All authors have read and agreed to the published version of the manuscript.

Funding: This research received no external funding.

Institutional Review Board Statement: The proposed research has no implication on patient treatment. Review board approval was not sought: the proposed image analysis was performed offline and thus did not change the current treatment protocol.

Informed Consent Statement: Informed consent was obtained from all subjects involved in the study.

Data Availability Statement: Data sharing not applicable.

Acknowledgments: Authors would like to thank Giovanni Borasi and Lucia M. Valastro for their crucial help in the management of the proposed study.

Conflicts of Interest: The authors declare no conflict of interest. The funders had no role in the design of the study; in the collection, analyses, or interpretation of data; in the writing of the manuscript; or in the decision to publish the results.

References

1. Moskvin, V.; DesRosiers, C.; Papiez, L.; Timmerman, R.; Randall, M.; DesRosiers, P.; Dittmer, P. Monte Carlo simulation of the Leksell Gamma Knife: I. Source modelling and calculations in homogeneous media. *Phys. Med. Biol.* **2002**, *47*, 301. [CrossRef]
2. Wu, A. Physics and dosimetry of the gamma knife. *Neurosurg. Clin. N. Am.* **1992**, *3*, 35–50. [CrossRef]
3. Khoo, V.S.; Joon, D.L. New developments in MRI for target volume delineation in radiotherapy. *Br. J. Radiol.* **2006**, *79*, S2–S15. [CrossRef]
4. Bol, G.H.; Kotte, A.N.T.J.; van der Heide, U.A.; Lagendijk, J.J.W. Simultaneous multi-modality ROI delineation in clinical practice. *Comput. Methods Programs Biomed.* **2009**, *96*, 133–140. [CrossRef] [PubMed]
5. Cuocolo, R.; Cipullo, M.B.; Stanzione, A.; Ugga, L.; Romeo, V.; Radice, L.; Brunetti, A.; Imbriaco, M. Machine learning applications in prostate cancer magnetic resonance imaging. *Eur. Radiol. Exp.* **2019**, *3*, 35. [CrossRef]
6. Comelli, A.; Terranova, M.C.; Scopelliti, L.; Salerno, S.; Midiri, F.; Lo Re, G.; Petrucci, G.; Vitabile, S. A kernel support vector machine based technique for Crohn's disease classification in human patients. In *Advances in Intelligent Systems and Computing*; Springer: Cham, Switzerland, 2018; Volume 611, pp. 262–273, ISBN 9783319615653.
7. Comelli, A.; Stefano, A.; Russo, G.; Bignardi, S.; Sabini, M.G.; Petrucci, G.; Ippolito, M.; Yezzi, A. K-nearest neighbor driving active contours to delineate biological tumor volumes. *Eng. Appl. Artif. Intell.* **2019**, *81*, 133–144. [CrossRef]
8. Comelli, A.; Stefano, A. A Fully Automated Segmentation System of Positron Emission Tomography Studies. In *Medical Image Understanding and Analysis*; Zheng, Y., Williams, B.M., Chen, K., Eds.; Communications in Computer and Information Science; Springer: Cham, Switzerland, 2020; Volume 1065, pp. 353–363.
9. Comelli, A.; Stefano, A.; Bignardi, S.; Coronnello, C.; Russo, G.; Sabini, M.G.; Ippolito, M.; Yezzi, A. Tissue Classification to Support Local Active Delineation of Brain Tumors. In *Medical Image Understanding and Analysis*; Zheng, Y., Williams, B.M., Chen, K., Eds.; Communications in Computer and Information Science; Springer: Cham, Switzerland, 2020; Volume 1065, pp. 3–14.
10. Gempt, J.; Bette, S.; Buchmann, N.; Ryang, Y.-M.; Förschler, A.; Pyka, T.; Wester, H.-J.; Förster, S.; Meyer, B.; Ringel, F. Volumetric Analysis of F-18-FET-PET Imaging for Brain Metastases. *World Neurosurg.* **2015**, *84*, 1790–1797. [CrossRef]
11. Stefano, A.; Vitabile, S.; Russo, G.; Ippolito, M.; Marletta, F.; D'Arrigo, C.; D'Urso, D.; Sabini, M.G.; Gambino, O.; Pirrone, R.; et al. An automatic method for metabolic evaluation of gamma knife treatments. In *Image Analysis and Processing—ICIAP 2015*; Lecture Notes in Computer Science; Springer: Cham, Switzerland, 2015; Volume 9279, pp. 579–589.
12. Weber, W.A.; Grosu, A.L.; Czernin, J. Technology Insight: Advances in molecular imaging and an appraisal of PET/CT scanning. *Nat. Clin. Pract. Oncol.* **2008**, *5*, 160–170. [CrossRef] [PubMed]
13. Fletcher, J.W.; Djulbegovic, B.; Soares, H.P.; Siegel, B.A.; Lowe, V.J.; Lyman, G.H.; Coleman, R.E.; Wahl, R.; Paschold, J.C.; Avril, N.; et al. Recommendations on the use of 18F-FDG PET in oncology. *J. Nucl. Med.* **2008**, *49*, 480–508. [CrossRef] [PubMed]
14. Stefano, A.; Porcino, N.; Banna, G.; Russoa, G.; Mocciaro, V.; Anile, G.; Gieri, S.; Cosentino, S.; Murè, G.; Baldari, S.; et al. Metabolic response assessment in non-small cell lung cancer patients after platinum-based therapy: A preliminary analysis. *Curr. Med. Imaging Rev.* **2015**, *11*, 218–227. [CrossRef]
15. Banna, G.L.; Anile, G.; Russo, G.; Vigneri, P.; Castaing, M.; Nicolosi, M.; Strano, S.; Gieri, S.; Spina, R.; Patanè, D.; et al. Predictive and Prognostic Value of Early Disease Progression by PET Evaluation in Advanced Non-Small Cell Lung Cancer. *Oncology* **2017**, *92*, 39–47. [CrossRef] [PubMed]
16. Cegla, P.; Kazmierska, J.; Gwozdz, S.; Czepczynski, R.; Malicki, J.; Cholewinski, W. Assessment of biological parameters in head and neck cancer based on in vivo distribution of 18F-FDG-FLT-FMISO-PET/CT images. *Tumori* **2019**, *106*, 33–38. [CrossRef]
17. Wahl, R.L.; Jacene, H.; Kasamon, Y.; Lodge, M.A. From RECIST to PERCIST: Evolving Considerations for PET response criteria in solid tumors. *J. Nucl. Med.* **2009**, *50* (Suppl. 1), 122S–150S. [CrossRef]
18. Borasi, G.; Russo, G.; Alongi, F.; Nahum, A.; Candiano, G.; Stefano, A.; Gilardi, M.C.; Messa, C. Radiotherapy and High Intensity Focused Ultrasound in Oncology: Competition or integration? A future scenario. *J. Ther. Ultrasound* **2013**, *1*, 6. [CrossRef]
19. Levivier, M.; Wikier, D.; Goldman, S.; David, P.; Metens, T.; Massager, N.; Gerosa, M.; Devriendt, D.; Desmedt, F.; Simon, S.; et al. Integration of the metabolic data of positron emission tomography in the dosimetry planning of radiosurgery with the gamma knife: Early experience with brain tumors. Technical note. *J. Neurosurg.* **2000**, *93* (Suppl. 3), 233–238. [CrossRef]
20. Stefano, A.L.; Gallivanone, F.; Messa, C.L.; Gilardi, M.C.L.; Castiglioni, I. Metabolic impact of Partial Volume Correction of [18F]FDG PET-CT oncological studies on the assessment of tumor response to treatment. *Q. J. Nucl. Med. Mol. Imaging* **2014**, *58*, 413–423. [PubMed]
21. D'Urso, D.; Stefano, A.; Romano, A.; Russo, G.; Cosentino, S.; Fallanca, F.; Gioe, M.; Attanasio, M.; Sabini, M.G.; Di Raimondo, F.; et al. Analysis of Metabolic Parameters Coming from Basal and Interim PET in Hodgkin Lymphoma. *Curr. Med. Imaging Rev.* **2017**, *14*, 533–544. [CrossRef]
22. van Velden, F.H.P.; Cheebsumon, P.; Yaqub, M.; Smit, E.F.; Hoekstra, O.S.; Lammertsma, A.A.; Boellaard, R. Evaluation of a cumulative SUV-volume histogram method for parameterizing heterogeneous intratumoural FDG uptake in non-small cell lung cancer PET studies. *Eur. J. Nucl. Med. Mol. Imaging* **2011**, *38*, 1636–1647. [CrossRef]
23. Nariai, T.; Tanaka, Y.; Wakimoto, H.; Aoyagi, M.; Tamaki, M.; Ishiwata, K.; Senda, M.; Ishii, K.; Hirakawa, K.; Ohno, K. Usefulness of L-[methyl-^{11}C] methionine—Positron emission tomography as a biological monitoring tool in the treatment of glioma. *J. Neurosurg.* **2005**, *103*, 498–507. [CrossRef] [PubMed]

24. Stefano, A.; Vitabile, S.; Russo, G.; Ippolito, M.; Sardina, D.; Sabini, M.G.; Gallivanone, F.; Castiglioni, I.; Gilardi, M.C. A Graph-Based Method for PET Image Segmentation in Radiotherapy Planning: A Pilot Study. In *Image Analysis and Processing—ICIAP 2013*; Lecture Notes in Computer Science; Springer: Berlin/Heidelberg, Germany, 2013; pp. 711–720.
25. Stefano, A.; Comelli, A.; Bravatà, V.; Barone, S.; Daskalovski, I.; Savoca, G.; Sabini, M.G.; Ippolito, M.; Russo, G. A preliminary PET radiomics study of brain metastases using a fully automatic segmentation method. *BMC Bioinform.* **2020**, *21*, 325. [CrossRef] [PubMed]
26. Miwa, K.; Matsuo, M.; Shinoda, J.; Aki, T.; Yonezawa, S.; Ito, T.; Asano, Y.; Yamada, M.; Yokoyama, K.; Yamada, J.; et al. Clinical Value of [11C]Methionine PET for Stereotactic Radiation Therapy With Intensity Modulated Radiation Therapy to Metastatic Brain Tumors. *Int. J. Radiat. Oncol.* **2012**, *84*, 1139–1144. [CrossRef] [PubMed]
27. Grosu, A.L.; Weber, W.a.; Riedel, E.; Jeremic, B.; Nieder, C.; Franz, M.; Gumprecht, H.; Jaeger, R.; Schwaiger, M.; Molls, M. L-(methyl-11C) methionine positron emission tomography for target delineation in resected high-grade gliomas before radiotherapy. *Int. J. Radiat. Oncol. Biol. Phys.* **2005**, *63*, 64–74. [CrossRef] [PubMed]
28. Grosu, A.L.; Weber, W.A.; Franz, M.; Stärk, S.; Piert, M.; Thamm, R.; Gumprecht, H.; Schwaiger, M.; Molls, M.; Nieder, C. Reirradiation of recurrent high-grade gliomas using amino acid PET (SPECT)/CT/MRI image fusion to determine gross tumor volume for stereotactic fractionated radiotherapy. *Int. J. Radiat. Oncol.* **2005**, *63*, 511–519. [CrossRef]
29. Tu, Z.; Mach, R.H. C-11 Radiochemistry in Cancer Imaging Applications. *Curr. Top. Med. Chem.* **2010**, *10*, 1060–1095. [CrossRef] [PubMed]
30. Drzymala, R.E.; Mohan, R.; Brewster, L.; Chu, J.; Goitein, M.; Harms, W.; Urie, M. Dose-volume histograms. *Int. J. Radiat. Oncol.* **1991**, *21*, 71–78. [CrossRef]
31. Stefano, A.; Vitabile, S.; Russo, G.; Ippolito, M.; Marletta, F.; D'Arrigo, C.; D'Urso, D.; Gambino, O.; Pirrone, R.; Ardizzone, E.; et al. A fully automatic method for biological target volume segmentation of brain metastases. *Int. J. Imaging Syst. Technol.* **2016**, *26*, 29–37. [CrossRef]
32. Soret, M.; Bacharach, S.L.; Buvat, I.I. Partial-volume effect in PET tumor imaging. *J. Nucl. Med.* **2007**, *48*, 932–945. [CrossRef] [PubMed]
33. El Naqa, I.; Grigsby, P.; Apte, A.; Kidd, E.; Donnelly, E.; Khullar, D.; Chaudhari, S.; Yang, D.; Schmitt, M.; Laforest, R.; et al. Exploring feature-based approaches in PET images for predicting cancer treatment outcomes. *Pattern Recognit.* **2009**, *42*, 1162–1171. [CrossRef] [PubMed]
34. Stefano, A.; Vitabile, S.; Russo, G.; D'Urso, D.; Ippolito, M.; Marletta, F.; Sabini, M.G.; Patti, I.V.; Pittera, S.; Sardina, D.; et al. Biological target volume segmentation for radiotherapy treatment planning. *Phys. Medica* **2016**, *32*, 64. [CrossRef]
35. Comelli, A.; Bignardi, S.; Stefano, A.; Russo, G.; Sabini, M.G.; Ippolito, M.; Yezzi, A. Development of a new fully three-dimensional methodology for tumours delineation in functional images. *Comput. Biol. Med.* **2020**, *120*, 103701. [CrossRef] [PubMed]
36. Comelli, A.; Stefano, A.; Russo, G.; Sabini, M.G.; Ippolito, M.; Bignardi, S.; Petrucci, G.; Yezzi, A. A smart and operator independent system to delineate tumours in Positron Emission Tomography scans. *Comput. Biol. Med.* **2018**, *102*, 1–15. [CrossRef] [PubMed]
37. Comelli, A.; Stefano, A.; Benfante, V.; Russo, G. Normal and Abnormal Tissue Classification in Positron Emission Tomography Oncological Studies. *Pattern Recognit. Image Anal.* **2018**, *28*, 106–113. [CrossRef]
38. Kang, S.R.; Song, H.C.; Byun, B.H.; Oh, J.R.; Kim, H.S.; Hong, S.P.; Kwon, S.Y.; Chong, A.; Kim, J.; Cho, S.G.; et al. Intratumoral Metabolic Heterogeneity for Prediction of Disease Progression After Concurrent Chemoradiotherapy in Patients with Inoperable Stage III Non-Small-Cell Lung Cancer. *Nucl. Med. Mol. Imaging (2010)* **2014**, *48*, 16–25. [CrossRef] [PubMed]
39. Takeshita, T.; Morita, K.; Tsutsui, Y.; Kidera, D.; Mikasa, S.; Maebatake, A.; Akamatsu, G.; Miwa, K.; Baba, S.; Sasaki, M. The influence of respiratory motion on the cumulative SUV-volume histogram and fractal analyses of intratumoral heterogeneity in PET/CT imaging. *Ann. Nucl. Med.* **2016**, *30*, 393–399. [CrossRef] [PubMed]
40. Stefano, A.; Gioè, M.; Russo, G.; Palmucci, S.; Torrisi, S.E.; Bignardi, S.; Basile, A.; Comelli, A.; Benfante, V.; Sambataro, G.; et al. Performance of Radiomics Features in the Quantification of Idiopathic Pulmonary Fibrosis from HRCT. *Diagnostics* **2020**, *10*, 306. [CrossRef] [PubMed]
41. Comelli, A.; Stefano, A.; Coronnello, C.; Russo, G.; Vernuccio, F.; Cannella, R.; Salvaggio, G.; Lagalla, R.; Barone, S. Radiomics: A New Biomedical Workflow to Create a Predictive Model. In *Medical Image Understanding and Analysis*; Communications in Computer and Information Science; Springer: Cham, Switzerland, 2020; pp. 280–293.

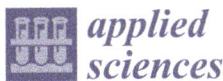

Article

ZFTool: A Software for Automatic Quantification of Cancer Cell Mass Evolution in Zebrafish

María J. Carreira [1,2,3,*], Nicolás Vila-Blanco [1,3], Pablo Cabezas-Sainz [3,4] and Laura Sánchez [3,4]

1. Centro Singular de Investigación en Tecnoloxías Intelixentes (CiTIUS), Universidade de Santiago de Compostela, 15782 Santiago de Compostela, Spain; nicolas.vila@usc.es
2. Departamento de Electrónica e Computación, Universidade de Santiago de Compostela, 15782 Santiago de Compostela, Spain
3. Instituto de Investigación Sanitaria de Santiago de Compostela (IDIS), 15706 Santiago de Compostela, Spain
4. Department of Zoology, Genetics and Physical Anthropology, Universidade de Santiago de Compostela, 27002 Lugo, Spain; pablo.cabezas@usc.es (P.C.-S.); lauraelena.sanchez@usc.es (L.S.)
* Correspondence: mariajose.carreira@usc.es

Abstract: Background: Zebrafish (*Danio rerio*) is a model organism for the study of human cancer. Compared with the murine model, the zebrafish model has several properties ideal for personalized therapies. The transparency of the zebrafish embryos and the development of the pigment-deficient "casper" zebrafish line give the capacity to directly observe cancer formation and progression in the living animal. Automatic quantification of cellular proliferation in vivo is critical to the development of personalized medicine. Methods: A new methodology was defined to automatically quantify the cancer cellular evolution. ZFTool was developed to establish a base threshold that eliminates the embryo autofluorescence, automatically measures the area and intensity of GFP (green-fluorescent protein) marked cells, and defines a proliferation index. Results: The proliferation index automatically computed on different targets demonstrates the efficiency of ZFTool to provide a good automatic quantification of cancer cell evolution and dissemination. Conclusion: Our results demonstrate that ZFTool is a reliable tool for the automatic quantification of the proliferation index as a measure of cancer mass evolution in zebrafish, eliminating the influence of its autofluorescence.

Keywords: xenotransplant; cancer cells; zebrafish image analysis; in vivo assay

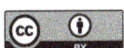

1. Introduction

Over the past 15 years, the zebrafish (*Danio rerio*) has emerged as a model system for the study of human cancer. The transparency of the zebrafish embryos and the development of the pigment-deficient "casper" zebrafish line allow scientists to observe cancer formation and progression directly in the living animal. The optical clarity of zebrafish can be exploited further by the use of fluorescent tags to label specific cell lineages to visualize tumor processes including initiation, progression, and regression. The zebrafish is experimentally amenable to transplantation assays that test the serial passage and malignant potential of fluorescently-labeled tumor cells as well as their capacity to disseminate and/or metastasize. Due to its fecundity and the optical clarity during embryonic development, the zebrafish has proven to be an excellent in vivo model system for high-throughput drug screening, because it allows the visual assessment of both drug efficacy and toxicity [1]. During recent years, the improvement of xenotransplantation of human cancer cells into zebrafish embryos has emerged as a powerful tool, complementary to murine models [2]. Mikut et al. [3] described the state of the art for automated processing of zebrafish imaging data and identified future challenges for zebrafish image analysis research. The zebrafish characteristics are exploited to address important questions in genetics, developmental biology, drug discovery, toxicology, and biomedical research. Zebrafish models exist for a broad range of human diseases, such as cardiovascular diseases [4], cancer [5], or movement disorders [6]. The present paper describes our research about measuring evolution on cancer cells on zebrafish. Although several articles have been published on zebrafish xenotransplantation [7–10], our aim is to optimize this technique for primary cultures originated from colorectal cancer patients in 48 h zebrafish embryos. Previously, RT qPCR and 2D imaging have been used to quantify both proliferation and migration. However, the techniques described so far do not provide an accurate measurement for both parameters. We propose accurate quantification on zebrafish embryos by temporal analysis of xenotransplanted cells marked with GFP (green-fluorescent protein). In the literature, some other works have conducted research on measuring the evolution of cancer cells and some of them developed an image analysis tool for it, such as ZebIAT [11], the Fiji distribution of the free software ImageJ, pioneer in bioimage analysis [12], or using commercial software [13]. A good revision of software for zebrafish image processing is in [3]. Nevertheless, these software tools are too specific, and none of them perform the analysis objective of our research, so we had to develop our own methodology.

2. Materials and Methods

2.1. Material

The images used in this paper were captured from zebrafish embryos, as described in the previous study for which this software was initially developed [14]. In the following, we resume those conditions.

Zebrafish embryos were obtained from mating adults according to standard procedures. The human colorectal cancer cell line HCT116 was obtained from American Type Culture Collection (ATCC, Manassas, VA, USA, Catalog No. CCL-247) and cultured using McCoy's 5A Medium containing 10% FBS (GIBCO, Invitrogen, Waltham, MA, USA) and 1% Pen/Strep (GIBCO, Invitrogen) at 37 °C with 5% CO_2 in a humidified atmosphere. The HCT116 cell line was transfected to express GFP constitutively. HCT116 cells were transduced using a lentiviral-driven GFP construct (Sigma, Darmstad, Germany, Mission TurboGFP, SHC003 V). Cells were placed 72 h postinfection under selective pressure using 10 μg/mL puromycin.

Two days postfertilization (dpf), zebrafish embryos were dechorionated (if needed) and anesthetized with 0.003% tricaine (Sigma). Cell injections were performed manually directly into the yolk of the embryo. Incorrectly injected embryos without cells inside the yolk or showing them in the circulation after xenotransplantation were discarded. After injection, 2 dpf embryos were incubated at 36 °C in 24-well plates with salt dechlorinate tap water (SDTW, chlorine free water obtained with a reverse osmosis filter system) for 72 h to check the proliferation of the cell line by ZFTool. Each embryo was photographed with an AZ-100 Nikon fluorescence stereomicroscope (same exposure times, gamma correction set to 1) at 0 h postinjection (hpi) and 72 hpi to be analyzed by ZFTool software. This software analyzes the green channel image. The gray image of the fish is used only for visualization purposes.

Figure 1 shows a typical image of both zebrafish and GFP mass at 0 hpi and 72 hpi. The GFP image is overlaid over the original embryo image just for positioning it over the zebrafish.

2.2. Methods

The objective of ZFTool is to automatize and improve the task of measuring the number and mean value of GFP pixels to compare them for 0 hpi and 24, 48, or 72 hpi (depending on the experiment) in order to quantify cancer mass evolution with time. ZFTool was developed as a Matlab toolbox and is available at https://gitlab.citius.usc.es/zebrafish/zftool. (Accessed on 22 August 2021). ZFTool eliminates the autofluorescence of the zebrafish through computation of the area with different intensity thresholds and automatically computing the autofluorescence threshold, which is established for both images at 0 hpi and 24, 48, or 72 hpi. ZFTool can establish a base threshold that eliminates embryo autofluorescence and measures the area of marked cells (GFP) and the intensity of those cells to define a proliferation index.

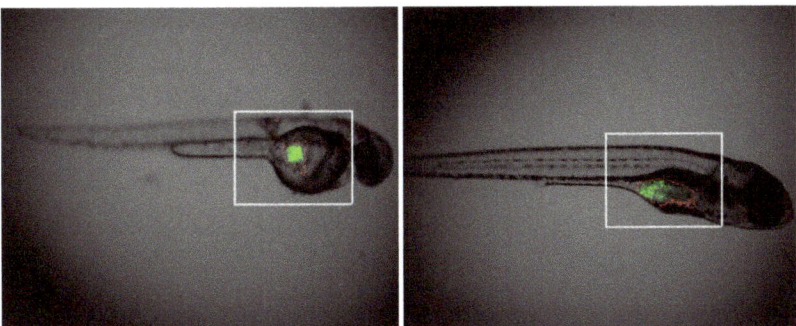

Figure 1. Example of segmentation over a characteristic image (zebrafish #8 at 0 hpi and 72 hpi) where the GFP value and the contour image are overlaid in green and red, respectively. The white rectangle will be the region of interest in the next figures.

The input to the system are two images at 0 hpi and two images at 24, 48, or 72 hpi (the user selects the time to measure the tumor evolution, ZFTool works with any of these values). The output is both numerical (final threshold, mean areas and GFP intensities, proliferation index) and graphical (GFP intensity and area evolution, threshold, and images with initial and final perimeter). As was stated before, zebrafish is ideal for quantification of GFP masses because of its transparency, but a problem arises caused by the variable autofluorescence of the fish, especially in the yolk area. In order to accurately quantify the GFP evolution, a preprocessing must be applied to eliminate the autofluorescence region from the count. This preprocessing is based on the observation of evolution of GFP area with a threshold from 0 (no threshold) to 50 in steps of 5 (see an example in Figure 2).

As was stated before, this autofluorescence is variable, depending of the fish and on the hpi, so this threshold must be adapted to each case. The ZFTool software evaluated the graph of GFP threshold with respect to the area and selected as threshold the point in which this area remains stable.

Once this autofluorescence is eliminated, some parameters are computed in order to measure the cancer mass evolution: the number of GFP pixels in the image (nGFP), which represents the area of the cells inside the yolk sac at two different times, and the GFP intensity Medium Value (GMV), which represents the medium intensity of the fluorescence inside the yolk. By multiplying the nGFP number by the GMV of each image, we determined the proliferation ratio between 0 hpi and 72 hpi to estimate the cell growth. The result obtained at 72 hpi was divided by that obtained at 0 hpi, yielding a proliferation index value (PI):

$$PI = \frac{nGFP_{72hpi} * GMV_{72hpi}}{nGFP_{0hpi} * GMV_{0hpi}} \quad (1)$$

A PI value = 1 means that cells remain stable during incubation, a PI slightly higher than 1 usually indicates a dissemination of cells (greater area, similar intensity), a PI near or over 2 indicates a proliferation of cells (greater area, greater intensity), and a PI lower than 1 indicates tumor cell death.

We must have in mind that, in order to compare these measures at 0 hpi and at 72 hpi, the threshold in both cases must be the same, so we will compute these two thresholds automatically and the biggest one will be applied to both images.

Due to zebrafish autofluorescence and the variability of capture conditions, the segmentation threshold will not be always the same. In order to design a methodology for automatic computation of this threshold, several tests were performed with a training set of 14 zebrafish, applying thresholds from 0 to 50 in 5 intervals and discarding regions with areas less than 10 pixels. Figure 3 shows the evolution of area and intensity for two characteristic zebrafish (#8 and #14), one with no proliferation of cell mass and another one with proliferation of cancer cell mass.

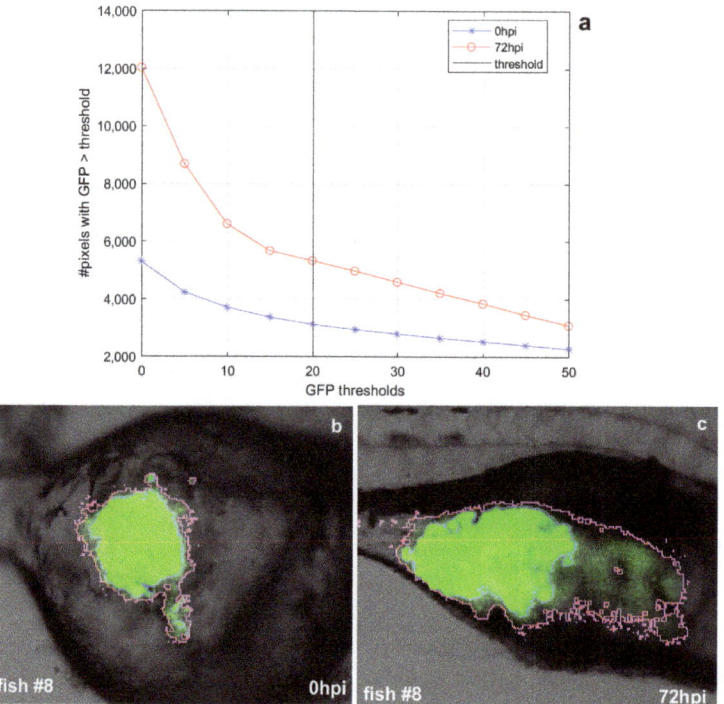

Figure 2. Example of autofluorescence in the yolk sac for fish #8 at 0 hpi and 72 hpi. (**a**) The graph shows the area evolution with respect to the GFP threshold in steps of 5. The abrupt decay in the area caused by the fish autofluorescence can be observed. When the area remains stable for 3 iterations, the threshold is fixed. (**b**) threshold at 0 hpi in magenta and final threshold (20 in this case) in blue. The GFP (green channel) was artificially enhanced in order to make visible the autofluorescence causing the initial contour. This is better seen in the image at 72 hpi (**c**). The original images are shown in Figure 3, where the autofluorescence cannot be appreciated.

After applying the whole algorithm to the test set, we can conclude that when the cancer cells disseminate over the fish, the GFP region area is greater but the mean GFP intensity becomes lower for 72 hpi than those values for 0 hpi. On the other hand, when there is cell multiplication, both the GFP area and GFP mean intensity achieve greater values, depending on the proliferation factor. This fact can be observed in Figure 3, where we can conclude dissemination of cells for fish #8 and proliferation for fish #14. For fish #8, the regions after applying the threshold can be seen in Figure 3 (middle), where it can be seen that the region is more irregular and the cells are disseminated over the region. For fish #14, we can observe in Figure 3 (bottom) a proliferation of cells, the GFP intensity is greater and the area is also greater.

As 2D images are more easily captured and do not require as expensive instrumentation as for 3D images (confocal microscope), we will work with 2D images for quantifying cancer mass evolution. We have previously conducted experimentation [15] in order to establish a correspondence between 2D and 3D image analysis. These results are resumed in Figure 4, where both 2D and a z-stack of 25 images were captured for fish #11 at 0 hpi and 72 hpi. 2D images were acquired under the same conditions of images in this manuscript

(AZ-100 microscope). The z-stack of 25 images separated by 1 µ was acquired using a confocal microscope. We used BioimageXD [16] to reconstruct the volume and compute the thresholded values to eliminate autofluorescence, as performed with 2D images.

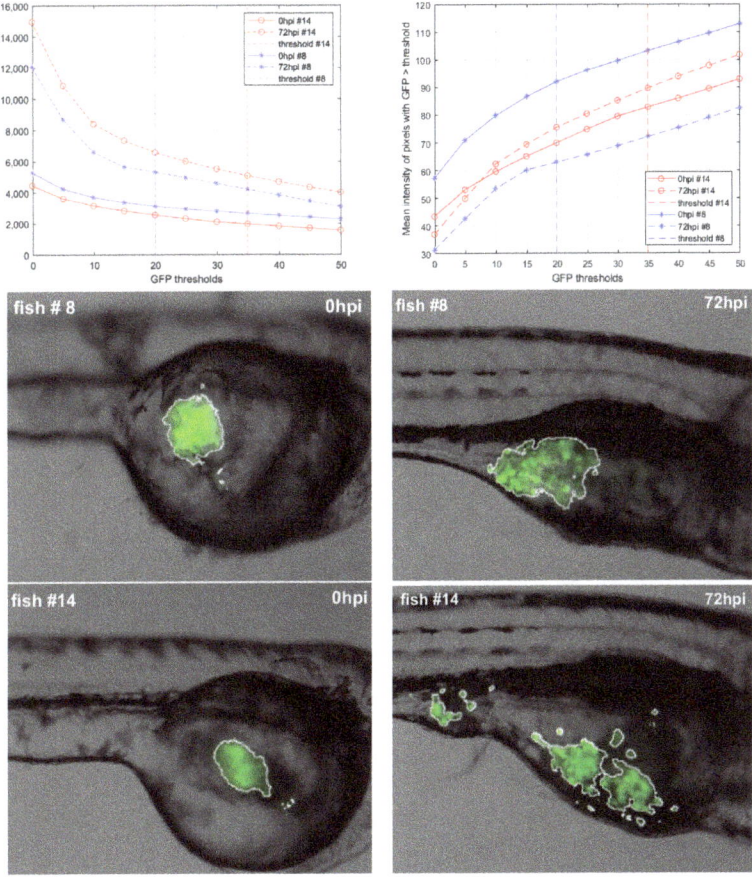

Figure 3. Characteristic zebrafish #8 and #14. **Up**: fish #8 (blue) presents greater area and lower intensity after 72 h while fish #14 (red) presents greater area and higher intensity after 72 h. Threshold final values for zebrafish #8 and #14 are 20 and 35, respectively. **Middle** and **bottom** rows: thresholded GFP regions for zebrafish #8 (**middle**) and zebrafish #14 (**bottom**) for 0 hpi (**left**) and 72 hpi (**right**).

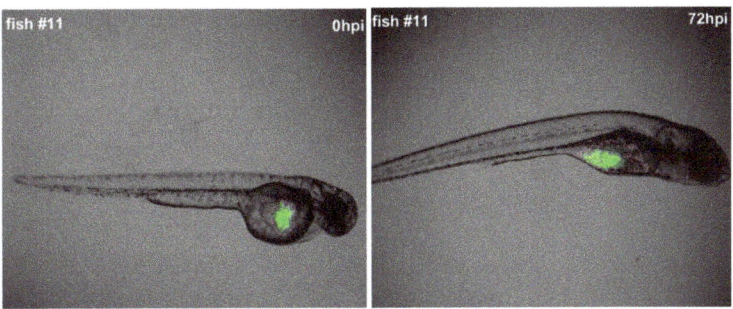

Figure 4. *Cont.*

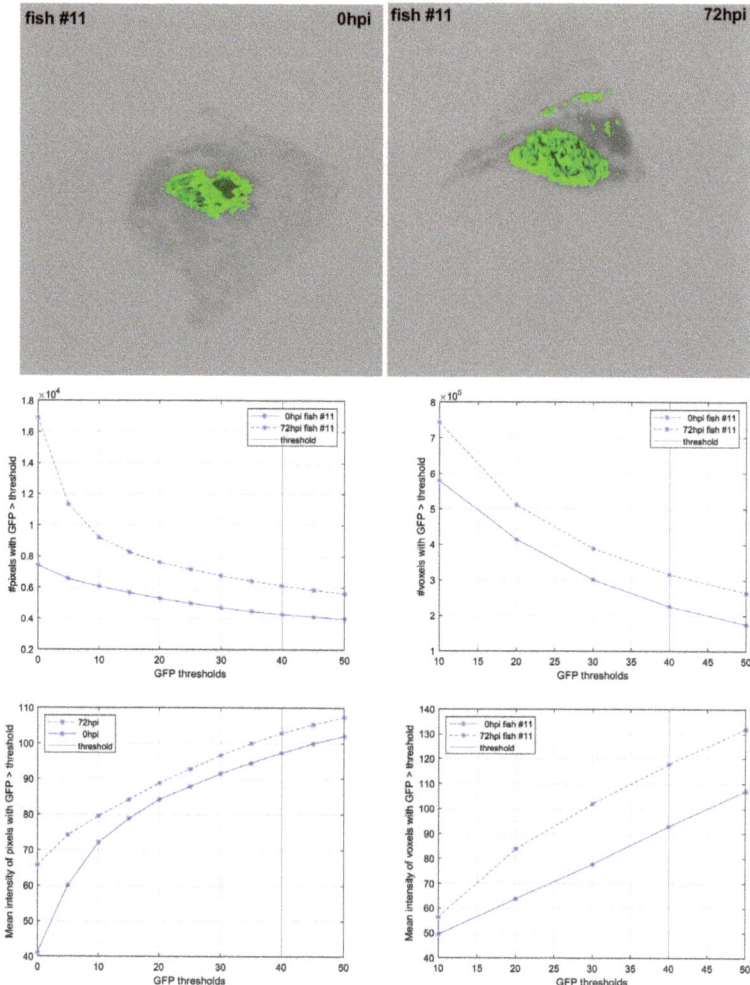

Figure 4. Comparison of 2D and 3D analyses for fish #11. First row: 2D analysis with ZFTool. Second row: 3D analysis with BioimageXD. Third row: # pixels evolution and # voxels evolution. Fourth row: GFP intensity evolution for pixels (**left**) and voxels (**right**).

As shown in Figure 4, the graphs follow the same evolution for 2D and 3D analysis, so we can use the 2D analysis of ZFTool as an estimation of the evolution of the tumor. The proliferation index obtained for fish #11 is 1.52 for 2D analysis and 1.77 for 3D analysis, concluding that there is a proliferation of cells (greater area and greater intensity) in both cases.

3. Results

To prove the algorithm and assess its performance, we analyzed images belonging to a test set. This test set is composed of 18 zebrafish with captures taken at 0 hpi and 72 hpi. Results confirmed the assumption made in the previous section that when area and intensity reach greater values, it is a symptom of proliferation, and when the area is greater and intensity is lower, it is a symptom of dissemination of cancer cells. The applied automatic threshold performs well in all cases and agrees with the expectations concluded by an expert. Table 1 shows the measurements for zebrafish #8, #11, and #14 and the final proliferation index.

Table 1. Final thresholds and measurements of areas and mean green value for zebrafish #8 (dissemination, PI around 1), #11 (proliferation, PI greater than 1), and #14 (proliferation and dissemination, PI greater than 2).

Zebrafish #	Threshold	$nGFP_{0hpi}$	GMV_{0hpi}	$nGFP_{72hpi}$	GMV_{72hpi}	PI
#8	20	3144	92.08	5349	63.07	1.16
#11	40	4279	97.25	6133	102.88	1.52
#14	35	1991	82.94	5106	89.72	2.77

4. Discussion and Conclusions

In this manuscript, we presented ZFTool, a software to quantify tumor evolution. Some issues to discuss are related with the correlation between 2D and 3D analysis, the affection of autofluorescence, and the biomarkers. Related to the first issue, although the relation between 2D and 3D measurements must be demonstrated, some previous experimentation conducted by the authors [15] explored the correlation between 2D and 3D tumor evolution, as shown in Figure 4 for fish #11, which obtained a similar value for the proliferation index (1.52 in 2D and 1.77 in 3D). With respect to autofluorescence, as ZFTool works directly with the channel green image, if another image (i.e., channel red) is provided, all the computations will work properly, as results do not depend on the channel being used. In case the fish do not have autofluorescence in that channel, the graphs of evolution shown in Figures 2 and 3 will have an almost horizontal tendency, so the value of the threshold will be almost indifferent; ZFTool will be able to work in this case also.

While working with different biomarkers, we decided to optimize the software with a permanent labeling of the cells, expressing GFP protein in the cytoplasm. In this way, cells were able to maintain the GFP intensity throughout the experiment, allowing to quantify the proliferation of the cells through the integrated density, leading to a proliferation index. Nevertheless, not all the xenograft assays are performed with this ideal labeling, requiring lipophilic dyes (DiI, DiD, DiO) to label the membrane of the cells. Using this approach, ZFTool functions as previously described, erasing the autofluorescence, which is important because working with a lypophilic dye could lead to an increase in autofluorescence or artifacts due to the lysis of the injected cells and the spread of the dye across areas of the zebrafish embryo. Even so, when a lipophilic dye is used, it is not possible to calculate a proliferation ratio, but a more accurate fold change between the conditions tested against the control.

Another issue is if it would be adequate to fix the autofluorescence of the fish previously to the injection. We have decided not to do this as the autofluorescence is dependent of each individual, by the stage of development and by the drugs under research. This is precisely why we fixed the threshold in this way: we computed the first possible threshold for each fish in each moment and fixed the greater value as the common threshold. As the graphs in Figures 2 and 3 show, this will be the first possible threshold, when the autofluorescence is eliminated, although selecting a subsequent threshold barely affected the mean area and intensity of the tumor.

In our research, a proliferation index was defined, as indicated in Equation (1). This parameter by itself should be an indicator of proliferation in most of the experiments. Nevertheless, there are different scenarios for the proliferation index, considering that if the dissemination is larger than the proliferation, the increase in the proliferation index could be due exclusively to spread instead of division of the cells. For this reason, ZFTool also offers as output both the intensity and area and, apart from that, the graphs and the images to be used as complementary diagnostics by the researchers. Although a nuclear marker could be used for quantifying cell proliferation, the quality of the images and its

2D character does not permit such exact counting, so we used the intensity of the GPF as an indicator of the number of superposed cells.

As a future perspective and projection of the software, once systematized, improved, and tested, it will help to automatize part of the xenograft procedure and conduct an in vivo assay screening that could help clinicians decide the best chemotherapy combinations for each patient through the injection of patient cancer cells into the zebrafish embryos. Although this objective could be achieved, there are many variables that this technique needs to take into consideration to evaluate the proliferation of the cancer cells and treatments, such as the microenvironment of the tumor and the matrix in the human body.

As a conclusion, in this work, we designed an algorithm to automatically perform the thresholding and computation of GFP area and mean intensity values. These values are characteristics that demonstrate the evolution of the injection of cancer cells into the yolk sac of a zebrafish embryo. This computation is of great interest for cancer research as zebrafish allow in vivo assays and we can perform a reliable, repeatable, and quick computation of characteristic features. We also defined a so-called proliferation index as a measure of the degree of dissemination or multiplication of tumor cells.

Author Contributions: Conceptualization, M.J.C. and L.S.; methodology, M.J.C. and N.V.-B.; software, M.J.C. and N.V.-B.; validation, P.C.-S. and L.S.; investigation, M.J.C., N.V.-B., P.C.-S., and L.S.; writing—original draft preparation, M.J.C. and N.V.-B.; writing—review and editing, M.J.C. and P.C.-S. All authors have read and agreed to the published version of the manuscript.

Funding: This work has received financial support from Consellería de Cultura, Educación e Ordenación Universitaria (accreditation 2019-2022 ED431G-2019/04) and the European Regional Development Fund (ERDF), which acknowledges the CiTIUS-Research Center in Intelligent Technologies of the University of Santiago de Compostela as a Research Center of the Galician University System.

Institutional Review Board Statement: The care, use, and treatment of zebrafish were performed in agreement with the Animal Care and Use Committee of the University of Santiago de Compostela and the standard protocols of Spain (Directive 2012-63-UE). The protocol was approved by the Animal Care and Use Committee of the University of Santiago de Compostela.

Informed Consent Statement: Not applicable.

Conflicts of Interest: The authors declare no conflict of interest.

Abbreviations

The following abbreviations are used in this manuscript:

5-FU	5-Fluorouracil
dpf	Days postfertilization
GFP	Green-Fluorescent Protein
GMV	GFP medium value
hpf	Hours postfecundation
hpi	Hours postinjection
nGFP	Number of GFP pixels

References

1. Ali, S.; Champagne, D.; Spaink, H.; Richardson, M. Zebrafish embryos and larvae: A new generation of disease models and drug screens. *Birth Defects Res. Part C Embryo Today* **2011**, *93*, 115–133. [CrossRef] [PubMed]
2. Drabsch, Y.; He, S.; Zhang, L.; Snaar-Jagalska, B.; Ten Dijke, P. Transforming growth factor-β signaling controls human breast cancer metastasis in a zebrafish xenograft model. *Breast Cancer Res.* **2013**, *15*, R106. [CrossRef]
3. Mikut, R.; Dickmeis, T.; Driever, W.; Geurts, P.; Hamprecht, F.; Kausler, B.; Ledesma-Carbayo, M.; Marée, R.; Mikula, K.; Pantazis, P.; et al. Automated Processing of Zebrafish Imaging Data: A Survey. *Zebrafish* **2013**, *10*, 401–421. [CrossRef]
4. Bakkers, J. Zebrafish as a model to study cardiac development and human cardiac disease. *Cardiovasc. Res.* **2011**, *91*, 279–288. [CrossRef]
5. Mione, M.; Trede, N. The zebrafish as a model for cancer. *Dis. Model. Mech.* **2010**, *3*, 517–523. [CrossRef] [PubMed]
6. Flinn, L.; Bretaud, S.; Lo, C.; Ingham, P.; Bandmann, O. Zebrafish as a new animal model for movement disorders. *J. Neurochem.* **2008**, *106*, 1991–1997. [CrossRef] [PubMed]

7. Bentley, V.; Veinotte, C.; Corkery, D.; Pinder, J.; LeBlanc, M.; Bedard, K.; Weng, A.; Berman, J.; Dellaire, G. Focused chemical genomics using zebrafish xenotransplantation as a preclinical therapeutic platform for T-cell acute lymphoblastic leukemia. *Haematologica* **2015**, *100*, 70–76. [CrossRef]
8. Jung, D.W.; Oh, E.S.; Park, S.H.; Chang, Y.T.; Kim, C.H.; Choi, S.Y.; Williams, D. A novel zebrafish human tumor xenograft model validated for anti-cancer drug screening. *Mol. Biosyst.* **2012**, *8*, 1930–1939. [CrossRef]
9. Konantz, M.; Balci, T.; Hartwig, U.; Dellaire, G.; André, M.; Berman, J.; Lengerke, C. Zebrafish xenografts as a tool for in vivo studies on human cancer. *Ann. N. Y. Acad. Sci.* **2012**, *1266*, 124–137. [CrossRef]
10. Veinotte, C.; Dellaire, G.; Berman, J. Hooking the big one: The potential of zebrafish xenotransplantation to reform cancer drug screening in the genomic area. *Dis. Model. Mech.* **2014**, *7*, 745–754. [CrossRef] [PubMed]
11. Annila, T.; Lihavainen, E.; Marques, I.; Williams, D.; Yli-Harja, O.; Ribeiro, A. ZebIAT, an image analysis tool for registering zebrafish embryos and quantifying cancer metastasis. *BMC Bioinform.* **2013**, *14*, S5. [CrossRef] [PubMed]
12. Teng, Y.; Xie, X.; Walker, S.; White, D.; Mumm, J.; Cowell, J. Evaluating human cancer cell metastasis in zebrafish. *BMC Cancer* **2013**, *13*, 453. [CrossRef] [PubMed]
13. Ghotra, V.; He, S.; de Bont, H.; van der Ent, W.; Spaink, H.; van de Water, B.; Snaar-Jagalska, B.; Danen, E. Automated whole animal bio-imaging assay for human cancer dissemination. *PLoS ONE* **2012**, *7*, e31281. [CrossRef] [PubMed]
14. Cabezas-Sainz, P.; Guerra-Varela, J.; Carreira, M.J.; Mariscal, J.; Roel, M.; Rubiolo, J.; Sciara, A.; Abal, M.; Botana, L.; López, R.; et al. Improving zebrafish embryo xenotransplantation conditions by increasing incubation temperature and establishing a proliferation index with ZFTool. *BMC Cancer* **2018**, *18*, 3. [CrossRef] [PubMed]
15. Guerra-Varela, J.; Terriente, J.; Mariscal, J.; Cabezas-Sainz, P.; Calzolari, S.; Dyballa, S.; Abal, M.; López, R.; Sánchez, L. Assessing proliferation and metastasis of human cancer cells trhough 3D imaging. In Proceedings of the 7th Zebrafish Disease Models Conference, Madison, WI, USA, 28 June–1 July 2014; 100–P1.
16. Kankaanpää, P.; Paavolainen, L.; Tiitta, S.; Karjalainen, M.; Päivärinne, J.; Nieminen, J.; Marjomäki, V.; Heino, J.; White, D. BioImageXD: An open, general-purpose and high-throughput image-processing platform. *Nat. Methods* **2012**, *9*, 683–689. [CrossRef] [PubMed]

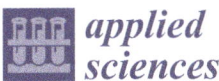

Article

Clinical Comparison of the Glomerular Filtration Rate Calculated from Different Renal Depths and Formulae

Wen-Ling Hsu [1,2], Shu-Min Chang [1] and Chin-Chuan Chang [1,2,3,4,5,*]

1. Department of Nuclear Medicine, Kaohsiung Medical University Hospital, No.100, Tzyou 1st Road, Kaohsiung 80756, Taiwan; unlin91@hotmail.com (W.-L.H.); shumin91@gmail.com (S.-M.C.)
2. Department of Medical Imaging and Radiological Sciences, Kaohsiung Medical University, Kaohsiung 80756, Taiwan
3. Department of Electrical Engineering, I-Shou University, Kaohsiung 84001, Taiwan
4. School of Medicine, College of Medicine, Kaohsiung Medical University, Kaohsiung 80756, Taiwan
5. Neuroscience Research Center, Kaohsiung Medical University, Kaohsiung 80756, Taiwan
* Correspondence: chinuan@gmail.com; Tel.: +886-7312-1101 (ext. 7147)

Abstract: A camera-based method using Technetium-99m diethylenetriaminepentaacetic acid (Tc-99m DTPA) is commonly used to calculate glomerular filtration rate (GFR), especially, as it can easily calculate split renal function. Renal depth is the main factor affecting the measurement of GFR accuracy. This study aimed to compare the difference of renal depths between three formulae and a CT scan, and, additionally, to calculate the GFRs by four methods. We retrospectively reviewed the medical records of patients receiving a renal dynamic scan. All patients underwent a laboratory test within one month, and a computed tomography (CT) scan within two months, before or after the renal dynamic scan. The GFRs were calculated by employing a renal dynamic scan using renal depth measured in three formulae (Tonnesen's, Itoh K's, and Taylor's), and a CT scan. The renal depths measured by the above four methods were compared, and the GFRs were compared to the modified estimated GFR (eGFR). Fifty-one patients were enrolled in the study. The mean modified eGFR was 60.5 ± 42.7 mL/min. The mean GFRs calculated by three formulae and CT were 45.3 ± 23.3, 54.7 ± 27.5, 56.5 ± 26.3, and 63.7 ± 30.0, respectively. All of them correlated well with the modified eGFR (r = 0.87, 0.87, 0.87, and 0.84, respectively). The Bland–Altman plot revealed good consistency between the calculated GFR by Tonnesen's and the modified eGFR. The renal depths measured using the three formulae were smaller than those measured using the CT scan, and the right renal depth was always larger than the left. In patients with modified eGFR > 60 mL/min, the GFR calculated by CT was the closest to the modified eGFR. The Renal depth measured by CT scan is deeper than that using formula, and it influences the GFR calculated by Gate's method. The GFR calculated by CT is more closely related to modified eGFR when modified eGFR > 60 mL/min.

Keywords: glomerular filtration rate; Gate's method; renal depth; computed tomography

Citation: Hsu, W.-L.; Chang, S.-M.; Chang, C.-C. Clinical Comparison of the Glomerular Filtration Rate Calculated from Different Renal Depths and Formulae. *Appl. Sci.* **2022**, *12*, 698. https://doi.org/10.3390/app12020698

Academic Editors: Francesco Garzott, Alessandro Stefano, Albert Comelli and Federica Vernuccio

Received: 19 November 2021
Accepted: 6 January 2022
Published: 11 January 2022

Publisher's Note: MDPI stays neutral with regard to jurisdictional claims in published maps and institutional affiliations.

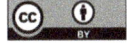

Copyright: © 2022 by the authors. Licensee MDPI, Basel, Switzerland. This article is an open access article distributed under the terms and conditions of the Creative Commons Attribution (CC BY) license (https://creativecommons.org/licenses/by/4.0/).

1. Introduction

Globally, people suffering from chronic kidney disease (CKD), acute kidney injury (AKI), and renal replacement therapy exceed 805 million in total [1]. Renal diseases are a notable public health issue and a leading, heavy, burden on the medical system. By 2040, CKD is predicted to become the fifth leading cause of death [2]. Renal diseases are not easily diagnosed, as they are asymptomatic in their early stages. Therefore, the accurate measurement of the glomerular filtration rate (GFR) is critical for detecting renal function and for clinical treatment.

Although inulin clearance has been the widely accepted gold standard [3] for measuring the GFR, this methodology is time-consuming, expensive, and not easily available, making it unsuitable for routine clinical use. Some equations such as Cockcroft–Gault

(CG) [4], modification of diet in renal disease (MDRD) [5], and CKD epidemiology collaboration (CKD-EPI) [6], which estimate GFRs based on serum creatinine measurement with ease and convenience, have been widely accepted for clinical use.

Among other techniques aimed to estimate GFR, the camera-based method with technetium-99m (Tc-99m) diethylenetriaminepentaacetic acid (DTPA) using modified Gate's method represent an easy way to estimate unilateral renal function. In addition, it can determine unilateral renal blood flow and distinguish between renal pelvic ectasia and post-renal obstruction. This is important clinical information for patients with unilateral renal disease, and for kidney donations. Unfortunately, some researchers have questioned the method [7,8].

The most important factor of Gate's method affecting the GFR is renal depth [9]. The more accurate the measurement of renal depth, the more accurate the GFR calculation will be. The renal depths have been measured by techniques such as ultrasound (US), lateral view in radionuclide renal scintigraphy, and the computed tomography (CT), with varied precisions [10,11]. The current study aimed to compare the renal depth measured by different formulae and a CT scan, and it additionally sought to compare the GFR calculated from different methods with the reference value.

2. Materials and Methods

2.1. Patients

This is a retrospective study that analyzed the medical records of patients from nuclear medicine databases from September 2019 to September 2020 in Kaohsiung Medical University Hospital. Patients were accepted if they fulfilled the following criteria: (i) had received radionuclide renal dynamic imaging; (ii) had received an abdominal CT scan within two months before or after the radionuclide renal scan; (iii) had undergone a laboratory test for plasma creatinine (Pcr) within a month; and (iv) were more than 20 years old. The study review process was approved by the Institutional Review Board of Kaohsiung Medical University Hospital. (KMUHIRB-E(I)-20210244).

2.2. Renal Dynamic Image

Thirty minutes before the exam, patients were encouraged to drink at least 300 mL of water. Each patient's age, sex, body weight, and body height were entered into the workstation. We noted the full syringe dose at the beginning and the empty syringe dose at the end of the examination. Patients were placed supine, and the procedure began immediately after the bolus intravenous injection of 6 mCi Tc-99m DTPA. The renal dynamic image was acquired in a 128 × 128 frame matrix for the ensuing 22 min using a Siemens E. CAM gamma camera (Siemens, Erlangen, Germany) equipped with a low-energy high-resolution collimator.

The regions of interest for each kidney were drawn manually by an experienced nuclear medicine radiographer. The background ROI for subtraction was drawn automatically by placing a semilunar region around the outer-lower aspect of each kidney (Figure 1). The GFRs were calculated by Gate's method using the following formula [9].

$$\text{Dual renal uptake (\%)} = [(Cr - Crb)/e^{-\mu RD} + (Cl - Clb/e^{-\mu LD})]/(\text{Full} - \text{Empty})$$

$$\text{GFR} = \text{dual renal uptake (\%)} \times 100 \times 9.8127 - 6.82519$$

where Cr: right kidney counts, Crb: right background counts, Cl: left kidney counts, Clb: left background counts, RD: right kidney depth, LD: left kidney depth, μ: attenuation coefficient of Tc-99m in soft tissue (0.153 cm^{-1}), e: Euler's number, Full: full syringe counts, Empty: empty syringe counts

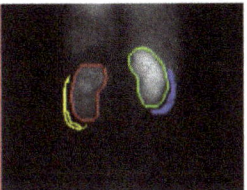

Figure 1. Demonstration of the region of interest (ROI) when calculating the glomerular filtration rate (GFR) by Gate's method from a 33-year-old woman. The ROIs for each kidney were drawn manually via the compression posterior image. Background subtraction was drawn by placing a semilunar ROI in the outer-lower of each kidney automatically.

The renal depth was estimated by the following three formulae (developed by Tonnesen, Itoh K, and Taylor, respectively) [12–14] and a CT scan.

2.3. Assessment of Renal Depth by Tonnesen's Formula

The right renal (dR) and left renal (dL) depths were estimated from the body height and weight using the following equations [12]:

$$dR = 13.3 \times (BW/BH) + 0.7$$

$$dL = 13.2 \times (BW/BH) + 0.7$$

where BW: body weight(kg), BH: body height(cm).

2.4. Assessment of Renal Depth by Itoh K's Formula

The right renal (dR) and left renal (dL) depths were estimated from body height and weight using the following equations [13]:

$$dR = 13.6361 \times (BW/BH)^{0.6996}$$

$$dL = 14.0285 \times (BW/BH)^{0.7554}$$

where BW: body weight(kg), BH: body height(cm).

2.5. Assessment of Renal Depth by Taylor's Formula

The right renal (dR) and left renal (dL) depths were estimated from the body height, body weight, and age using the following equations [14]:

$$dR = 15.31 \times (BW/BH) + 0.022 \times age + 0.077$$

$$dL = 16.17 \times (BW/BH) + 0.027 \times age - 0.94$$

where BW: body weight (kg), BH: body height (cm), age: patient's age (year).

2.6. Assessment of Renal Depth by CT

The CT scan was performed in the supine position with a 5 mm slice thickness spiral scan covering the whole abdomen (Figure 2). We chose the axial views, including the middle point of the long axis of each kidney, and the renal depth was defined as the distance from the middle point of the anteroposterior diameter to the body surface on the back in each view.

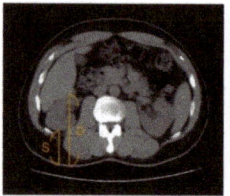
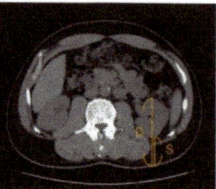

Figure 2. Demonstration of measuring the renal depth via CT image. Two axial slices including the middle of each kidney were collected. The point of deepest (D) and superficial (S) to back body surface were drawn. The renal depth was calculated as (D + S)/2.

2.7. Estimated GFR (eGFR)

The eGFR was a creatinine-based equation and was modified with CKD patients in Chinese patients. The GFRs were calculated with renal depth assessed by three formulae and a CT scan, and they were compared with the eGFR estimated using the following equations [15]:

$$\text{eGFR (mL/min/1.73 m}^2) = 175 \times (\text{Pcr})^{-1.234} \times (\text{Age})^{-0.179} \ (\times 0.79 \text{ if female})$$

where Pcr was in unit of mg/dL; Age was in years.

2.8. Modified Estimated GFR (Modified eGFR)

We use the body surface area (BSA) according to Du Bois to modify the estimated GFR [16]:

$$\text{Modified eGFR(ml/min)} = \text{eGFR} \times (\text{BSA}/1.73)$$

$$\text{BSA (m}^2) = 0.20247 \times \text{BH}^{0.725} \times \text{BW}^{0.425}$$

where BH: body height (m); BW: body weight (kg).

2.9. Statistical Analysis

Continuous variables of measurement data were expressed as mean ± standard deviation (SD). A regression test was performed to compare the correlations between the calculated GFRs and modified eGFR. The Bland–Altman, boxplots, and data were analyzed using the MedCalc Statistical Software, version 20.014 (MedCalc Software Ltd., Ostend, Belgium; https://www.medcalc.org; lasted accessed on 17 November 2021). A *p*-value < 0.05 was considered statistically significant.

3. Results

A total of 51 patients, consisting of 21 males and 30 females with a mean age of 60.5 years (range 25–86 years), were enrolled in this study (Table 1). Among them, ten patients were diagnosed with comorbid diabetes mellitus. Clinical manifestations of these patients included hydronephrosis and renal calculus (*n* = 32, 62.7%), renal tumors (*n* = 10, 19.6%), urinary tract infection (*n* = 2, 3.9%), acute kidney injury (*n* = 1, 2.0%), and some other or undetermined diagnosis (*n* = 6, 11.8%). Plasma creatinine level ranged from 0.48 mg/dL to 6.12 mg/dL, and the mean value was 1.8 ± 1.3 mg/dL. The average modified eGFR was 60.5 ± 42.7 mL/min. The mean GFRs calculated by Tonnesen's formula, Itoh K's formula, Taylor's formula, and CT were 45.3 ± 23.3, 54.7 ± 27.5, 56.5 ± 26.3, and 63.7 ± 30.0, respectively.

Table 1. Clinical characteristics of 51 patients enrolled in this study.

Variable	Values [a]
Age	60.5 ± 13.3
Sex	
Male	21 (41)
Female	30 (59)
Height (cm)	160.6 ± 8.3
Weight (kg)	63.4 ± 10.9
BMI (kg/m^2)	24.5 ± 3.5
Plasma creatinine (mg/dL)	1.8 ± 1.3
Modified eGFR (ml/min)	60.5 ± 42.7
Tonnesen's GFR (ml/min)	45.3 ± 23.3
Itoh K's GFR (ml/min)	54.7 ± 27.5
Taylor's GFR (ml/min)	56.5 ± 26.3
CT GFR (ml/min)	63.7 ± 30.0

Abbreviations: BMI, body mass index; modified eGFR, estimated GFR by modified abbreviated modification of diet in renal disease study equation and modify by body surface area; GFR, glomerular filtration rate; SD, standard deviation; CT, computed tomography. [a] Values are presented as No. (%) or mean ± SD.

The scatter plot and regression lines are seen in Figure 3. The correlation coefficient of the calculated GFRs (Tonnesen's, Itoh K's, Taylor's, and CT) and modified eGFR were 0.87, 0.87, 0.87, and 0.84, respectively. All were statistically significant with a *p*-value < 0.001. The Bland–Altman plot showed good agreement between GFRs calculated by Tonnesen's (*p* = 0.0001) and the modified eGFRs. However, no statistical difference was observed between the GFRs calculated by Itoh K's (*p* = 0.0818), Taylor's (*p* = 0.2355) methods, and by a CT scan (*p* = 0.3402) and the modified eGFR (Figure 4).

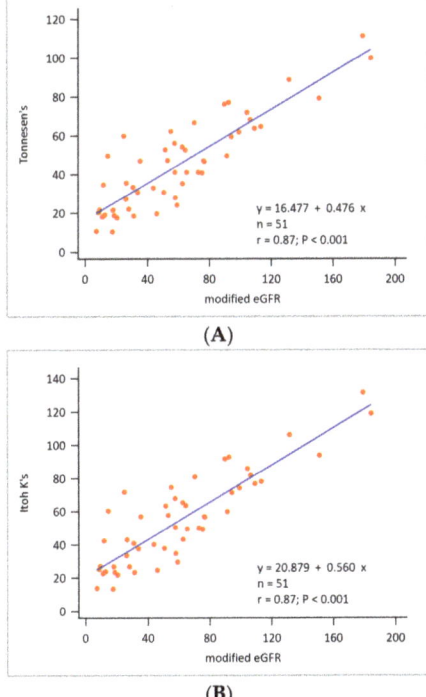

Figure 3. *Cont.*

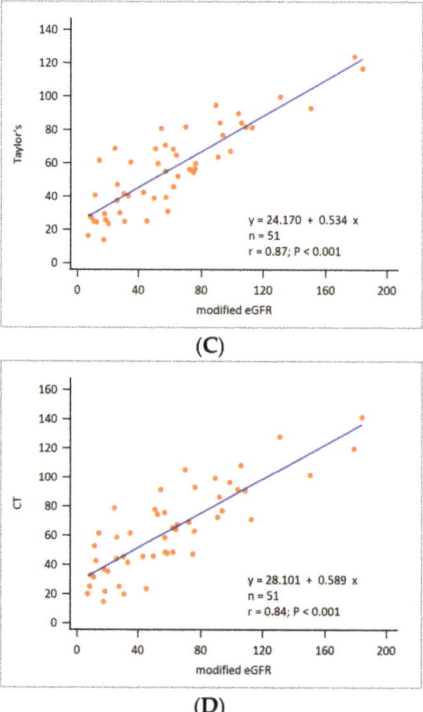

(C)

(D)

Figure 3. The correlation between GFRs calculated using renal depth by four ways and modified eGFR. (**A**), the GFR calculated using the renal depth estimated by Tonnesen's formula (r = 0.87, y = 0.476x + 16.477). (**B**), the GFR calculated using the renal depth estimated by Itoh K's formula (r = 0.87, y = 0.560x + 20.879). (**C**), the GFR calculated using the renal depth estimated by Taylor's formula (r = 0.87, y = 0.534x + 24.170). (**D**), the GFR calculated using the renal depth estimated by CT (r = 0.84, y = 0.589x + 28.101).

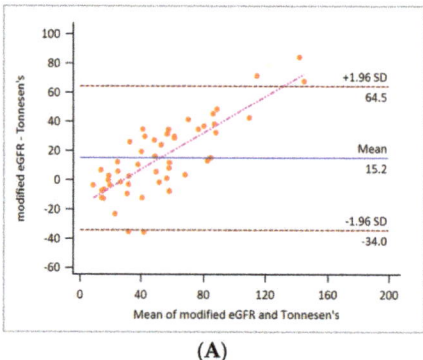

(A)

Figure 4. *Cont.*

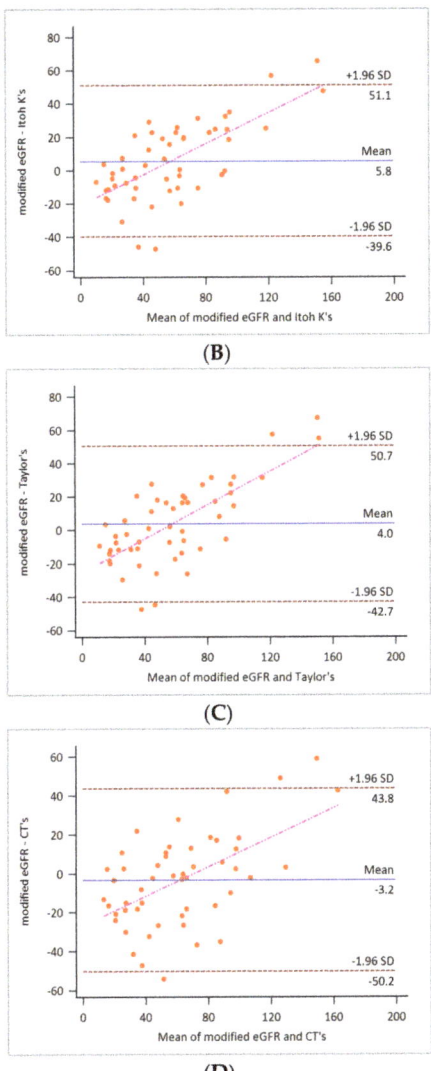

Figure 4. The Bland–Altman plot for GFRs calculated through four methods and the modified eGFR. (**A**), GFR calculated by Tonnesen's formula ($p = 0.0001$). (**B**), GFR calculated by Itoh K's formula ($p = 0.0818$). (**C**), GFR calculated by Taylor's formula ($p = 0.2355$). (**D**), GFR calculated by CT scan ($p = 0.3402$).

The renal depth, when estimated by the three formulae, was significantly smaller than that estimated by a CT scan (all for $p < 0.05$), and the right side was somewhat larger than the left side ($p < 0.05$; Figure 5). On the contrary, the deeper right renal depth was found only in 63% of the patients when estimated by CT scans. In patients with modified eGFR > 60 mL/min, the GFRs calculated using Tonnesen's formula were obviously low, leading to the underestimation of the GFR in the clinical setting. The GFRs calculated using CT scans were closer when the modified eGFR was more than 60 mL/min (Figure 6).

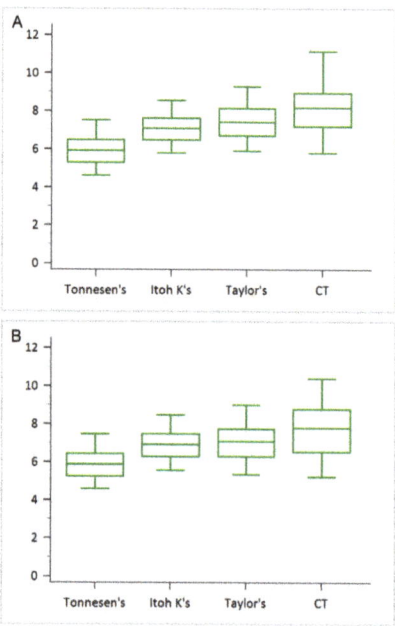

Figure 5. The boxplots for comparison of the bilateral renal depth measured by three formulas (Tonnesen's, Itoh K's, and Taylor's) and the CT scan. (**A**), right renal depth. (**B**), left renal depth.

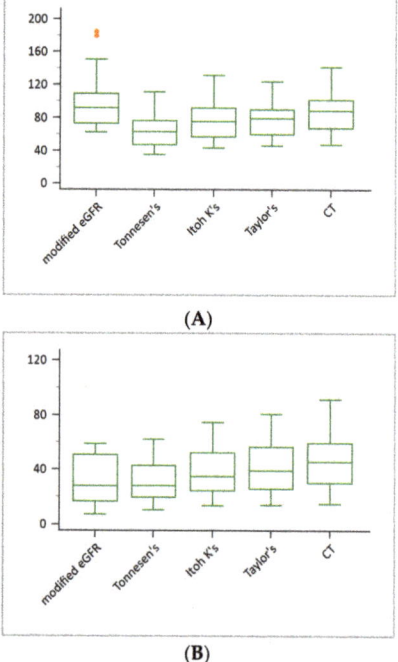

Figure 6. The boxplots for comparison of the GFRs calculated by Tonnesen's, Itoh K's, Taylor's formula, CT scan, and the modified eGFR. (**A**), patients with modified eGFR more than 60 mL/min. (**B**), patients with modified eGFR less than 60 mL/min.

4. Discussion

This is a retrospective study that analyzed and compared how the renal depth influences the GFR. As previously mentioned, renal depth is the main factor affecting Gate's method [9]. In our study, we found that the GFR calculated by four methods (three formulae and the CT scan) were all well correlated to the modified eGFR. However, the depths of both kidneys measured by CT were significantly deeper than those measured by the other three formulae. Further, in the current study we noticed that, in the patients with a modified eGFR over 60 mL/min, the GFR calculated by Tonnesen's is underestimated due to the smallest renal depths. Moreover, the GFR calculated by CT renal depth is closest to the modified eGFR. The result is compatible with that described in the previous studies, in which it was stated that Gate's method underestimated GFR because Tonnesen's formula underestimated the renal depth [14,17,18].

The plasma creatinine equation and creatinine clearance have been used widely in estimating the GFR, and, thus, were used as the reference in the current study. It is a simple method in clinical practice, but there are some limitations. First, the separate renal GFR cannot be assessed and calculated. Second, it is not suitable in some patient groups, such as obese individuals, children, pregnant women, and patients without CKD. It has been reported to overestimate GFR in malnourished patients [4], and underestimate it in healthy people [5].

Nowadays, Gate's method is still the method most preferred in the clinical evaluation of the GFR. It has the advantage of providing total GFR while also calculating the separate renal GFR at the same time. In clinical practice, patients who received the renal dynamic imaging may have various conditions of unilateral renal disease, e.g., urinary tract obstruction, tumor, renal artery anomaly, congenital renal abnormality, and pyelonephritis, etc. Measuring the renal depths accurately is crucial, but it is not always easy in calculating the GFR. Some previous studies reported that the depth of the right kidney is deeper than that of the left side [12–14]; however, in the current study, only 63% of patients had deeper right kidney than left side. The exact reason for this finding is not certain, but we speculate that there may be selection bias due to different clinical backgrounds and relatively smaller patient populations. We need to consider this situation when we estimate unilateral renal function. It will help improve the accuracy of clinical diagnosis.

Acquiring the lateral view when conducting the dynamic renal imaging is simple and clinically feasible without additional radiation exposure for accurate GFR measurement [19]. However, in patients with clinical situations such as hydronephrosis and tumor, radiotracers cannot be detected completely and, therefore, this decreases the scanning validity. Based on the attenuation coefficient of Tc-99m in soft tissue of 0.153, even a 1-cm error (either positive or negative) in the renal depth measurement will lead to a 14–16% error, either under or over-estimation, in the calculation of the GFR [20,21]. In the current study, 82.3% of patients had hydronephrosis, renal calculi, and/or renal tumor, so we did not use lateral view acquiring for renal depth evaluation.

With respect to the CT scan, the advantage is found in the clear anatomic depiction. It measures objective renal depth while also providing information of renal location and morphology, and, thus, it helps to raise the accuracy when evaluating the GFR. The multidetector CT had been used to measure unilateral renal GFR [22,23]. Kwon et al., reported that unilateral GFR measured by contrast enhanced CT was reproducible and it agreed well with the iothalamate clearance [22]. An additional article by You et al. reported that, with a renal dynamic image as the reference, the unilateral renal GFR measured by CT revealed a well and significant correlation [23]. We have found similar results in the current study, especially for patients with modified eGFR over 60 mL/min. However, there is a disadvantage pertaining to additional radiation exposure during the CT scan, and this should be taken into consideration in clinical settings.

Dynamic contrast-enhanced magnetic resonance imaging (DCE-MRI), based on the intrarenal kinetics of contrast, is another clinical technique for evaluating the GFR, and this has now been studied [24,25]. The best advantage of using DCE-MRI to measure

GFR is that patients receive no ionizing radiation exposure. However, the accuracy of the technique has not yet been validated with the standard reference. Additionally, checking renal function before administrating the contrast agents in patients with renal function impairment is also important.

The current study compared the clinical roles of three formulae, and CT scans, on evaluating bilateral renal depths and calculating the GFR. There are some limitations in the current study. First, it was a retrospective study design with relatively smaller patient population. Second, the patients' background was relatively diverse although more than half of the patients displayed clinical symptoms of urinary tract obstruction and/or hydronephrosis. Further prospective studies dealing with larger patient populations and similar clinical settings may be conducted.

5. Conclusions

According to our results, it is found that the renal depth estimated by CT scans is evidently deeper than that measured by the three formulae. The value of the GFR calculated by CT scans is closer to the modified eGFR in patients with modified eGFR over 60 mL/min. It is potentially valuable for us to take these findings into consideration when clinically dealing with the GFR.

Author Contributions: Conceptualization, W.-L.H. and C.-C.C.; Data curation, S.-M.C.; Formal analysis, W.-L.H.; Investigation, C.-C.C.; Methodology, W.-L.H. and C.-C.C.; Resources, S.-M.C.; Supervision, C.-C.C.; Writing—original draft, W.-L.H.; and Writing—review and editing, C.-C. All authors have read and agreed to the published version of the manuscript.

Funding: This research received no external funding.

Institutional Review Board Statement: The study was conducted according to the guidelines of the 221 Declaration of Helsinki, and approved by the Institutional Review Board of Kaohsiung Medical University Hospital (KMUHIRB-E(I)-20210244, approved on 28 October 2021).

Informed Consent Statement: Patient consent was waived due to clinical data were retrospectively collected by the chart reviewing.

Acknowledgments: We would like to thank our medical and non-medical staff including nephrologists, urologist, nurses and secretaries for their efforts.

Conflicts of Interest: The authors declare no conflict of interest existed.

References

1. Jager, K.J.; Kovesdy, C.; Langham, R.; Rosenberg, M.; Jha, V.; Zoccali, C. A single number for advocacy and communication-worldwide more than 850 million individuals have kidney diseases. *Nephrol. Dial. Transpl.* **2019**, *34*, 1803–1805. [CrossRef]
2. Luyckx, V.A.; Al-Aly, Z.; Bello, A.K.; Bellorin-Font, E.; Carlini, R.G.; Fabian, J.; Garcia-Garcia, G.; Iyengar, A.; Sekkarie, M.; van Biesen, W. Sustainable Development Goals relevant to kidney health: An update on progress. *Nat. Rev. Nephrol.* **2021**, *17*, 15–32. [CrossRef]
3. Price, M. Comparison of creatinine clearance to inulin clearance in the determination of glomerular filtration rate. *J. Urol.* **1972**, *107*, 339–340. [CrossRef]
4. Cockcroft, D.W.; Gault, H. Prediction of creatinine clearance from serum creatinine. *Nephron* **1976**, *16*, 31–41. [CrossRef]
5. Levey, A.S.; Bosch, J.P.; Lewis, J.B.; Greene, T.; Rogers, N.; Roth, D. A more accurate method to estimate glomerular filtration rate from serum creatinine: A new prediction equation. *Ann. Intern. Med.* **1999**, *130*, 461–470. [CrossRef]
6. Levey, A.S.; Stevens, L.A.; Schmid, C.H.; Zhang, Y.L.; Castro, A.F., 3rd; Feldman, H.I.; Kusek, J.W.; Eggers, P.; Van Lente, F.; Greene, T.; et al. A new equation to estimate glomerular filtration rate. *Ann. Intern. Med.* **2009**, *150*, 604–612. [CrossRef]
7. Chen, L.-I.; Kuo, M.-C.; Hwang, S.-J.; Chen, Y.-W.; Wu, K.-D.; Chen, H.-C. Comparisons of technetium-99m diethylenetriamine-pentaacetic acid plasma clearance and renal dynamic imaging with inulin clearance. *Am. J. Kidney Dis.* **2011**, *58*, 1043–1045. [CrossRef]
8. De Santo, N.G.; Anastasio, P.; Cirillo, M.; Santoro, D.; Spitali, L.; Mansi, L.; Celentano, L.; Capodicasa, D.; Cirillo, E.; Del Vecchio, E. Measurement of Glomerular FiltrationRate by the 99mTc-DTPA Renogram Is Less Precise than Measured and Predicted Creatinine Clearance. *Nephron* **1999**, *81*, 136–140. [CrossRef] [PubMed]
9. Gates, G.F. Glomerular filtration rate: Estimation from fractional renal accumulation of 99mTc-DTPA (stannous). *Am. J. Roentgenol.* **1982**, *138*, 565–570. [CrossRef] [PubMed]

10. Granerus, G.; Moonen, M. Effects of extra-renal background subtraction and kidney depth correction in the measurement of GFR by gamma camera renography. *Nucl. Med. Commun.* **1991**, *12*, 519–527. [CrossRef] [PubMed]
11. Maneval, D.C.; Magill, H.L.; Cypess, A.M.; Rodman, J.H. Measurement of skin-to-kidney distance in children: Implications for quantitative renography. *J. Nucl. Med.* **1990**, *31*, 287–291.
12. Tonnesen, K. Influence on the radiorenogram of variation in skin to kidney distance and the clinical importance hereof. In *Radionuclides in Nephrology*; Thieme: Stuttgart, Germany, 1975; pp. 79–86.
13. Itoh, K.; Arakawa, M. Re-estimation of renal function with 99m Tc-DTPA by the Gates' method. *Kaku Igaku* **1987**, *24*, 389–396. [PubMed]
14. Taylor, A.; Lewis, C.; Giacometti, A.; Hall, E.C.; Barefield, K.P. Improved formulas for the estimation of renal depth in adults. *J. Nucl. Med.* **1993**, *34*, 1766–1769. [PubMed]
15. Ma, Y.-C.; Zuo, L.; Chen, J.-H.; Luo, Q.; Yu, X.-Q.; Li, Y.; Xu, J.-S.; Huang, S.-M.; Wang, L.-N.; Huang, W.; et al. Modified glomerular filtration rate estimating equation for Chinese patients with chronic kidney disease. *J. Am. Soc. Nephrol.* **2006**, *17*, 2937–2944. [CrossRef]
16. DuBois, D. A formula to estimate the approximate surface area if height and body mass be known. *Arch. Intern. Med.* **1916**, *17*, 863–871. [CrossRef]
17. Liu, Y.; Zhao, A.; Lu, X.; Wang, Q.; Yang, L.; Zhang, Y.; Yan, A.; Tian, P.; Xue, J. Renal depth measured by CT optimize the glomerular filtration rate using the Gates method in living donor kidney transplantation. *Chin. J. Organ Transpl.* **2019**, *12*, 195–199.
18. Xue, J.; Deng, H.; Jia, X.; Wang, Y.; Lu, X.; Ding, X.; Li, Q.; Yang, A. Establishing a new formula for estimating renal depth in a Chinese adult population. *Medicine* **2017**, *96*, e5940. [CrossRef]
19. Sugawara, S.; Ishii, S.; Kojima, Y.; Ito, H.; Suzuki, Y.; Oriuchi, N. Feasibility of gamma camera-based GFR measurement using renal depth evaluated by lateral scan of 99mTc-DTPA renography. *Ann. Nucl. Med.* **2020**, *34*, 349–357. [CrossRef] [PubMed]
20. Awdeh, M.; Kouris, K.; Hassan, I.M.; Abdel-Dayem, H.M. Factors affecting the Gates' measurement of glomerular filtration rate. *Am. J. Physiol. Imaging* **1990**, *5*, 36–41.
21. Gruenewald, S.; Collins, L.; Fawdry, R. Kidney depth measurement and its influence on quantitation of function from gamma camera renography. *Clin. Nucl. Med.* **1985**, *10*, 398–401. [CrossRef] [PubMed]
22. Kwon, S.H.; Saad, A.; Herrmann, S.M.; Textor, S.C.; Lerman, L.O. Determination of single-kidney glomerular filtration rate in human subjects by using CT. *Radiology* **2015**, *276*, 490–498. [CrossRef] [PubMed]
23. You, S.; Ma, X.W.; Zhang, C.Z.; Li, Q.; Shi, W.W.; Zhang, J.; Yuan, X.D. Determination of single-kidney glomerular filtration rate (GFR) with CT urography versus renal dynamic imaging Gates method. *Eur. Radiol.* **2018**, *28*, 1077–1084. [CrossRef] [PubMed]
24. Buckley, D.L.; Shurrab, A.E.; Cheung, C.M.; Jones, A.P.; Mamtora, H.; Kalra, P.A. Measurement of single kidney function using dynamic contrast-enhanced MRI: Comparison of two models in human subjects. *J. Magn. Reson. Imaging Off. J. Int. Soc. Magn. Reson. Med.* **2006**, *24*, 1117–1123. [CrossRef] [PubMed]
25. Tipirneni-Sajja, A.; Loeffler, R.B.; Oesingmann, N.; Bissler, J.; Song, R.; McCarville, B.; Jones, D.P.; Hudson, M.; Spunt, S.L.; Hillenbrand, C.M. Measurement of glomerular filtration rate by dynamic contrast-enhanced magnetic resonance imaging using a subject-specific two-compartment model. *Physiol. Rep.* **2016**, *4*, e12755. [CrossRef]

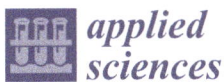

Article

Left Atrial Flow Stasis in Patients Undergoing Pulmonary Vein Isolation for Paroxysmal Atrial Fibrillation Using 4D-Flow Magnetic Resonance Imaging

Hana Sheitt [1,2,3,4,5], Hansuk Kim [3,4,6], Stephen Wilton [1,4], James A White [1,3] and Julio Garcia [1,2,3,4,5,*]

1. Department of Cardiac Sciences, University of Calgary, Calgary, AB T2N 1N4, Canada; hana.sheitt@ucalgary.ca (H.S.); sbwilton@ucalgary.ca (S.W.); jawhit@ucalgary.ca (J.A.W.)
2. Department of Radiology, University of Calgary, Calgary, AB T2N 1N4, Canada
3. Stephenson Cardiac Imaging Centre, University of Calgary, Calgary, AB T2N 1N4, Canada; hansuk.kim@ucalgary.ca
4. Libin Cardiovascular Institute, University of Calgary, Calgary, AB T2N 1N4, Canada
5. Alberta Children's Hospital Research Institute, University of Calgary, Calgary, AB T2N 1N4, Canada
6. Biomedical Engineering, University of Calgary, Calgary, AB T2N 1N4, Canada
* Correspondence: julio.garciaflores@ucalgary.ca

Featured Application: Left atrial stasis is a useful metric to evaluate hemodynamic recovery of the left atrial after pulmonary vein ablation.

Abstract: Atrial fibrillation (AF) is associated with systemic thrombo-embolism and stroke events, which do not appear significantly reduced following successful pulmonary vein (PV) ablation. Prior studies supported that thrombus formation is associated with left atrial (LA) flow alterations, particularly flow stasis. Recently, time-resolved three-dimensional phase-contrast (4D-flow) showed the ability to quantify LA stasis. This study aims to demonstrate that LA stasis, derived from 4D-flow, is a useful biomarker of LA recovery in patients with AF. Our hypothesis is that LA recovery will be associated with a reduction in LA stasis. We recruited 148 subjects with paroxysmal AF (40 following 3–4 months PV ablation and 108 pre-PV ablation) and 24 controls (CTL). All subjects underwent a cardiac magnetic resonance imaging (MRI) exam, inclusive of 4D-flow. LA was isolated within the 4D-flow dataset to constrain stasis maps. Control mean LA stasis was lower than in the pre-ablation cohort (30 ± 12% vs. 47 ± 18%, $p < 0.001$). In addition, mean LA stasis was reduced in the post-ablation cohort compared with pre-ablation (36 ± 15% vs. 47 ± 18%, $p = 0.002$). This study demonstrated that 4D flow-derived LA stasis mapping is clinically relevant and revealed stasis changes in the LA body pre- and post-pulmonary vein ablation.

Keywords: atrial fibrillation; 4D-flow; stasis; pulmonary vein ablation

1. Introduction

Atrial fibrillation (AF) is the most common arrhythmia associated with high morbidity and thrombo-embolism mortality [1]. At age 40 and older, AF lifetime risks increase for both men and women [2]. Previous studies have suggested that reduced flow velocity, i.e., flow stasis, in the left atria (LA) and LA appendage among subjects with paroxysmal AF in sinus rhythm can be an independent predictor of thrombus formation and stroke [3–5]. The complex 3-dimensional nature of LA flow can be explored using four-dimensional flow (4D-flow) by magnetic resonance imaging (MRI), which has proved to effectively assess LA stasis [6–8]. Furthermore, 4D-flow facilitates the visualization of flow patterns [9,10], vortex formation [8], and other advanced hemodynamic biomarkers [9,10]. In patients where rate control and anti-arrhythmic drugs are insufficient, pulmonary vein (PV) ablation therapy is used to maintain sinus rhythm. Therefore, the assessment of LA stasis changes due to ablation therapy requires further exploration.

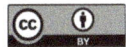

This study aims to demonstrate that LA stasis, derived from 4D-flow, is a useful biomarker of LA recovery in patients with AF undergoing PV ablation. Our hypothesis is that LA recovery will be associated with a reduction in LA stasis.

2. Materials and Methods

2.1. Study Population

A total of 172 subjects were recruited prospectively. This included a control cohort ($n = 24$), a pre-ablation cohort ($n = 108$) with paroxysmal AF with an over 2-year duration of the first-time diagnosis, and a post-ablation cohort ($n = 40$) with PV ablation therapy performed 3–6 months prior to imaging exam. A commercial software (Acuity®, Cohesic Inc., Calgary, AB, Canada) was used for the delivery of informed consent, health questionnaires, and collection of MRI-related variables.

Pre-ablation and post-ablation patients were required to be ≥ 18 years of age and have sinus rhythm at the time of imaging, with no more than mild mitral valve insufficiency, no cardiomyopathy, or complex congenital heart disease. Patients with implantable devices, severe renal impairment (eGFR ≤ 30 mL/min/1.73 m^2), or other recognized contraindications to MRI were excluded. Control subjects were required to be ≥ 18 years of age and have no history of cardiovascular disease, diabetes, or uncontrolled hypertension.

2.2. Risk Score

In all patients, the CHA$_2$DS$_2$-VASc risk score was calculated following current AF guidelines [11,12]. In addition, medical records obtained prior to MRI exam were used to document clinical risk factors for stroke/thrombo-embolism. Patients were given a single point for congestive heart failure/left ventricular (LV) systolic dysfunction, hypertension, diabetes mellitus, vascular disease, age 65–74, female gender, and two points for age ≥ 75 and prior stroke/transient ischemic attack thrombo-embolism [12].

2.3. Cardiac Magnetic Resonance Imaging Protocol

Cardiac imaging examination was performed using 3T MRI scanners (Skyra and Prima, Siemens, Germany). All subjects underwent a standardized clinical imaging protocol inclusive of retrospective electrocardiographic gating, time-resolved balanced steady-state free precession (SSFP) cine imaging in four-chamber, three-chamber, two-chamber, and short-axis views of LV at end-expiration. Contrast usage of gadolinium contrast volume of 0.2 mmol/kg (Gadovist®, Bayer Inc., Mississauga, ON, Canada) was administrated to acquire a contrast-enhanced 3D magnetic resonance angiogram (MRA) of the pulmonary veins in all subjects for assessing LA structure. Time-resolved three-dimensional phase-contrast MRI with three-directional velocity encoding (4D-flow, Siemens WIP 785A) was performed for 5–10 min, following contrast administration to measure in-vivo blood flow velocities within the whole heart. We have previously reported this whole-heart protocol [8,13]. Briefly, 4D-flow data was acquired during free breathing using navigator gating of diaphragmatic motion; sequence parameters were as follows: flip angle = 15 degrees, spatial resolution = $2.0 - 3.5 \times 2.0 - 3.5 \times 2.5 - 3.5$ mm; temporal resolution = 39–48 ms; and velocity sensitivity = 150–200 cm/s. Total acquisition time varies between 8–12 min, depending on heart rate and respiratory navigator efficiency. The number of phases was adjusted to 25.

2.4. Standard Cardiac Imaging Analysis

Standard cardiac images were analyzed by a blinded reader to the study, using dedicated software (cvi^{42}, Circle Cardiovascular Imaging Inc., Calgary, AB, Canada) to determine LV end-diastolic and LV end-systolic volume, LV ejection fraction, LV mass, and LA maximum volume.

2.5. 4D-Flow Data Analysis

4D-flow data were pre-processed for Maxwell terms, eddy current-induced phase offset, and velocity aliasing (if present), Figure 1A. A 3D phase-contrast magnetic resonance angiogram was generated for each subject and used to perform a LA segmentation using an in-house program based on Matlab (Matlab, Mathworks, Natick, MA, USA), Figure 1B. Then, the 4D-flow data set was masked to calculate velocity magnitude and stasis maps, Figure 1C. Velocity magnitude was calculated as follows:

$$V_{mag} = \sqrt{V_x^2 + V_y^2 + V_z^2} \tag{1}$$

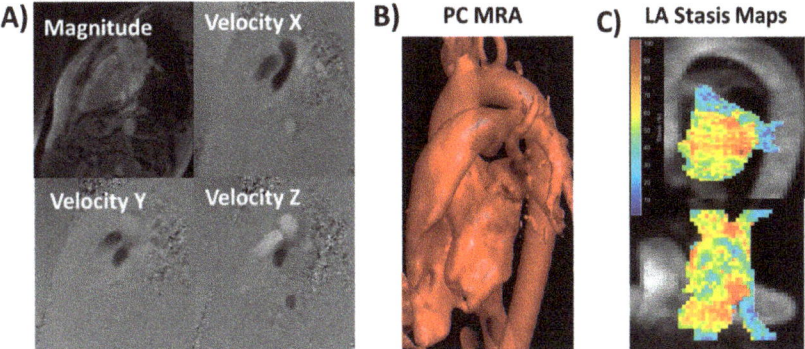

Figure 1. Data processing and analysis workflow. Panel (**A**) shows an example of corrected 4D-flow images. Panel (**B**) illustrates a time-average phase-contrast (PC) magnetic resonance angiogram (MRA) with an optimal threshold for visualizing left atrial (LA) anatomy. The LA was manually segmented using slice-by-slice, isolating the LA volume. Panel (**C**) shows the calculated LA stasis maps within the LA volume using a sagittal and a top-view maximum intensity projection. Red areas represent high stasis; blue areas represent low stasis.

Velocity magnitude from all voxels inside the isolated LA volume at all cardiac timeframes was used to create a velocity histogram [6,14]. Local peak velocity was obtained by averaging the top 5% of all velocity magnitude values. Local mean and standard deviation velocity were obtained. The relative amount of flow stasis (in percent) was calculated for each voxel by determining the incidence of voxels < 0.1 m/s among the total number of time frames [7,8]. Mean LA stasis was obtained by averaging the relative amount of flow stasis of voxels in the segmented LA volume. Volumetric LA stasis mapping was used to characterize stasis distribution visually.

2.6. Statistical Analysis

Shapiro-Wilk test was used to determine if parameters were normally distributed. To compare parameters within groups, 1-way analysis of variance or Kruskal-Wallis was used. Since AF prevalence increases with age, subjects were divided into three groups (<50 years, between 50 to 60 years, and >60 years) to assess age effect on LA stasis. Tukey's test or Mann-Whitney U-test were performed for multiple comparisons. Bonferroni correction was used to adjust for multiple comparisons and the differences were considered significant if $p < 0.0166$. Pearson correlation was calculated to investigate relationships between parameters. Statistical analysis was performed using SPSS 25 (SPSS, Chicago, IL, USA).

3. Results
3.1. Patient Characteristics

Patient baseline demographics are summarized in Table 1. The mean age of the pre-ablation cohort was 58 ± 10 years with 76% of men; the post-ablation cohort was 58 ± 11 years with 80% of men. Both cohorts were significantly older than the control cohort, 38 ± 15 years with 71% of men ($p < 0.001$). Similar differences were found for weight, body surface area, and diastolic blood pressure ($p = 0.001$). The mean CHA_2DS_2-VASc risk score of the pre-ablation patient population was 1.83 ± 0.98 (versus 0.33 ± 0.48 in controls, $p < 0.001$; and versus 0.81 ± 0.88 in post-ablation patients, $p < 0.001$). In pre-ablation patients, 2 (1.8%) having a risk score of 0, 47 (43.5%) having a risk score of 1, 34 (31.5%) having a risk score of 2, 18 (16.7%) having a risk score of 3, and 7 (6.5%) having a risk score of ≥4. Post-ablation patients showed a lower average risk score than pre-ablation (0.81 ± 0.88, $p < 0.001$), with 21 (52.5%) having a risk score of 0, 10 (25%) having a risk score of 1, 8 (20%) having a risk score of 2, and 1 (2.5%) having a risk score of 3. Cohorts showed a significant difference in LA volume ($p < 0.001$), with higher pre-ablation LA volume than controls (88 ± 29 mL vs. 66 ± 15 mL, $p < 0.001$), and lower post-ablation LA volume than pre-ablation (74 ± 20 mL vs. 88 ± 15 mL, $p = 0.018$). LV function remained similar pre- and post-ablation, however, controls differed, showing lower end-systolic volume than pre-ablation cohort (54 ± 11 mL vs. 69 ± 20 mL, $p = 0.002$). Ejection fraction was reduced in AF cohorts ($p < 0.004$), with similar values pre- and post-ablation.

Table 1. Data baseline.

	Control ($n = 24$)	Pre-Ablation ($n = 108$)	Post-Ablation ($n = 40$)	p-Value
Demographics				
Age (years)	38 ± 15	58 ± 10	58 ± 11	<0.001
Sex n (% women)	7 (29)	26 (24)	8 (20)	0.707
Height (m)	1.73 ± 0.10	1.78 ± 0.09	1.79 ± 0.07	0.064
Weight (Kg)	75 ± 19	90 ± 18	87 ± 16	0.001
Body Surface Area (m^2)	1.89 ± 0.28	2.11 ± 0.25	2.07 ± 0.21	0.001
Heart Rate (bpm)	65 ± 11	62 ± 13	65 ± 13	0.541
Systolic Blood Pressure (mmHg)	114 ± 15	119 ± 14	117 ± 26	0.479
Diastolic Blood Pressure (mmHg)	64 ± 12	71 ± 10	67 ± 7	0.011
Stroke Risk Score				
CHA_2DS_2-VASc Score	0.33 ± 0.48	1.83 ± 0.98	0.81 ± 0.88	<0.001
Score 0 (n)	16	2	21	
Score 1 (n)	8	47	10	
Score 2 (n)	0	34	8	
Score 3 (n)	0	18	1	
Score 4 (n)	0	6	0	
Score 5 (n)	0	1	0	
Left Atrium				
Left Atrial Volume (mL)	66 ± 15	88 ± 29	74 ± 20	<0.001
Left Ventricle				
End-Diastolic Volume (mL)	154 ± 31	171 ± 35	158 ± 30	0.026
End-Systolic Volume (mL)	54 ± 11	69 ± 20	65 ± 16	0.003
Ejection Fraction (%)	65 ± 4	60 ± 7	59 ± 6	0.004
Left Ventricle Mass (g)	100 ± 29	114 ± 29	113 ± 23	0.07

3.2. Left Atrial Hemodynamic Assessment

Control mean LA stasis was lower than in the pre-ablation cohort (30 ± 12% vs. 47 ± 18%, $p < 0.001$). Mean LA stasis was reduced in the post-ablation cohort as compared with pre-ablation (36 ± 15% vs. 47 ± 18%, $p = 0.002$), Figure 2A. Both pre- and post-ablation cohorts showed elevated standard deviation LA stasis as compared with controls (23 ± 5% vs. 17 ± 3%, $p < 0.001$; 22 ± 5% vs. 17 ± 3%, $p = 0.001$, Figure 2B). Similarly, mean LA velocity and standard deviation also decreased, Figure 2C,D.

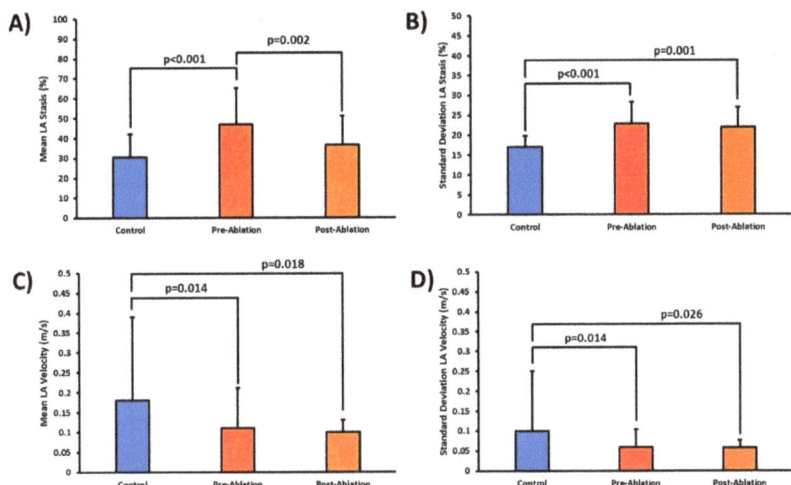

Figure 2. Left atrial stasis and velocity in controls, pre-ablation, and post-ablation patients. Panel (**A**) shows the comparison of all cohorts for mean left atrial (LA) stasis. Panel (**B**) shows the comparison of standard deviation LA stasis. Panels (**C**) and (**D**) show the comparison for all cohorts for mean and standard deviation LA velocity.

When comparing age groups, subjects older than 60-year-old showed an increased LA volume compared with the younger group of 50-year-old (88 ± 29% vs. 73 ± 19%, $p = 0.01$, Figure 3A). Standard deviation LA stasis increased with age when considering all subjects ($p < 0.001$, Figure 3B). Subjects between 50 and 60 years showed an increment of 13% in standard deviation LA stasis as compared with the younger cohort of 50-year-old ($p = 0.008$). Similarly, an increment of 21% was observed in the older cohort of >60-year-old ($p < 0.001$). LA volume was >100 mL in 20% of subjects with an increased stasis compared with a lower LA volume of 60 mL, which included 45 subjects (23 ± 6% vs. 20 ± 5%, $p = 0.033$). Overall, subjects with risk score > 2 ($n = 26$) showed more increased standard deviation LA stasis than those with a risk score of 0 ($n = 122$) (24 ± 5% vs. 21 ± 5%, $p = 0.031$). No association was found with LA peak velocity, mean velocity, or standard deviation velocity.

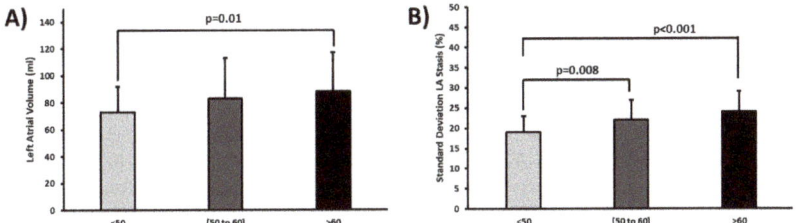

Figure 3. Age comparison for left atrial volume and standard deviation stasis. Panel (**A**) shows the comparison of age groups for left atrial (LA) volume. Panel (**B**) indicates the comparison of age groups for standard deviation LA stasis.

4. Discussion

This study illustrates the usefulness of 4D-flow to quantify and assess LA stasis. The main findings of our study were: (1) LA stasis can be substantially reduced after PV ablation; (2) Standard deviation LA stasis and atrial volume significantly increase with age;

(3) Standard deviation LA stasis was higher in patients with risk score > 2 pre-ablation and was reduced post-ablation.

Virchow's triad is widely accepted and defines the main factors leading to thrombogenesis [15]. These factors include abnormal stasis or reduced blood flow, endothelial/endocardial injury or dysfunction, and hypercoagulability. Time-resolved 4D-flow provides a non-invasive characterization of LA hemodynamics and has been used to assess AF patients pre-ablation [7,8,16]. As derived from 4D-flow, LA stasis may serve as an essential biomarker that characterizes the predisposition to atrial thrombogenesis to that of regular risk predictors (e.g., CHA_2DS_2-VASc Score). Despite the comprehensive assessment obtained by 4D-flow, an accurate 3D segmentation is required. In our study, semi-manual segmentation was obtained. A careful selection of intensity threshold can facilitate the appropriate visualization of PV and LA appendage. Fluckiger et al. reported comparable mean flow velocity in the LA between paroxysmal AF patients and controls [14]. In our study, the mean LA velocity was significantly reduced in pre-ablation and post-ablation, which aligned with a more extensive study conducted by Lee et al. [17]. The latter was supported by other recent studies [6,8,16]. Significant inverse relationships between LA mean/peak velocity and risk score were reported in previous studies [6,17]. In our study, no significant associations were found for LA mean/peak and standard deviation velocities. Much of the attention has been given to the LA appendage as the primary source of thrombus formation in AF. A previous study from Markl et al. suggested that atrial flow dynamics are disrupted in AF patients, even during coordinated activity, thus suggesting an AF component that may be unrecognized [6]. In one of our recent studies, we demonstrated that vortex formation within the LA is influenced by pulmonary vein inflow velocities and LA remodeling with a higher prevalence of stasis [8]. There may be an interplay between the functional (LA volume, pressure overload, and dilation) and hemodynamic features (stasis, vortex formation, energetics, and flow patterns). The associations between these factors are complex and may have compensatory effects. However, identifying irreversible recovery should warn for earlier detection of complications or adverse outcomes [18,19]. Despite the lack of significant change in LA velocities between the pre-ablation and post-ablation cohort, we were able to detect an improvement via mean LA stasis. Note that LV and LA standard metrics also failed to detect a significant change pre- and post-ablation.

Overall, these findings put in context new evidence characterizing paroxysmal AF complex hemodynamics. However, current guidelines rely on clinical factors and co-morbidities, with the exclusion of AF burden, atrial size, flow hemodynamics, and other factors that may suggest more advanced atrial disease and this higher risk of thromboembolic events [20]. Therefore, including the above-mentioned factors may help to improve long-term LA recovery outcomes.

This study has some limitations, including limited patients matching pre and post-ablation, follow-up of AF recurrence, age-matching, and manual static segmentation. Our study excluded patients with more than mild mitral insufficiency, given that it is anticipated to be a potential confounder to LA hemodynamics and baseline characteristics. Clinical background decision for ablation referral was not individually investigated. Our segmentations did not separate LA volume from the LA appendage, which can be useful for a better characterization of LA stasis. However, LA appendage measurements may be affected by the high noise levels and the influence of low spatial resolution. For all subjects, we used an optimized 4D-flow WIP sequence for Siemens scanners. However, this sequence is based on average data over multiple heart cycles, which is known to limit the assessment of arrhythmic effects. The latter justifies, in part, that all our subjects were in sinus rhythm. Recent developments are leading towards multi-dimensional and self-gated acquisition frameworks that may allow better to explore heart variability and its hemodynamics [21]. However, these developments are still in the early stage, require high computational cost, and are not widely accessible for clinical application.

5. Conclusions

This study demonstrated that 4D-flow could characterize relevant LA blood flow stasis changes in patients with AF undergoing PV isolation.

Author Contributions: Conceptualization, H.S., S.W., J.A.W., and J.G.; methodology, H.S., J.G.; software, H.S., H.K., J.G.; validation, S.W., J.A.W. and J.G.; formal analysis, H.S., J.G.; investigation, J.G.; resources, J.G.; data curation, H.S., H.K., and J.G.; writing—original draft preparation, H.S., J.G.; writing—review and editing, H.S., H.K., S.W., J.A.W.; visualization, J.G.; supervision, J.G.; project administration, J.G.; funding acquisition, J.G. All authors have read and agreed to the published version of the manuscript.

Funding: This research was funded by The University of Calgary, URGC SEM #1054341; J.G. start-up funding; H.S. received support from The Libin Cardiovascular Institute, H.K. from the Biomedical Engineering graduate program. We acknowledge the support of the Natural Science and Engineering Research Council of Canada/Conseil de recherche en science naturelles et en génie du Canada, RGPIN-2020-04549 and DGECR-2020-00204.

Institutional Review Board Statement: The study was conducted according to the guidelines of the Declaration of Helsinki and approved by the Conjoint Health Research Ethics Board of University of Calgary (REB13-0902 approved on 6/18/2014; and currently active MOD11 approved on 10/5/2020).

Informed Consent Statement: Written informed consent was obtained from all subjects involved in the study.

Data Availability Statement: The anonymized data presented in this study are available on request from the corresponding author. The data are not publicity available due to privacy and ethical restrictions.

Acknowledgments: We thank Easter Prosia for her assistance in verifying heart volume measurements and Sandra Rivest for English editing revision.

Conflicts of Interest: The authors declare no conflict of interest.

References

1. Fuster, V.; Rydén, L.E.; Cannom, D.S.; Crijns, H.J.; Curtis, A.B.; Ellenbogen, K.A.; Halperin, J.L.; Kay, G.N.; Le Huezey, J.-Y.; Lowe, J.E.; et al. ACCF/AHA/HRS focused updates incorporated into the ACC/AHA/ESC 2006 guidelines for the management of patients with atrial fibrillation: A report of the American College of Cardiology Foundation/American Heart Association Task Force on practice guidel. *Circulation* **2011**, *123*, e269–e367. [CrossRef] [PubMed]
2. Lloyd-Jones, D.M.; Wang, T.J.; Leip, E.P.; Larson, M.; Levy, D.; Vasan, R.S.; D'Agostino, R.B.; Massaro, J.M.; Beiser, A.; Wolf, P.A.; et al. Lifetime Risk for Development of Atrial Fibrillation. *Circulation* **2004**, *110*, 1042–1046. [CrossRef] [PubMed]
3. Goldman, M.E.; Pearce, L.A.; Hart, R.G.; Zabalgoitia, M.; Asinger, R.W.; Safford, R.; Halperin, J.L. Pathophysiologic correlates of thromboembolism in nonvalvular atrial fibrillation: I. Reduced flow velocity in the left atrial appendage (The Stroke Prevention in Atrial Fibrillation [SPAF-III] study). *J. Am. Soc. Echocardiogr.* **1999**, *12*, 1080–1087. [CrossRef]
4. Zabalgoitia, M.; Halperin, J.L.; Pearce, L.A.; Blackshear, J.L.; Asinger, R.W.; Hart, R.G. Transesophageal echocardiographic correlates of clinical risk of thromboembolism in nonvalvular atrial fibrillation. Stroke Prevention in Atrial Fibrillation III Investigators. *J. Am. Coll. Cardiol.* **1998**, *31*, 1622–1626. [CrossRef]
5. Fyrenius, L.; Wigström, T.; Ebbers, M.; Karlsson, J.; Engvall, A.; Bolger, F. Three dimensional flow in the human left atrium. *Heart* **2001**, *86*, 448–455. Available online: http://www.ncbi.nlm.nih.gov/pubmed/11559688 (accessed on 14 April 2021). [CrossRef]
6. Markl, M.; Lee, D.; Furiasse, N.; Carr, M.; Foucar, C.; Ng, J.; Carr, J.; Goldberger, J.J. Left Atrial and Left Atrial Appendage 4D Blood Flow Dynamics in Atrial Fibrillation. *Circ. Cardiovasc. Imaging* **2016**, *9*, e004984. [CrossRef]
7. Markl, M.; Lee, D.C.; Ng, J.; Carr, M.; Carr, J.; Goldberger, J.J. Left Atrial 4-Dimensional Flow Magnetic Resonance Imaging: Stasis and Velocity Mapping in Patients With Atrial Fibrillation. *Investig. Radiol.* **2016**, *51*, 147–154. [CrossRef]
8. Garcia, J.; Sheitt, H.; Bristow, M.S.; Lydell, C.; Howarth, A.G.; Heydari, B.; Prato, F.S.; Drangova, M.; Thornhill, R.E.; Nery, P.; et al. Left atrial vortex size and velocity distributions by 4D flow MRI in patients with paroxysmal atrial fibrillation: Associations with age and CHA2 DS2-VASc risk score. *J. Magn. Reson. Imaging* **2020**, *51*, 871–884. [CrossRef]
9. Dyverfeldt, P.; Bissell, M.; Barker, A.J.; Bolger, A.F.; Carlhäll, C.-J.; Ebbers, T.; Francios, C.J.; Frydrychowicz, A.; Geiger, J.; Giese, D.; et al. 4D flow cardiovascular magnetic resonance consensus statement. *J. Cardiovasc. Magn. Reson.* **2015**, *17*, 72. [CrossRef]
10. Garcia, J.; Barker, A.J.; Markl, M. The Role of Imaging of Flow Patterns by 4D Flow MRI in Aortic Stenosis. *JACC Cardiovasc. Imaging* **2019**, *12*. [CrossRef]

11. January, C.T.; Wann, L.S.; Alpert, J.S.; Calkins, F.H.; Cigarroa, J.E.; Cleveland, J.C.; Conti, J.B.; Ellinor, P.T.; Ezekowitz, M.D.; Field, M.E.; et al. 2014 AHA/ACC/HRS guideline for the management of patients with atrial fibrillation: Executive summary: A report of the American College of Cardiology/American Heart Association Task Force on practice guidelines and the Heart Rhythm Society. *Circulation* **2014**, *130*, 2071–2104. [CrossRef]
12. Lip, G.Y.H.; Nieuwlaat, R.; Pisters, R.; Lane, D.A.; Crijns, H.J.G.M. Refining clinical risk stratification for predicting stroke and thromboembolism in atrial fibrillation using a novel risk factor-based approach: The euro heart survey on atrial fibrillation. *Chest* **2010**, *137*, 263–272. [CrossRef]
13. Garcia, J.; Beckie, K.; Hassanabad, A.F.; Sojoudi, A.; White, J.A. Aortic and mitral flow quantification using dynamic valve tracking and machine learning: Prospective study assessing static and dynamic plane repeatability, variability and agreement. *JRSM Cardiovasc. Dis.* **2021**, *10*, 204800402199990. [CrossRef]
14. Fluckiger, J.U.; Goldberger, J.J.; Lee, D.; Ng, J.; Lee, R.; Goyal, A.; Markl, M. Left atrial flow velocity distribution and flow coherence using four-dimensional FLOW MRI: A pilot study investigating the impact of age and Pre- and Postintervention atrial fibrillation on atrial hemodynamics. *J. Magn. Reson. Imaging* **2013**, *38*, 580–587. [CrossRef]
15. Watson, T.; Shantsila, E.; Lip, G.Y. Mechanisms of thrombogenesis in atrial fibrillation: Virchow's triad revisited. *Lancet* **2009**, *373*, 155–166. [CrossRef]
16. Demirkiran, A.; Amier, R.P.; Hofman, M.B.M.; van der Geest, R.J.; Robbers, L.F.H.J.; Hopman, L.H.G.A.; Mulder, M.J.; van de Ven, P.; Allaart, C.P.; van Rossum, A.C.; et al. Altered left atrial 4D flow characteristics in patients with paroxysmal atrial fibrillation in the absence of apparent remodeling. *Sci. Rep.* **2021**, *11*, 5965. [CrossRef] [PubMed]
17. Lee, D.C.; Markl, M.; Ng, J.; Carr, M.; Benefield, B.; Carr, J.C.; Goldberger, J.J. Three-dimensional left atrial blood flow characteristics in patients with atrial fibrillation assessed by 4D flow CMR. *Eur. Hear. J. Cardiovasc. Imaging* **2016**, *17*, 1259–1268. [CrossRef] [PubMed]
18. Burstein, B.; Nattel, S. Atrial fibrosis: Mechanisms and clinical relevance in atrial fibrillation. *J. Am. Coll. Cardiol.* **2008**, *51*, 802–809. [CrossRef]
19. Shen, M.J.; Arora, R.; Jalife, J. Atrial Myopathy. *JACC Basic Transl. Sci.* **2019**, *4*, 640–654. [CrossRef]
20. January, C.T.; Wann, L.S.; Calkins, H.; Chen, L.Y.; Cigarroa, J.E.; Cleveland, J.C.; Ellinor, P.T.; Ezekowitz, M.D.; Field, M.E.; Furie, K.L. 2019 AHA/ACC/HRS Focused Update of the 2014 AHA/ACC/HRS Guideline for the Management of Patients With Atrial Fibrillation: A Report of the American College of Cardiology/American Heart Association Task Force on Clinical Practice Guidelines and the Heart R. *Circulation* **2019**, *140*, e125–e151. [CrossRef]
21. Ma, L.; Yerly, J.; Di Sopra, L.; Piccini, D.; Lee, J.; DiCarlo, A.; Passman, R.; Greenland, P.; Kim, D.; Stuber, M.; et al. Using 5D flow MRI to decode the effects of rhythm on left atrial 3D flow dynamics in patients with atrial fibrillation. *Magn. Reson. Med.* **2021**, *85*, 3125–3139. [CrossRef]

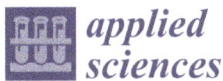

Article

Fundus Image Registration Technique Based on Local Feature of Retinal Vessels

Roziana Ramli [1,*], Khairunnisa Hasikin [2,*], Mohd Yamani Idna Idris [1], Noor Khairiah A. Karim [3] and Ainuddin Wahid Abdul Wahab [1]

[1] Department of Computer System and Technology, Faculty of Computer Science and Information Technology, Universiti Malaya, Kuala Lumpur 50603, Malaysia; yamani@um.edu.my (M.Y.I.I.); ainuddin@um.edu.my (A.W.A.W.)

[2] Department of Biomedical Engineering, Faculty of Engineering, Universiti Malaya, Kuala Lumpur 50603, Malaysia

[3] Regenerative Medicine Cluster/Imaging Unit, Advanced Medical & Dental Institute, Universiti Sains Malaysia, Kepala Batas 13200, Malaysia; drkhairiah@usm.my

* Correspondence: roziana.ramli@um.edu.my (R.R.); khairunnisa@um.edu.my (K.H.)

Citation: Ramli, R.; Hasikin, K.; Idris, M.Y.I.; A. Karim, N.K.; Wahab, A.W.A. Fundus Image Registration Technique Based on Local Feature of Retinal Vessels. *Appl. Sci.* **2021**, *11*, 11201. https://doi.org/10.3390/app112311201

Academic Editors: Alessandro Stefano, Albert Comelli and Federica Vernuccio

Received: 30 September 2021
Accepted: 19 November 2021
Published: 25 November 2021

Publisher's Note: MDPI stays neutral with regard to jurisdictional claims in published maps and institutional affiliations.

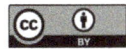

Copyright: © 2021 by the authors. Licensee MDPI, Basel, Switzerland. This article is an open access article distributed under the terms and conditions of the Creative Commons Attribution (CC BY) license (https://creativecommons.org/licenses/by/4.0/).

Abstract: Feature-based retinal fundus image registration (RIR) technique aligns fundus images according to geometrical transformations estimated between feature point correspondences. To ensure accurate registration, the feature points extracted must be from the retinal vessels and throughout the image. However, noises in the fundus image may resemble retinal vessels in local patches. Therefore, this paper introduces a feature extraction method based on a local feature of retinal vessels (CURVE) that incorporates retinal vessels and noises characteristics to accurately extract feature points on retinal vessels and throughout the fundus image. The CURVE performance is tested on CHASE, DRIVE, HRF and STARE datasets and compared with six feature extraction methods used in the existing feature-based RIR techniques. From the experiment, the feature extraction accuracy of CURVE (86.021%) significantly outperformed the existing feature extraction methods ($p \leq 0.001$*). Then, CURVE is paired with a scale-invariant feature transform (SIFT) descriptor to test its registration capability on the fundus image registration (FIRE) dataset. Overall, CURVE-SIFT successfully registered 44.030% of the image pairs while the existing feature-based RIR techniques (GDB-ICP, Harris-PIIFD, Ghassabi's-SIFT, H-M 16, H-M 17 and D-Saddle-HOG) only registered less than 27.612% of the image pairs. The one-way ANOVA analysis showed that CURVE-SIFT significantly outperformed GDB-ICP ($p = 0.007$*), Harris-PIIFD, Ghassabi's-SIFT, H-M 16, H-M 17 and D-Saddle-HOG ($p \leq 0.001$*).

Keywords: image registration; fundus image; feature extraction

1. Introduction

Retinal fundus image registration (RIR) is an essential tool in facilitating the diagnosis and treatment of retinal diseases [1]. RIR aligns fundus images according to geometrical transformation estimated from correspondence between fixed and moving images. Existing RIR techniques can be grouped based on the type of correspondence utilized in estimating the geometrical transformation, namely, intensity-based and feature-based.

The intensity-based RIR technique searches the similarity between the intensity patterns in fixed and moving images to estimate the geometrical transformation. The similarity between the intensity patterns is established using a similarity metric such as mutual information [2], cross-correlation [3] and phase correlation [4,5]. However, the registration performance of the intensity-based RIR technique is limited in the presence of non-uniform intensity distribution and homogenous texture [6], which is commonly observed in fundus images. Furthermore, the intensity patterns from the non-overlapping area can mislead the similarity metric in estimating inaccurate geometrical transformation.

Generally, the feature-based RIR technique is more reliable and robust in registering fundus images compared to the intensity-based RIR technique. This is because the feature-based RIR technique estimates the geometrical transformation according to the correspondence of local features such as feature points. However, the feature-based RIR technique requires the feature points to be extracted from reliable information to ensure accurate registration. Reliable information is distributed throughout an image and repeatable despite the changes in viewpoint or intensity [7]. The feature-based RIR technique is mainly comprised of feature extraction, feature descriptor, matching and estimating geometrical transformation. Feature extraction plays a crucial role in ensuring the feature points are detected and selected from reliable information by examining the local patches.

The feature extraction method in the existing feature-based RIR techniques extracts feature points from retinal vessels [8], vessel bifurcations [9], corner [10], extrema [11–13] or distinctive structure information [14]. Among this information, the retinal vessel is the most reliable because it can be found throughout the fundus image and is repeatable despite the changes in viewpoint or intensity. Additionally, the appearance of the retinal vessels within the local patches are consistent as a continuous line in 2-dimensional, and curvature shape in 3-dimensional, despite its size and contrast. However, the noises such as the retinal nerve fiber layer, underlying choroidal vessels, microaneurysm and exudates can also appear as curvature shapes in the local patches.

Therefore, this paper introduces a new feature extraction method based on the local feature of retinal vessels (CURVE). The proposed CURVE extracts feature points throughout the fundus image with the ability to discriminate the aforementioned noises. To register the fundus images, a feature-based RIR technique framework (CURVE-SIFT) is described where CURVE is paired with the scale-invariant feature transform (SIFT) descriptor [15].

The remainder of this paper is organized as follows. Section 2 highlights and discusses the issues of the feature extraction method in the existing feature-based RIR techniques. Section 3 describes the methodology of the CURVE-SIFT technique. The experimental settings in developing and evaluating the CURVE-SIFT technique are presented in Section 4. Section 5 reports and discusses the experimental results. Finally, the conclusion and future work are given in Section 6.

2. Related Works

The majority of the existing feature-based RIR techniques [13,16–18] mainly utilized the SIFT detector [15] to extract the feature points. SIFT detector finds extrema from local patches in a hierarchical difference of Gaussian (DoG) scale-space to allow feature points to be found based on the structure of various sizes. Then, the extrema that are low contrast and on edges are rejected to ensure the final feature points are distinctive and repeatable. However, the retinal vessels exhibit inconsistent contrast levels throughout the fundus image. Therefore, Ghassabi et al. [11] utilized robust uniform SIFT (UR-SIFT) [19] to overcome this issue.

The UR-SIFT is an improvement of the SIFT detector, where the feature points are selected according to the strength of the texture surrounding the points. This enables UR-SIFT to be more efficient in extracting feature points on retinal vessels compared to the standard SIFT detector. Furthermore, UR-SIFT ensures the extracted feature points are distributed throughout the hierarchical DoG scale space. The distribution is set in reverse from the scale coefficients of the scale space. This results in more feature points being extracted in the lower part of the hierarchical DoG scale space where the images are larger and finer. Opposite to this, fewer feature points are extracted in the upper part of the hierarchical DoG scale space where the images are smaller and coarser.

Ghassabi et al. further improved their work by introducing a stability score as part of the selection criterion [8]. The stability score incorporates Frangi's vesselness measure (FVM) [20], a vessel enhancement filter that suppresses noise in the image. Incorporating FVM enabled the ability of [8] to discriminate between retinal vessels and noises.

Extracting feature points on retinal vessels from the underexposed region in the fundus image is addressed in [12], where the illumination invariant Difference of Gaussian (*ii*DoG) operator was incorporated into the hierarchical scale space [21]. *ii*DoG operator is composed of normalized difference of Gaussian (*n*DoG) and DoG operators based on a piecewise function. The combination of these operators increases the visibility of the underexposed region while leaving the correctly exposed region unchanged. This work utilized a similar approach as in SIFT detector to extract extrema from the hierarchical *ii*DoG scale space. A threshold is introduced to discard the extrema on the retinal surface before the final feature points are selected. The threshold is based on the distribution of the intensity in the local patch.

Other than SIFT, the existing feature-based RIR techniques [10,22–24] extract geometric corner [25], Harris corner [26] and speeded up robust features (SURF) [27,28]. Meanwhile, Ramli et al. [14] introduced D-Saddle to extract feature points from the low-quality region based on distinctive structural information.

There are several issues that can be outlined from the highlighted feature extraction methods. First, feature enhancement algorithms such as DoG and *ii*DoG operators are mainly incorporated in building the hierarchical scale space. These operators increase the visibility of the retinal vessels as well as the noises, which make it more challenging for the feature extraction method to discriminate between them.

Second, the feature extraction methods are mainly without a proper selection module to select feature points on retinal vessels. A proper selection module should consider both retinal vessels and noise information as they may appear similarly within a local patch. Therefore, considering both in the selection module allows for more robust discrimination between retinal vessels and noises.

3. Methodology

The CURVE-SIFT technique constitutes five main stages, as shown in Figure 1. Stage 1 converts the input images to grayscale. The proposed CURVE in Stage 2 extracts feature points from the input grayscale images, which also highlights the main contribution of this paper. Stage 3 computes the SIFT descriptor to describe the surrounding region of each CURVE feature point. From the computed descriptors, matches are established, and outliers are removed in Stage 4. Finally, Stage 5 estimates the geometrical transformation between fixed and moving images. The details of these stages are explained in the following sub-sections. The mathematical symbols and notation used in this section are listed in Appendix A (Table A1).

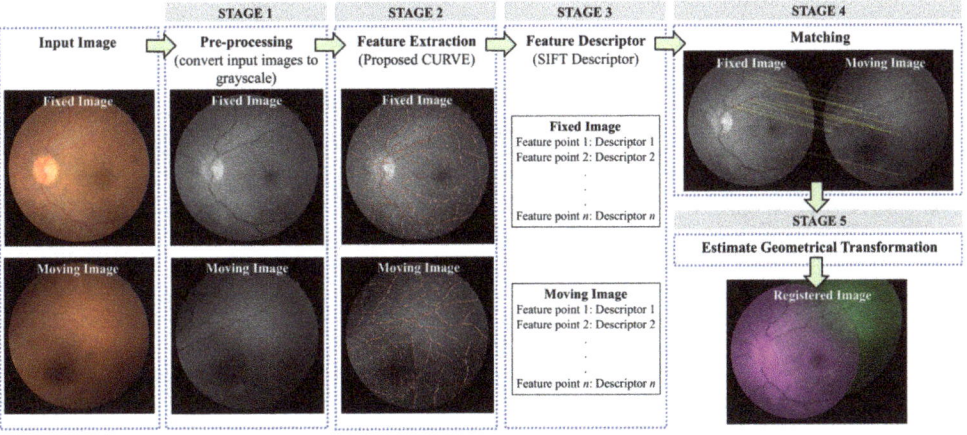

Figure 1. A general framework of the CURVE-SIFT technique.

3.1. STAGE 1: Pre-Processing

The conversion of the input images from color to grayscale follows the calculation of luminance in Recommendation ITU-R BT.601-7 [29] given below:

$$I = 0.2989\mathcal{R} + 0.587\mathcal{G} + 0.1140\mathcal{B} \qquad (1)$$

where, I is the input image in grayscale, $\mathcal{R}$ is the red channel, $\mathcal{G}$ is the green channel and $\mathcal{B}$ is the blue channel. The grayscale conversion based on luminance was chosen for this study because it has been shown to be superior to other grayscale conversions in terms of highlighting texture visibility [30] and trade-off between accuracy and processing cost.

3.2. STAGE 2: Feature Extraction

This sub-section describes the proposed CURVE to extract feature points on retinal vessels. CURVE is composed of feature detection and feature selection modules. The feature detection module detects candidate feature points according to the curvature shape of the retinal vessels. The curvature shape of the retinal vessels is observed when its grayscale image is depicted in 3D (see Table A2 in Appendix B). However, the detected candidate feature points are located on retinal vessels as well as noises. Therefore, the feature selection module removes the detected candidate feature points associated with noises by considering the unique characteristics of both retinal vessels and noises in intensity profiles. Then, the final feature points are chosen based on the strength of the retinal vessels. The steps in the feature detection and feature selection modules are summarized in Figure 2.

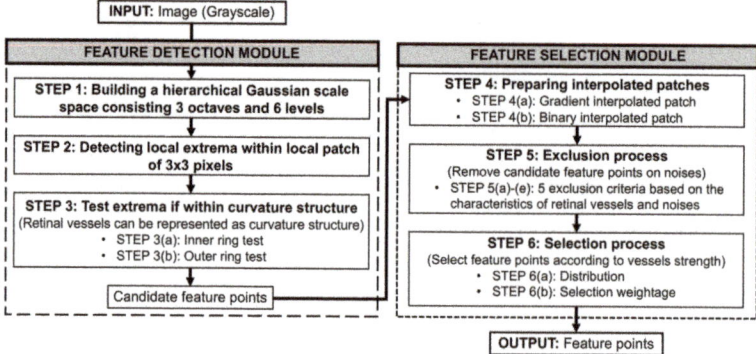

Figure 2. Overview of CURVE feature extraction in Stage 2. CURVE is composed of a feature detection module and feature selection module.

3.2.1. Feature Detection Module

The feature detection module examines local patches in the images of the hierarchical Gaussian scale space to detect extrema within the curvature shape of various sizes. This module involves three main steps, as explained below.

(a) STEP 1: Building a hierarchical Gaussian scale space

The initial step of the feature detection module is to build a hierarchical Gaussian scale space. The hierarchical Gaussian scale space enables the detection of the candidate feature points on various sizes of retinal vessels at the lower octave as the images are larger and finer with detailed information. At the higher octave, the candidate feature points are detected on thicker retinal vessels as the images are smaller and coarser with prominent information.

Building the hierarchical Gaussian scale space (G) involves generating three octaves ($P = 3 \mid p = 0, \ldots, P-1$) and six levels ($Q = 6 \mid q = -1, \cdots, Q-2$) per octave, as in [15,31].

The initial Gaussian image $G_{p,q}$ at $p = 0$ and $q = -1$ is created through convolution of input image I with width of relative Gaussian kernel $\check{\sigma}_{p,q}$ at $p = 0$ and $q = -1$ as follows:

$$G_{0,-1} = I * \check{\sigma}_{0,-1} \tag{2}$$

with, $\check{\sigma}_{0,-1}$ is denoted by:

$$\check{\sigma}_{0,-1} = \sqrt{\sigma_{0,-1}^2 - \sigma_s^2} \tag{3}$$

The width of the relative Gaussian kernel $\check{\sigma}_{p,q}$ assumes the input image I is pre-filtered with a sampling Gaussian kernel $\sigma_s \geq 0.5$ [15]. Thus, $\sigma_{0,-1}$ can be expressed as in [15,31]:

$$\sigma_{0,-1} = \sigma_0 \cdot 2^{-1/Q-3} \tag{4}$$

where, $\sigma_0 = 1.6$ is the base width of the Gaussian kernel.

$$\check{\sigma}_{0,-1} = \sqrt{\sigma_{0,-1}^2 - \sigma_s^2} \tag{5}$$

To obtain $G_{p,-1}$ at higher octave $p \in [1, \ldots, P-1]$, $G_{p-1,2}$ is downsampled by half. The subsequent $G_{p,q}$ at $p \in [0, \ldots, P-1]$ and $q \in [0, \ldots, Q-2]$ can be obtained from the convolution between $G_{p,-1}$ in the respective octave with the relative Gaussian kernel of width $\check{\sigma}_q$ given by:

$$\check{\sigma}_q = \sigma_0 \cdot \sqrt{2^{2q/Q-3} - 1} \tag{6}$$

(b) STEP 2: Detecting local extrema

The feature detection module continues with the detection of extrema within the local patches of 3×3 pixels. An extremum represents the maximum or minimum intensity value of the center pixel compared to the eight immediate neighbors in the local patch. The local patches across the image are overlapped by $1/3$ of its size. The extrema found near the border of the field of view (FOV) are excluded from further processing using a mask image.

(c) STEP 3: Test extrema if within curvature structure

The retinal vessels generally exhibit curvature shape in 3-dimensions. Therefore, the extrema are tested if they are within the curvature structure by performing two tests as reported in [32]. These tests are the inner ring test and outer ring test.

- STEP 3(a): Inner ring test

The inner ring test considers eight pixels surrounding an extremum ($a_j \mid j \in [1, \ldots, 8]$), as depicted in Figure 3a. Four out of eight pixels are tested at a time for patterns $\times$ and $+$, as shown in Figure 3b–e. These patterns are formed when the intensities of two opposing pixels are brighter (dark green dot) than the other two opposing pixels in orthogonal (pink dot). The extrema can pass this test with one or two patterns. Then, the central intensity value β is estimated by taking the median value of four pixels if the extremum passes with one pattern, and eight pixels if it passes with two patterns. The extrema that failed the inner ring test are eliminated.

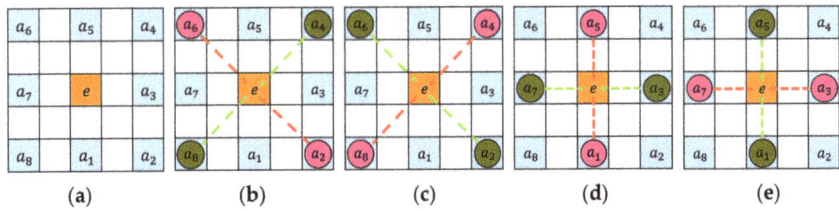

Figure 3. Inner ring test. (**a**) Eight pixels denoted by a_j, $j \in [1, \ldots, 8]$ surrounding an extremum, e. (**b**,**c**) Patterns in the shape of $\times$. (**d**,**e**) Patterns in the shape of $+$. Pixels with a dark green dot have higher intensity values than pixels with a pink dot.

- STEP 3(b): Outer ring test

A circumference of 16 pixels surrounding an extremum that passes the inner ring test forms the outer ring pixels ($b_l \mid l \in [1,\ldots, 16]$) as shown in Figure 4a. These pixels are divided into groups of *low*, *middle* and *high* as defined below:

$$\begin{aligned} \text{Group low (red dot)} &: I_{b_l} < \beta - \varepsilon \\ \text{Group middle (purple dot)} &: \beta - \varepsilon \le I_{b_l} \le \beta + \varepsilon \\ \text{Group high (green dot)} &: I_{b_l} > \beta + \varepsilon \end{aligned} \qquad (7)$$

where, I_{b_l} is the intensity of the outer ring pixels and ε is the offset. The offset ε is set to 0.0010 as the intensity value of the pixels is in the range of [0, 1] [14].

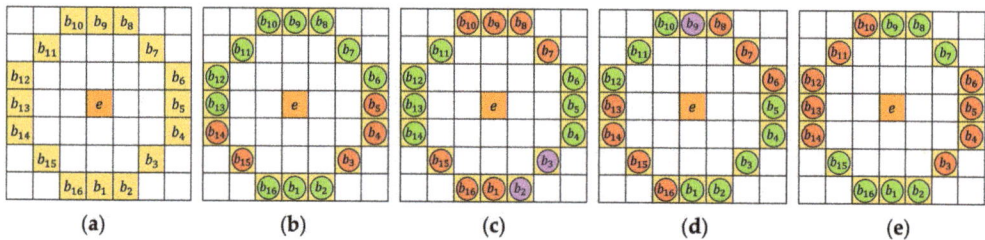

Figure 4. Outer ring test. (a) Sixteen pixels denoted by $b_l, l \in [1,\ldots, 16]$ surrounding an extremum, *e*. (b–e) Examples of outer ring patterns. Pixels with red dot are from group *low*, pixels with purple dot are from group *medium* and pixels with green dot are from group *high*.

Then, the extrema are tested for the outer ring patterns consisting of consecutive and alternating arcs from groups *low* and *high*. The length of each arc can be between 2 to 8 pixels. These arcs can also be separated by pixels from group *middle* up to two pixels. Examples of the outer ring patterns are depicted in Figure 4b–e. The extrema that pass the outer ring test are the extrema found within the curvature structure, as shown in Figure 5. These extrema are assigned as candidate feature points and included in the feature selection module.

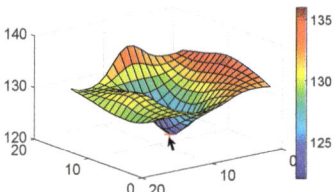

Figure 5. Example of candidate feature point (pointed by black arrow) from feature detection module. The candidate feature point is an extremum within a curvature structure.

3.2.2. Feature Selection Module

The feature selection module includes exclusion and selection processes. The exclusion process discards the candidate feature points associated with noises while the selection process selects the final feature points according to the strength of the retinal vessels. These processes require gradient and binary interpolated patches as input.

(a) STEP 4: Preparing gradient and binary interpolated patches

The initial step of the feature selection module is to extract a square patch with the size of $s_p \times s_p$ pixels for each candidate feature point from the respective $G_{p,q}$. The size of the patch is varied depending on the octave position (p) of the candidate feature point to ensure the retinal vessel can be captured within the patch despite the image size of $G_{p,q}$. The side length (s_p) of the patch is an odd number computed as follows:

$$s_p = s_{initial} - 4(p+1) \qquad (8)$$

where, $s_{initial}$ is the initial side length. There are three possible values for $s_{initial}$ as defined in (9). $s_{initial}$ is set by referring to the size of the initial Gaussian image $G_{0,-1}$. These values are determined by observing the retinal vessels with the thickest width on the fundus images from five datasets; CHASE_DB1 [33,34], DRIVE [35,36], HRF [37,38], STARE [39,40] and Fundus Image Registration (FIRE) dataset [41]. Furthermore, by considering scale or zoom less than 1.5 [8]. The $s_{initial}$ is suitable for input images larger than that of the largest image used to determine $s_{initial}$ (10 megapixels). This is because hierarchical Gaussian scale space down-sampled the input image by half as the level increased and reduced the image details as the octave increased, allowing the vessels of varying sizes to fit in the square patch even for input images larger than 10 megapixels.

$$s_{initial} \begin{cases} 35 \text{ pixels} & \text{if } G_{0,-1} > 1000 \times 1000 \text{ pixels} \\ 25 \text{ pixels} & \text{if } G_{0,-1} \leq 1000 \times 1000 \text{ pixels} > 600 \times 600 \text{ pixels} \\ 21 \text{ pixels} & \text{if } G_{0,-1} \leq 600 \times 600 \text{ pixels} \end{cases} \qquad (9)$$

The extracted gradient patch is up-sampled using cubic interpolation with a refinement factor of two to smooth the region around the vessel edges. Then, this interpolated patch is converted to a binary image as depicted in Figure 6(aii,bii). These patches are used as input for exclusion and selection processes.

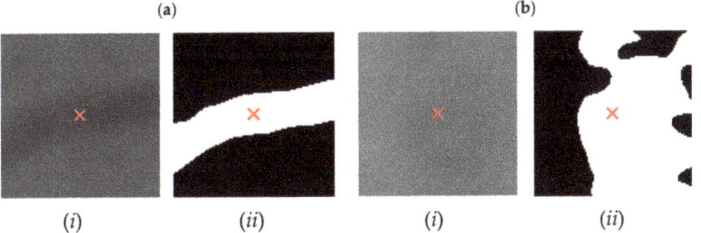

Figure 6. Examples of the (*i*) gradient and (*ii*) binary interpolated patches extracted from (**a**) retinal vessel and (**b**) noise. Red '×' represents the position of the candidate feature point on the patch.

(b) STEP 5: Exclusion process

The curvature structure in the local patch represents retinal vessels of various sizes as well as noises such as the retinal nerve fiber layer, underlying choroidal vessels, microaneurysm and exudates. Therefore, five exclusion criteria specifying the characteristics of the retinal vessels and noises on the sum of intensity profiles are presented to discard candidate feature points on noises.

The intensity profile is the intensity value of the pixels extracted from a cross-sectional line running through the patch. In this study, the intensity profiles extracted from multiple cross-sectional lines are summed to distinctively highlight the characteristics of the retinal vessels and noises in the interpolated patch. The intensity profiles are extracted from a total of L_{total} cross-sectional lines that parallel each other with $L_{distance}$ distance between the lines. These cross-sectional lines are positioned either along or perpendicular to the main orientation of the interpolated patch. The main orientation is the angle between the *x*-axis and major axis of the ellipse on the prominently connected region of the binary interpolated patch.

The L_{total}, $L_{distance}$ and orientation of the cross-sectional lines are set according to the exclusion criteria as summarized in Table 1. The length of the cross-sectional lines in the pixel can be determined from L_{total} and $L_{distance}$ to ensure the lines do not exceed the size of the interpolated patch in any orientation as follows:

$$L_{length} = s_{bin} - (L_{distance} \cdot L_{total}) \tag{10}$$

where, L_{length} is the length of the cross-sectional lines, s_{bin} is the side length of the binary interpolated patch, $L_{distance}$ is the distance between the parallel cross-sectional lines and L_{total} is the total cross-sectional lines.

Table 1. Settings and details of exclusion criteria in STEP 5.

		STEP 5(a): Exclusion Criterion 1	STEP 5(b): Exclusion Criterion 2	STEP 5(c): Exclusion Criterion 3	STEP 5(d): Exclusion Criterion 4	STEP 5(e): Exclusion Criterion 5
		Settings to extract the sum of intensity profiles from interpolated patches				
Interpolated Patch		Binary	Gradient	–	–	Binary and gradient
Cross-sectional lines	L_{total}	5	7	–	–	7
	$L_{distance}$	3 pixels	5 pixels	–	–	5 pixels
	Orientation	Along main orientation	Perpendicular to main orientation	–	–	Perpendicular to main orientation
		Details of exclusion criteria				
Input		Sum of intensity profiles from binary interpolated patch	Sum of intensity profiles from gradient interpolated patch	Valley with maximum depth from STEP 5(b)	Valley with maximum depth and global minimum from STEP 5(c)	Sums of intensity profiles from binary and gradient interpolated patches
Candidate feature point	On Vessels	A horizontal line. Figure 7(aii)	With at least a valley. Figure 8(aii)	Is global minimum. Figure 9(aii,bii)	At-axis. Figure 10a,b	Intersected when overlaid. Figure 11(aiii)
	On Noise	With at least a peak. Figure 7(bii)	Without valley. Figure 8(bii)	Is local minimum. Figure 9(cii)	At 1st or 4th section on x-axis. Figure 10c	Apart from each other when overlaid. Figure 11(biii)

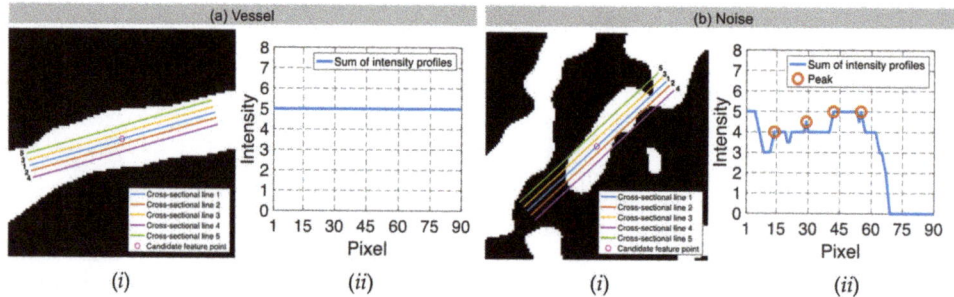

Figure 7. Exclusion criterion 1. (*i*) Cross-sectional lines and (*ii*) sum of intensity profiles for binary interpolated patch with (**a**) retinal vessel and (**b**) noise. A candidate feature point is discarded if any peak is found on the sum of intensity profiles from binary interpolated patch as in (**b**)(*ii*).

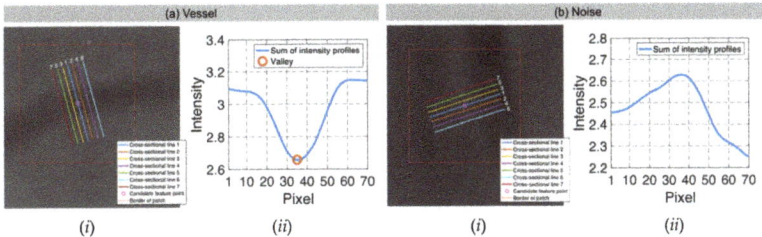

Figure 8. Exclusion criterion 2. (*i*) Cross-sectional lines and (*ii*) sum of intensity profiles for gradient interpolated patch with (**a**) retinal vessel and (**b**) noise. A candidate feature point is discarded if the sum of intensity profiles from gradient interpolated patch is without any valley as in (**b**)(*ii*).

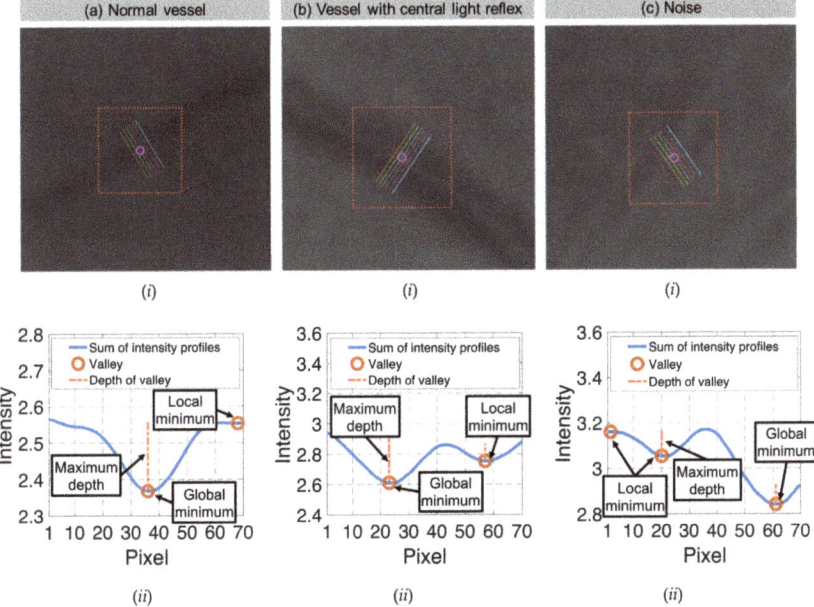

Figure 9. Exclusion criterion 3. (*i*) Cross-sectional lines and (*ii*) sum of intensity profiles for gradient interpolated patch with (**a**) normal retinal vessel, (**b**) retinal vessel with central light reflex and (**c**) noise. A candidate feature point is discarded when the valley with the maximum depth is a local minimum as in (**c**)(*ii*).

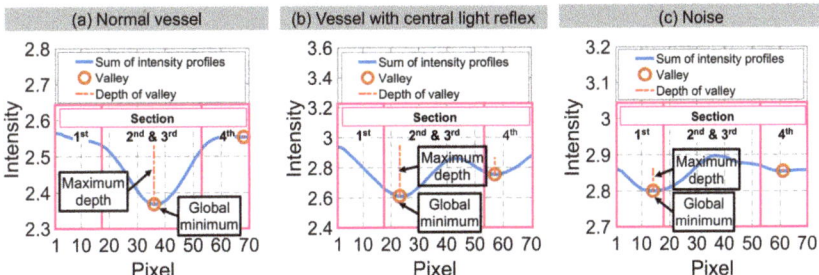

Figure 10. Exclusion criterion 4. (**a**,**b**) The valley with the maximum depth is on the 2nd or 3rd section for retinal vessels. (**c**) The valley with the maximum depth is on the 1st or 4th section for noise. A candidate feature point is discarded when the valley with the maximum depth is at the 1st or 4th section, as in (**c**).

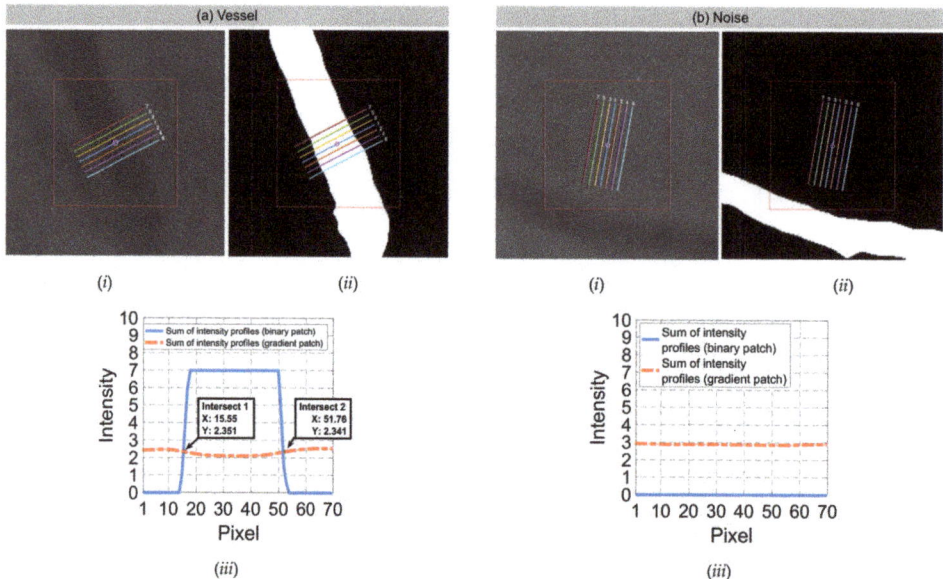

Figure 11. Exclusion criterion 5. Cross-sectional lines on (*i*) gradient and (*ii*) binary interpolated patches for (**a**) retinal vessel and (**b**) noise. (*iii*) The intersection between sums of intensity profiles from (*i*) and (*ii*). A candidate feature point is discarded when the overlaid sums of intensity profiles are apart from each other, as in (**b**)(*iii*).

$L_{total} L_{distance} \text{At} x$

- STEP 5(a): Exclusion criterion 1

  Retinal vessel in a binary interpolated patch forms a nearly straight and wide connected region, as depicted in Figure 7(a*i*). This characteristic can be represented by the sum of the intensity profiles extracted from five cross-sectional lines positioned along the main orientation of the patch. The L_{total}, $L_{distance}$ and orientation for these cross-sectional lines are chosen to best express the retinal vessel of various sizes in the patch. For retinal vessels, the sum of the intensity profiles appears as a horizontal line, as depicted in Figure 7(a*ii*). Contrarily, the noise comprises an inconsistent connected region, as shown in Figure 7(b*i*), which results in the detection of peaks in the sum of intensity profiles. Therefore, a candidate feature point with peaks on the sum of intensity profiles is discarded.

- STEP 5(b): Exclusion criterion 2

  For the gradient interpolated patch associated with the retinal vessel as in Figure 8(a*i*), the cross-sectional lines with $L_{total} = 7$, $L_{distance} = 5$ and positioned perpendicular to the main orientation are fully intersected by the vessel. Therefore, the sum of the intensity profiles from these cross-sectional lines will consist of at least a valley, as depicted in Figure 8(a*ii*). In opposite, no valley can be found on the sum of the intensity profiles extracted from the patch associated with noise, as shown in Figure 8(b*ii*). Thus, this candidate feature point is discarded from further processing.

- STEP 5(c): Exclusion criterion 3

  The valleys discovered in STEP 5(b) are further examined for their depth and positioned on the y-axis. For a candidate feature point located on a retinal vessel, the valley with the maximum depth is at the lowest position of the y-axis or global minimum, as shown in Figure 9(a*ii*,b*ii*). Therefore, a candidate feature point is discarded if the valley with the maximum depth is a local minimum, such as in Figure 9(c*ii*).

- STEP 5(d): Exclusion criterion 4

The valley with maximum depth and global minimum from STEP 5(c) is examined for its position on the *x*-axis. The sum of the intensity profiles is divided into four sections of equal size. The valley with the maximum depth is expected to be at the second or third section on the *x*-axis if a candidate feature point on a retinal vessel is either normal or with central light reflex as shown in Figure 10a,b Therefore, a candidate feature point is excluded if the valley with the maximum depth is located at the first and fourth sections, as in Figure 10c.

- STEP 5(e): Exclusion criterion 5

This criterion overlaid the sum of the intensity profiles from gradient and binary interpolated patches. The intersection can be found when a candidate feature point is located on a retinal vessel and vice versa, as depicted in Figure 11. Thus, the candidate feature point is discarded when the overlaid sums of the intensity profiles are apart from each other.

(c) STEP 6: Selection process

The exclusion process removes the majority of the candidate feature points detected on noises. However, the remaining candidate feature points may include points detected on noises with a high structural similarity as the retinal vessels in the interpolated patches. Therefore, the selection process includes two main steps to select the final feature points, namely, distribution and selection weightage. The distribution will ensure the final feature points are selected throughout the image, while the selection weightage highlights the strength of the retinal vessel in the patch for each candidate feature point.

- STEP 6(a): Distribution

The distribution of the feature points all over the image is vital to ensure a high registration accuracy [42]. There are two procedures involved in distributing the feature points. First, the feature points are distributed across the hierarchical Gaussian scale space by computing the maximum number of feature points ($N_{p,q}$) for each Gaussian image $G_{p,q}$. $N_{p,q}$ is set proportionally inverse to the width of the Gaussian kernels used when building the scale space as described in [8,11,19]:

$$N_{p,q} = N_{total} \cdot F_{p,q} \quad (11)$$

The proportion of the feature points $F_{p,q}$ is given by:

$$F_{p,q} = \frac{f_0}{\mu^{(Q)p+q+1}} \quad (12)$$

The proportion in the initial image of the scale space f_0 and the constant factor μ can be expressed as:

$$f_0 = \frac{\mu^{P(Q)-1}}{\sum_{n=1}^{P(Q)} \mu^{n-1}} \quad (13)$$

$$\mu = 2^{\frac{1}{Q}} \quad (14)$$

where, P is the total octave with index $p \in [1, \ldots, P-1]$, Q is the total level with index $q \in [-1, \ldots, Q-2]$, n is the index of the images in the hierarchical Gaussian scale space and N_{total} is the total feature points in the hierarchical Gaussian scale space. In this study, N_{total} is set to 4500 points, which empirically shows to provide a reasonable amount of feature points to perform image registration. However, if the candidate feature points are detected at less than 4500 points, N_{total} is set to 90% of the total candidate feature points.

The second procedure distributes $N_{p,q}$ across partitioned grids in each Gaussian image $G_{p,q}$. This operation begins by partitioning $G_{p,q}$ into rectangle grids of 150 × 150 pixels. The maximum number of feature points N_u in a grid image of index u is computed as follows:

$$N_u = DC_u \cdot N_{p,q} \quad (15)$$

The distribution coefficient for a grid image (DC_u) represents a combination of three factors. These factors are entropy [43], peak deviation nonuniformity [44] and total candidate feature points detected in the grid image.

The first factor of the entropy (EG) [43] defines the texture of the grayscale grid image. The grid image with high contrast retinal vessels, regardless of the sizes, will yield a large entropy value and vice versa. However, the entropy value presents a minimal distinction between the grid image with low contrast retinal vessels and with only noises or retinal surface.

Therefore, peak deviation nonuniformity (UG) [44] is included as the second factor. This factor is sensitive to the changes in the grayscale level. Thus, it is beneficial in distinguishing between the grid image containing low contrast vessels and the grid image with only noises.

In the coarser grid image, particularly at the higher octave, fewer candidate feature points are detected compared to the finer grid image. However, the values of the entropy and peak deviation nonuniformity measured from the coarser and finer grid images only show a minimal difference. To compensate for these factors, the total candidate feature points detected in the grid image (TG) is considered as the third factor.

The distribution coefficient DC_u for a grid image u can be expressed as the combination of the three factors:

$$DC_u = W_{EG}\frac{EG}{\sum_u^U EG} + W_{UG}\frac{UG}{\sum_u^U UG} + W_{TG}\frac{TG}{\sum_u^U TG} \quad (16)$$

where, W_{EG} is the weight factor for the entropy, W_{UG} is the weight factor for the peak deviation nonuniformity, W_{TG} is the weight factor for the total candidate feature points, u is the index of the grid image with $u \in [1, \cdots, U]$ and U is the total grid in a Gaussian image $G_{p,q}$. The weight factors are empirically set to $W_{EG} = 0.3$, $W_{UG} = 0.3$ and $W_{TG} = 0.4$ to give a distinctive representation in describing the grid image.

- STEP 6(b): Selection weightage

The selection process is continued by computing selection weightage for each candidate feature point. The selection weightage highlights the strength of the retinal vessels indicated by entropy, area of the intersected region and the mean histogram of gradient orientation at the vessel edges.

The entropy (EP) is computed as in [43] to describe the texture in the gradient interpolated patch. Next, the area of the intersected region (AP) is determined between the sums of intensity profiles from the gradient and binary interpolated patches in STEP 5(e), as depicted in Figure 12. The lowest intersection point on the y-axis is used as the reference level to approximate the area of the intersected region using the trapezoidal rule. The area of the intersected region expresses the strength of the retinal vessels in terms of size and contrast. For example, the intersected region has a larger area for a thicker and high contrast retinal vessel. The area decreases as the size and contrast of the retinal vessel decreases.

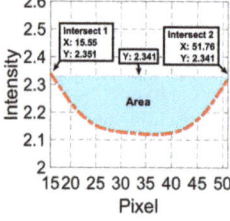

Figure 12. Area of intersected region between the sums of the intensity profiles from *exclusion criterion 5*.

The mean histogram of the gradient orientation at the vessel edges (HP) is estimated using both gradient and binary interpolated patches. Initially, the partial derivative is performed on the gradient interpolated patch to obtain gradient orientation for each pixel. The partial derivative is approximated using the central difference as it gives a more accurate approximation compared to other techniques, such as forward and backward approximations.

Then, the binary interpolated patch is used to obtain the vessel edges by performing binary dilation to increase the thickness of the edges. Once the pixels on the vessel edges are identified, the gradient orientation is extracted. The gradient orientation for these pixels is organized into a histogram of 36 bins, as shown in Figure 13. In this histogram, the non-zero frequencies are averaged to represent the mean histogram of the gradient orientation at the vessel edges. The mean histogram will yield a high value for a high contrast retinal vessel as the edges are thicker and the gradient orientation is more uniform. In contrast, the mean histogram will yield a low value for the low contrast retinal vessel as the edges are thinner and the gradient orientation is less uniform.

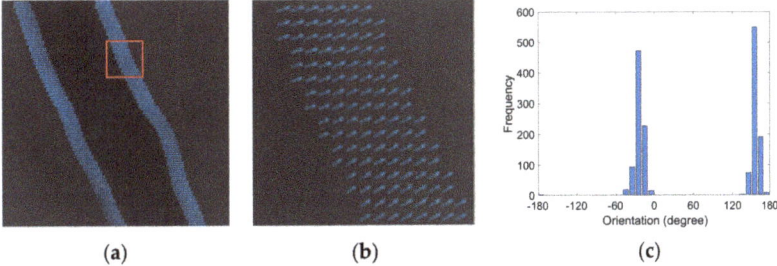

Figure 13. (a) Example of gradient orientation at the edges of the retinal vessel in a gradient interpolated patch. (b) Close-up from the red rectangle region. (c) Histogram of 36 bins generated for the gradient orientation in (a). The frequency in the histogram signifies the total occurrence of the gradient orientation within the respective bin.

The selection weightage denoted by SW_i is computed for each candidate feature point (i) to highlight the strength of the retinal vessels as expressed below:

$$SW_i = W_{EP} \frac{EP}{\sum_i^{TC} HP} + W_{AP} \frac{AP}{\sum_i^{TC} AP} + W_{HP} \frac{HP}{\sum_i^{TC} HP} \qquad (17)$$

where, W_{EP} is the weight factor for the entropy, W_{AP} is the weight factor for the area of the intersected region, W_{HP} is the weight factor for the mean histogram of the gradient orientation at the vessel edges, i is the index of the candidate feature point with $i \in [1, \cdots, TC]$ and TC is the total candidate feature point in a Gaussian image $G_{p,q}$. The weight factors are empirically set to $W_{EP} = 0.3$, $W_{AP} = 0.4$ and $W_{HP} = 0.3$ to distinctively highlight the strength of the retinal vessels.

Finally, a total of N_u candidate feature points with the highest value of the selection weightage SW are selected as feature points in each grid image. Then, the positions of the selected feature points are refined to sub-pixel accuracy at the respective $G_{p,q}$, as in [15,45]. The feature points with refined positions are converted from the position at the respective scale space to the coordinate system of the initial Gaussian image $G_{0,-1}$ follows:

$$K_m = 2^p . K_{m,p,q} \qquad (18)$$

where, K_m is the feature point of index m in the coordinate system of the initial Gaussian image $G_{0,-1}$ and $K_{m,p,q}$ is the feature point of index m in the coordinate system at the respective octave p and level q.

3.3. STAGE 3: Feature Descriptor

SIFT descriptor [15] is assigned to each feature point extracted from fixed and moving images. VLFeat toolbox [46] with default settings is used to compute the SIFT descriptor.

3.4. STAGE 4: Matching

The matches are obtained by establishing pairwise distances between SIFT descriptors. The distances are computed using the sum of squared differences (SSD). The outliers in the matches are eliminated using M-estimator SAmple Consensus (MSAC) algorithm [47]. MSAC eliminates the outliers when the distance between the matches in the fixed image and the projected matches from the moving image exceeds a specified threshold. The projection is performed according to the non-reflective similarity transformation and estimated from two randomly selected matches. The distance threshold is set between 1 and 100 with an increasing step of 0.1. The random trial is repeated 5000 times, and the desired confidence is set to 99%.

3.5. STAGE 5: Geometrical Transformation

Similarity and local weighted mean transformations [48] are estimated for each image pair from the established inliers. Only the transformation that gives the best registration accuracy is chosen for evaluation. The radius of influence for local weighted mean transformation is set in the range of 10 to the total inliers with an increasing step of two.

4. Experimental Setup

The CURVE-SIFT was implemented in MATLAB R2016b running on a virtual machine from Google Cloud Engine with specifications of Intel Xeon® E5 2.6GHz (24 vCPUs) and 40 GB of RAM. Toolboxes employed were Image Processing, Computer Vision, Signal Processing and VLFeat [46].

The evaluation was divided into two parts. First, CURVE was evaluated in extracting feature points on retinal vessels. The performance of CURVE was compared with five feature extraction methods from the existing feature-based RIR techniques, namely, Harris corner [26], SIFT [15], SURF [27,28], Ghassabi's [8] and D-Saddle [14]. Then, CURVE-SIFT was evaluated in registering image pairs from three retinal image registration applications and compared with five existing feature-based RIR techniques; GDB-ICP [13], Harris-PIIFD [10], Ghassabi's-SIFT [8], H-M 16 [16], H-M 17 [9] and D-Saddle-HOG [14]. In the experiment, these five existing feature-based RIR techniques were utilized exactly as they are. H-M 16, H-M 17 and D-Saddle-HOG were originally developed using FIRE dataset for super-resolution, image mosaicking and longitudinal study applications, while Ghassabi's-SIFT, GDB-ICP and Harris-PIIFD were developed for image mosaicking and low-quality image using other datasets.

4.1. Datasets

A total of five public datasets at the original image size were employed in the evaluation. The original image size was used in the experiment as decreasing the spatial resolution of the fundus image can degrade its quality and led to an inaccurate diagnosis and treatment of retinal diseases [49]. Four of the datasets evaluated the feature extraction performance, namely, CHASE_DB1 [33,34], DRIVE [35,36], HRF [37,38] and STARE [39,40]. These datasets contain fundus images affected by pathological cases. The provided ground truth images are in the form of the segmented vessels performed by experts. This enables the evaluation of the extracted feature points on the retinal vessels. The details of CHASE_DB1, DRIVE, HRF and STARE datasets are described in Table 2.

Table 2. Descriptions of CHASE_DB1, DRIVE, HRF and STARE datasets for evaluating feature extraction performance.

Descriptions	Datasets			
	CHASE_DB1	DRIVE	HRF	STARE
Total images	28	40	45	20
Image size (pixels)	999 × 960	564 × 584	3504 × 2336	605 × 700
Total patients	14	40	45	20
Age (Years)	9–10	25–90	N/A	N/A
Pathological cases	Vessel tortuosity	33 images without sign of diabetic retinopathy 7 images with mild early diabetic retinopathy	15 images of healthy patients 15 images of diabetic retinopathy 15 images of glaucomatous	Abnormalities that obscure the blood vessel appearance, such as hemorrhaging, etc.
Field of view	30°	45°	45°	35°
Year	2012	2004	2009	2000
Ground truth images	56	60	45	40
Intensity distribution [1]	22.6136	49.3307	34.9433	49.5126

[1] Described by peak deviation nonuniformity intensity. Values close to 0 indicates non-uniform intensity distribution in the image.

The registration performance of CURVE-SIFT is evaluated in the Fundus Image Registration dataset (FIRE) [41]. This dataset is the only public fundus image registration dataset with ground truth annotation. The FIRE dataset consists of 134 image pairs divided into super-resolution, image mosaicking and longitudinal study applications, as described in Table 3. All image pairs are affected by diabetic retinopathy where vessel tortuosity, microaneurysms and cotton-wool are visible on the images. Each image pair includes 10 corresponding ground truth annotations identified by experts.

Table 3. Descriptions of FIRE dataset for evaluating registration performance.

Descriptions	Retinal Image Registration Applications		
	Super-Resolution	Image Mosaicking	Longitudinal Study
Total images	71	49	14
Image size (pixels)		2912 × 2912	
Total patients		39	
Age (Years)		19–67	
Pathological cases		Diabetic retinopathy	
Field of view		45°	
Year		2006 to 2015	
Ground truth images		10 corresponding points for each image pair	
Anatomical differences [1]	No	No	Yes
Scale	≈1	≈1	≈1
Overlapping area (%)	86–100	17–89	95–100
Rotation (°)	0°–12°	6°–52°	1°–4°

[1] Anatomical differences observed between fixed and moving images.

Registering image pairs from super-resolution, image mosaicking and longitudinal study applications involve a combination of several challenges, namely, overlapping area and rotation. The overlapping area is an intersection region between fixed and moving images. A small overlapping area limits the amount of similar information between images, which can be insufficient to estimate an accurate geometrical transformation. The rotation in the fundus image is introduced to access part of the retina or due to involuntary movement by the patient. The rotation alters the orientation of similar information between images. This alteration can be challenging for the feature-based RIR technique to establish correspondences.

The super-resolution application combines multiple fundus images with a large overlapping area and small rotation. The super-resolution application is performed to increase the density of the spatial sampling, which can resolve the blurred edges of the retinal vessels caused by patient movements or improper imaging setup.

The image mosaicking application aligns multiple fundus images to generate an image with a wider view of the retina. The wide view image of the retina can be used to view the full extent of the retinal disease in one big picture during diagnosis [50,51] and during the preparation of eye laser treatment for diabetic retinopathy [52]. However, registering image pairs from the image mosaicking application can be challenging as it involves a combination of small overlapping areas and large rotation.

The longitudinal study application combines multiple fundus images that are acquired at different screening sessions. Therefore, the anatomical changes due to progression or remission of retinopathy such as increased vessel tortuosity, microaneurysms and cotton-wool spots can be observed between fixed and moving images. The longitudinal study application is essential in monitoring the progression of retinal diseases, such as glaucoma and age-related macular degeneration, which usually undergoes a long degeneration process [53].

4.2. Evaluation Metrics

4.2.1. Feature Extraction Performance

(a) Extraction accuracy

The extraction accuracy expresses the ability of a feature extraction method to extract feature points on retinal vessels. The extraction accuracy for an image can be computed by:

$$ExAc = \frac{total\ feature\ points\ extracted\ on\ vessels}{total\ feature\ points} \times 100\% \qquad (19)$$

where, $ExAc$ is the extraction accuracy in percentage.

The extraction accuracy for an image is set to 0% when the feature points extracted are below the minimum requirement of three points to perform a transformation. One-way Analysis of Variance (ANOVA) with Tukey's post hoc was performed to compare the extraction accuracy between methods.

(b) Factors influencing the extraction accuracy

Two factors influencing the feature extraction accuracy were investigated. These factors are changes in image size and intensity distribution throughout the image. The relations were investigated using Spearman's rank-order correlation. The image size and the intensity distribution of the fundus images in CHASE, DRIVE, HRF and STARE datasets are summarized in Table 2. The intensity distribution is described by peak deviation nonuniformity [44].

4.2.2. Registration Performance

(a) Success rate

Success rate measures the ability of a feature-based RIR technique to register image pairs and meet the specified requirement of target registration error (TRE). TRE is the mean distance in pixel between the ground truth annotations in a fixed image to the transformed ground truth annotations from the moving image. A perfect registration for an image pair is represented by TRE values equal to 0.

However, achieving a perfect registration can be challenging in a real-world application. Thus, the registration for an image pair is considered successful if the obtained TRE is below one pixel for super-resolution applications and five pixels for image mosaicking and longitudinal study applications [54]. The success rate can be computed as given below:

$$Success\ rate = \frac{total\ image\ pairs\ with\ successful\ registration}{total\ image\ pairs} \times 100\% \qquad (20)$$

The one-way ANOVA with Tukey's post hoc was performed to compare the success rate between the feature-based RIR techniques.

(b) Factors influencing the success rate

Factors of overlapping area and rotation were investigated for their influence on the success rate using Spearman's rank-order correlation. It should be noted that for this evaluation, the successful registration was set below five pixels for all image pairs despite its registration application. As the details of the overlapping area and rotation are not initially provided by the FIRE dataset, this information is measured as follows.

The overlapping area in percentage is obtained from the overlap area between the fixed image and transformed moving image. The moving image is transformed to the orientation of the fixed image using affine transformation inferred from the corresponding ground truth annotations. The rotation for an image pair is measured from the average angle between corresponding ground truth annotations without considering the effect of translation, as in [14]. Thus, results were in the larger angle of rotation. The range of overlapping area and rotation in the FIRE dataset is provided in Table 3.

5. Results
5.1. Feature Extraction Performance

CURVE extracts an average of 2482 feature points from the CHASE, DRIVE, HRF and STARE datasets, where 2149 of them are accurately associated with retinal vessels. This constitutes an average feature extraction accuracy of 86.021% with a variation of 9.199% between images, as outlined in Table 4. Furthermore, the one-way ANOVA analysis shows that the feature extraction accuracy of CURVE was significantly outperformed by all existing feature extraction methods ($p < 0.001*$). CURVE obtained the biggest accuracy difference with SIFT detector (69.857%) and the smallest difference with Harris corner (44.408%). Examples of CURVE feature points extracted from four datasets are depicted in Figure 14.

Table 4. Overall feature extraction accuracy (%) in CHASE_DB1, DRIVE, HRF and STARE datasets.

Feature Extraction Method	Total Images	Mean	Standard Deviation	Min	Max
Harris corner	133	41.613	21.317	0.000	92.857
SIFT detector	133	16.164	5.411	5.241	30.299
SURF	133	18.929	4.206	9.502	30.412
Ghassabi's	133	28.280	5.975	17.055	44.197
D-Saddle	133	20.509	4.791	12.221	31.273
CURVE	133	86.021	9.199	59.677	97.842

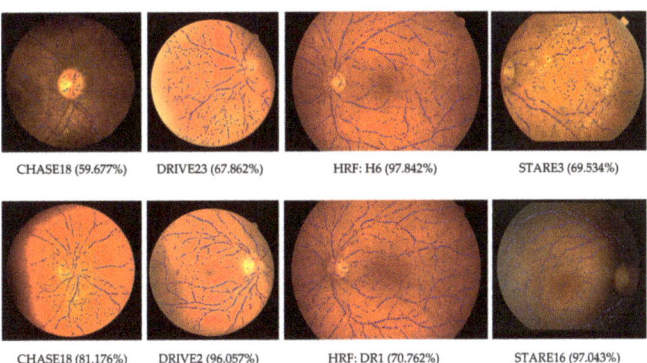

Figure 14. Examples of feature points extracted by CURVE. Top row: Images with the lowest extraction accuracy in each dataset. Bottom row: Images with the highest extraction accuracy in each dataset.

The high feature extraction accuracy of CURVE is contributed to by the utilization of both the retinal vessels and noise characteristics in the feature detection and selection modules. Thus, enabling accurate discrimination between the retinal vessels and noises. Contrarily, Ghassabi's and D-Saddle enhanced the fundus image to increase the visibility of the retinal vessels. However, this enhancement also increases the visibility of the noise, which led both methods to yield low feature extraction accuracy. The extracted feature points located on the noises for these methods were observed to be on the edge of the optic disc, retinal nerve fiber layer, underlying choroidal vessels and macula. The other feature extraction methods such as Harris corner, SIFT detector and SURF are without a specific feature selection module to extract feature points on retinal vessels. These feature extraction methods were used in the existing feature-based RIR techniques [10,13,16], where the authors focused on the development of the feature descriptor and transformation model.

Other than that, the minimal usage of rigid thresholds or variables allows CURVE to accurately extract feature points from fundus images with varying sizes. This is shown by the smallest Spearman's rho among all methods and insignificant correlation between the changes in image size and the extraction accuracy of CURVE ($r_s = -0.032$, $p = 0.712$) as presented in Table 5. Furthermore, the extraction accuracy of D-Saddle ($r_s = -0.138$, $p = 0.114$) and Ghassabi's ($r_s = -0.142$, $p = 0.104$) exhibit insignificant correlation with the changes in image size but their correlations are stronger than CURVE. In contrast, SIFT detector is very sensitive to the changes in image size among all methods where its feature extraction accuracy decreases in larger images ($r_s = -0.649$, $p < 0.001*$).

Table 5. Correlation between extraction accuracy and factors.

Feature Extraction Method	Image Size		Intensity Distribution	
	r_s	p-Value	r_s	p-Value
Harris corner	−0.178	0.041 *	0.360	<0.001 **
SIFT detector	−0.649	<0.001 **	0.138	0.113
SURF	0.590	<0.001 **	−0.398	<0.001 **
Ghassabi's	−0.142	0.104	0.314	<0.001 **
D-Saddle	−0.138	0.114	0.386	<0.001 **
CURVE	**−0.032**	**0.712**	0.342	<0.001 **

r_s: Spearman's rho. **: Correlation is significant at the 0.01 level (2-tailed). *: Correlation is significant at the 0.05 level (2-tailed).

However, CURVE performance is significantly affected in the presence of non-uniform intensity distribution in the image ($r_s = 0.342$, $p < 0.001*$). CURVE is sensitive towards the non-uniform intensity distribution because it highly depends on the intensity changes to locate the curvature of the retinal vessels in the feature detection module. Furthermore, CURVE does not incorporate any feature enhancement algorithm. The feature enhancement algorithms, such as DoG and iiDoG operators, can suppress the non-uniform intensity distribution and increase the visibility of the retinal vessels but at the cost of increasing the visibility of the noises. Thus, it is avoided in the proposed CURVE. Contrarily, the correlation between SIFT detector and the intensity distribution is not significant and the weakest among all feature extraction methods ($r_s = 0.138$, $p = 0.113$).

5.2. Registration Performance

The evaluation continues by accessing the registration performance of CURVE-SIFT and six existing feature-based RIR techniques [8–10,13,14,16]. From the experimental results outlined in Table 6, CURVE-SIFT successfully registered a total of 59 image pairs in the FIRE dataset with a success rate of 44.030%. The one-way ANOVA analysis shows that the success rate of CURVE-SIFT significantly outperformed GDB-ICP at $p = 0.007*$, whereas Harris-PIIFD, Ghassabi's-SIFT, H-M 16, H-M 17 and D-Saddle-HOG at $p < 0.001*$. The biggest success rate difference was observed between CURVE-SIFT and Harris-PIIFD (40.299%), while the smallest difference was with GDB-ICP (16.418%).

Table 6. Success rate (%) in the FIRE dataset.

Feature-Based RIR Technique	Total Image Pairs [1]	Mean	Standard Deviation	TRE (Pixels) Min	TRE (Pixels) Max
Overall					
GDB-ICP	37	27.612	44.875	2.354	10.416
Harris-PIIFD	5	3.731	19.024	3.319	1486.255
Ghassabi's-SIFT	17	12.687	33.407	3.082	322.616
H-M 16	22	16.418	37.183	2.857	410.087
H-M 17	26	19.403	39.694	2.920	60.875
D-Saddle-HOG	16	11.940	32.548	4.583	27.266
CURVE-SIFT	59	**44.030**	49.829	1.928	1016.330
Super-resolution					
GDB-ICP	17	23.944	42.978	0.486	4.575
Harris-PIIFD	2	2.817	16.663	0.785	12.850
Ghassabi's-SIFT	13	18.310	38.950	0.665	15.798
H-M 16	18	25.352	43.812	0.554	13.903
H-M 17	20	28.169	45.302	0.489	5.696
D-Saddle-HOG	10	14.085	35.034	0.748	9.327
CURVE-SIFT	28	**39.437**	49.219	0.613	9.696
Image Mosaicking					
GDB-ICP	16	32.653	47.380	1.946	6.323
Harris-PIIFD	0	0.000	0.000	10.041	3870.632
Ghassabi's-SIFT	0	0.000	0.000	7.358	578.494
H-M 16	0	0.000	0.000	7.976	129.658
H-M 17	1	2.041	14.286	3.327	41.192
D-Saddle-HOG	2	4.082	19.991	3.082	366.401
CURVE-SIFT	26	**53.061**	50.423	1.787	19.799
Longitudinal Study					
GDB-ICP	4	28.571	46.881	2.354	10.416
Harris-PIIFD	3	21.429	42.582	3.319	1486.255
Ghassabi's-SIFT	4	28.571	46.881	3.082	322.616
H-M 16	4	28.571	46.881	2.857	410.087
H-M 17	5	**35.714**	49.725	2.920	60.875
D-Saddle-HOG	4	28.571	46.881	4.583	27.266
CURVE-SIFT	5	**35.714**	49.725	1.928	1016.330

[1] Total image pairs with successful registration.

Moreover, the overall success rate of D-Saddle-HOG (14.085%) reported in this study is much lower than in [14] because this study evaluates D-Saddle performance on the FIRE dataset at the original image size of 2912 × 2912 pixels. Contrarily, the work presented in [14] evaluates D-Saddle-HOG performance on the FIRE dataset at the smaller image size of 583 × 583 pixels. The extraction accuracy of D-Saddle is insignificantly correlated to the changes in image size, as shown in Table 5. However, D-Saddle-HOG employed a Histogram of Oriented Gradients (HOG) descriptor [55] in its framework where a larger image can decrease the number of correct matches or inliers established between the computed HOG descriptor [56]. Insufficient amounts of the established inliers can lead to the estimation of inaccurate geometrical transformation.

The most noticeable performance of CURVE-SIFT is observed in the image mosaicking application. The image pairs from the image mosaicking application involved the combination of smaller overlapping areas (17–89%) and larger rotation (6°–52°) in the dataset. Despite these challenges, the success rate of CURVE-SIFT (53.061%) is significantly outperformed for all existing feature-based RIR techniques ($p < 0.001*$). This performance is contributed to by CURVE's ability to accurately extract feature points on retinal vessels and distribute them throughout the image to increase the chances of the inliers being established within the overlapping area. Furthermore, the employed SIFT descriptor has the ability to establish over 60% of inliers when the rotation is below 90° [57]. These abilities are also expressed in the established Spearman's rank-order correlations in Table 7, where CURVE-SIFT yields smaller Spearman's rho values indicating weaker correlations with the overlapping area and rotation compared to Harris-PIIFD, Ghassabi's, H-M 16, H-17 and D-Saddle. In contrast, the existing feature-based RIR techniques recorded a much lower success rate with less than 32.653%, whereas Harris-PIIFD, Ghassabi's and H-M 16 were unable to register any of the image pairs in the image mosaicking application.

Table 7. Correlation between success rate and factors.

Feature-Based RIR Technique	Overlapping Area		Rotation	
	r_s	p-Value	r_s	p-Value
GDB-ICP	0.443	<0.001 **	−0.380	<0.001 **
Harris-PIIFD	0.732	<0.001 **	−0.723	<0.001 **
Ghassabi's-SIFT	0.795	<0.001 **	−0.766	<0.001 **
H-M 16	0.785	<0.001 **	−0.763	<0.001 **
H-M 17	0.773	<0.001 **	−0.765	<0.001 **
D-Saddle-HOG	0.769	<0.001 **	−0.745	<0.001 **
CURVE-SIFT	0.415	<0.001 **	−0.382	<0.001 **

r_s: Spearman's rho. **: Correlation is significant at the 0.01 level (2-tailed).

The image pairs from the super-resolution application are the least challenging in the FIRE dataset as they involve a large overlapping area (86–100%) and small rotation (0°–12°). However, the super-resolution application requires a very accurate registration with a TRE of less than one pixel. For this reason, CURVE-SIFT only recorded a success rate of 39.437% in this application, where the TRE of the failed registration ranged between 1.003 pixels to 9.696 pixels. The success rate of CURVE-SIFT outperformed all existing feature-based RIR techniques evaluated in this study but only significant with Harris-PIIFD ($p < 0.001*$), Ghassabi's-SIFT ($p = 0.030*$) and D-Saddle-HOG ($p = 0.004*$).

The image pairs from the longitudinal study application are the most challenging for CURVE-SIFT to register, where it obtained the lowest success rate (35.714%) among the applications in the FIRE dataset. Furthermore, no significant difference can be noted between the success rate of CURVE-SIFT and existing feature-based RIR techniques. This shows that the registration performance of CURVE-SIFT is affected when the anatomical appearance is varied between images in the pair. Particularly, CURVE-SIFT failed to register image pairs when the prominent differences of vessel thickness and tortuosity were observed between images. The difference in vessel thickness between fixed and moving images leads to different descriptors being computed for local features at the same part of the vessels. As a result, these local features were unable to establish a correspondence, resulting in low registration accuracy. In the event of increased tortuosity, the corresponding local features were appropriately established. However, the tortuosity causes the vessels to bend and alters the actual physical position of the vessels on the eyeball. Consequently, the registration was performed between local features on the same part of the vessels but at different physical positions, which resulted in high TRE. For existing feature-based RIR techniques, the invariant features utilized in their works were extracted throughout the image. Thus, minimize the impact of vessel thinning and tortuosity compared to our work. Examples of registered image pairs for CURVE-SIFT in each application are depicted in Figure 15.

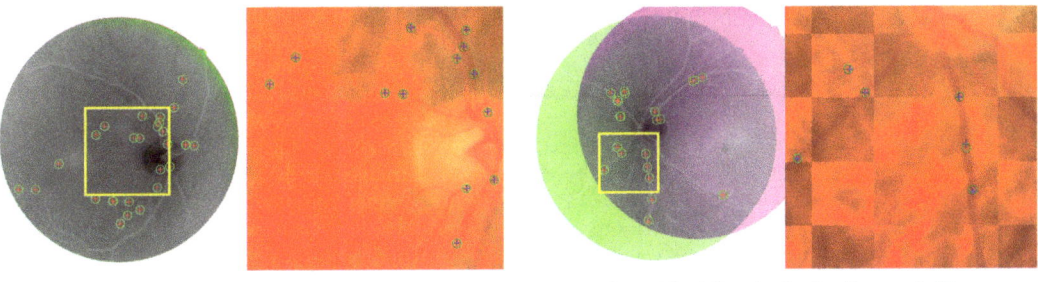

Super-resolution Application (Image pair $\mathcal{S}52$)   Image Mosaicking Application (Image pair $\mathcal{P}7$)

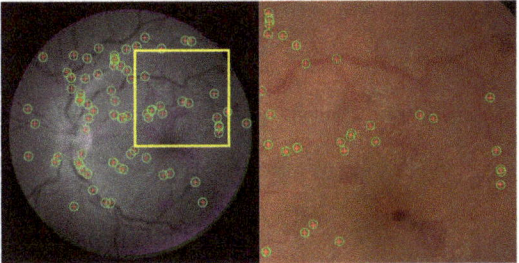

Longitudinal Study Application (Image pair $\mathcal{A}12$)

Figure 15. Examples of the successfully registered image pairs for CURVE-SIFT in the FIRE dataset. The green markers are inliers on the fixed image, while red/blue markers are inliers on moving image. Right images: Close-up for yellow square area as checkerboard image containing alternating rectangular regions from fixed image and moving image.

6. Conclusions

This paper introduces a new feature extraction method known as CURVE for the feature-based RIR technique. The proposed CURVE aims to extract feature points on retinal vessels and throughout the fundus image, which is important to ensure accurate registration of fundus images. However, in the local patches, the noises, such as retinal nerve fiber layer, underlying choroidal vessels, microaneurysm and exudates can also appear similar to retinal vessels. Therefore, CURVE incorporates both characteristics of the retinal vessels and noises in its modules to enable accurate discrimination between them.

The ability of CURVE to extract feature points on retinal vessels was demonstrated on the CHASE_DB1 [33,34], DRIVE [35,36], HRF [37,38] and STARE [39,40] datasets. Then, the CURVE performance was compared with five feature extraction methods from the existing feature-based RIR techniques, namely, Harris corner [26], SIFT detector [15], SURF [27,28], Ghassabi's [8] and D-Saddle [14]. From the experiment, CURVE accurately extracts an average of 86.021% of the feature points on retinal vessels and significantly outperformed the existing feature extraction methods ($p < 0.001^*$). Further analysis shows that the impact of image size on CURVE performance is minimal ($r_s = -0.032$, $p = 0.712$) but significantly affected in the presence of non-uniform intensity distribution in the image ($r_s = 0.342$, $p < 0.001^*$).

The registration performance when utilizing CURVE feature points in the feature-based RIR technique was demonstrated on the FIRE dataset. CURVE was paired with the SIFT descriptor [41], and the registration performance of CURVE-SIFT was compared with five existing feature-based RIR techniques; GDB-ICP [13], Harris-PIIFD [10], Ghassabi's-SIFT [8], H-M 16 [16], H-M 17 [9] and D-Saddle-HOG [14]. Overall, CURVE-SIFT successfully registered 44.030% of the image pairs in the FIRE dataset, while the success rate of the existing feature-based RIR techniques is less than 27.612%. The one-way ANOVA analysis showed that CURVE-SIFT is significantly outperformed GDB-ICP at $p = 0.007^*$ whereas Harris-PIIFD, Ghassabi's-SIFT, H-M 16, H-M 17 and D-Saddle-HOG at $p < 0.001^*$. CURVE-

SIFT obtained the highest success rate (53.061%) in the image mosaicking application, while the success rates of the existing feature-based RIR techniques were only between 0% to 32.653%. The image mosaicking application consists of image pairs with smaller overlapping areas compared to other applications in the FIRE dataset. Thus demonstrating the ability of CURVE to extract feature points on retinal vessels throughout the image. This is crucial to increase the chances of the inliers being established within the overlapping area to estimate an accurate geometrical transformation. In the future, we will focus our efforts to improve CURVE in extracting feature points from fundus images with non-uniform intensity distribution. Moreover, we will explore the possibility of a fusion strategy to combine deep convolutional neural network (CNN) with local feature point for feature extraction [58]. However, at the time of this study, the size of the public RIR dataset was small, which may result in model overfitting or underfitting [59]. The study will begin once a larger dataset or suitable pre-trained model for RIR is available publicly.

Author Contributions: Conceptualization, R.R. and N.K.A.K.; methodology, R.R. and M.Y.I.I.; software, R.R. and A.W.A.W.; validation, R.R. and K.H.; investigation, R.R., M.Y.I.I., K.H., A.W.A.W. and N.K.A.K.; writing—original draft preparation, R.R. and M.Y.I.I.; writing—review and editing, R.R. and K.H. All authors have read and agreed to the published version of the manuscript.

Funding: This research was funded by Fundamental Research Grant Scheme (FRGS) (FP003-2021).

Institutional Review Board Statement: Not applicable.

Informed Consent Statement: Not applicable.

Data Availability Statement: The data presented in this study namely, CHASE_DB1 [31,32], DRIVE [33,34], HRF [35,36], STARE [37,38] and (FIRE) [39] are openly available at https://blogs.kingston.ac.uk/retinal/chasedb1/ (10 February 2019), https://drive.grand-challenge.org/ (10 February 2019), https://www5.cs.fau.de/research/data/fundus-images/ (10 February 2019), https://cecas.clemson.edu/~ahoover/stare/ (10 February 2019) and https://projects.ics.forth.gr/cvrl/fire/ (10 February 2019).

Conflicts of Interest: The authors declare no conflict of interest. The funders had no role in the design of the study; in the collection, analyses, or interpretation of data; in the writing of the manuscript, or in the decision to publish the results.

Appendix A

Table A1. Mathematical symbols and notation.

No.	Symbol	Description	No.	Symbol	Description
1	$\breve{\sigma}_{p,q}$	Relative Gaussian kernel at octave p and level q.	28	$L_{distance}$	Distance between the parallel cross-sectional lines. Exclusion criterion 1 : $L_{distance} = 3$ pixels. Exclusion criterion 2, 5 : $L_{distance} = 5$ pixels.
2	β	Central intensity value.	29	L_{length}	Length of the cross-sectional lines.
3	ε	Offset, $\varepsilon = 0.0010$.	30	L_{total}	Total of the cross-sectional lines, an odd number. Exclusion criterion 1 : $L_{total} = 5$ pixels. Exclusion criterion 2, 5 : $L_{total} = 7$ pixels.
4	μ	Constant factor.	31	m	Index of the feature point.
5	σ_0	Base width of Gaussian kernel, $\sigma_0 = 1.6$.	32	n	Index of the images in the hierarchical Gaussian scale space.
6	σ_s	Sampling Gaussian kernel, $\sigma_s = 0.5$.	33	N_{total}	Total feature points in the hierarchical Gaussian scale space, $N_{total} = 4500$ points.
7	$\sigma_{p,q}$	Absolute Gaussian kernel at octave p and.	34	$N_{p,q}$	The maximum number of feature points in $G_{p,q}$.
8	a_j	Pixel for inner ring test.	35	N_u	The
9	AP	Area of the intersected region between the sums of intensity profiles from the gradient and binary interpolated patches.	36	p	Octave index, $p \in [0, \ldots, P-1]$.
10	b_l	Pixel for outer ring test.	37	P	Total octave in the scale space, $P = 3$.

Table A1. Cont.

No.	Symbol	Description	No.	Symbol	Description
11	$\mathcal{B}$	The blue channel.	38	q	Level index within an octave, $q \in [-1, \ldots, Q-2]$.
12	DC_u	Distribution coefficient for a grid of index u.	39	Q	Total level in each octave, $Q = 6$.
13	e	Extremum.	40	$\mathcal{R}$	The red channel.
14	EG	Entropy of a grid image.	41	s_{bin}	Side length of the binary interpolated patch.
15	EP	Entropy of a gradient interpolated patch.	42	$s_{initial}$	Initial side length of the patch in pixels. $s_{initial}$ is set according to the image size of the initial Gaussian image $G_{0,-1}$. $s_{initial} \begin{cases} 35 \text{ pixels} & \text{if } G_{0,-1} > 1000 \times 1000 \text{ pixels} \\ 25 \text{ pixels} & \text{if } G_{0,-1} \leq 1000 \times 1000 \text{ pixels} \\ & \phantom{\text{if } G_{0,-1}} > 600 \times 600 \text{ pixels} \\ 21 \text{ pixels} & \text{if } G_{0,-1} \leq 600 \times 600 \text{ pixels} \end{cases}$
16	f_0	Proportion of the feature points at the initial Gaussian image $G_{0,-1}$.	43	s_p	Side length of the patch at octave p.
17	$F_{p,q}$	Proportion of the feature points at $G_{p,q}$.	44	SW_i	Selection weightage for a candidate feature point of index i.
18	$\mathcal{G}$	The green channel.	45	TG	Total candidate feature points detected in a grid image.
19	G	Hierarchical Gaussian scale space.	46	u	Index of the grids in $G_{p,q}$.
20	$G_{p,q}$	Gaussian image at octave p and.	47	U	Total grids in a Gaussian image $G_{p,q}$.
21	i	Index of the candidate feature point in a Gaussian image.	48	UG	Peak deviation nonuniformity of a grid image.
22	I	Input image in grayscale.	49	W_{AP}	Weight factor for the area of the intersected region, $W_{AP} = 0.4$.
23	I_{a_j}	Intensity of inner ring pixel a_j in grayscale, $I_{a_j} \in [0, 1]$.	50	W_{EG}	Weight factor for the entropy, $W_{EG} = 0.3$.
24	I_{b_l}	Intensity of outer ring pixel b_l in grayscale $I_{b_l} \in [0, 1]$.	51	W_{EP}	Weight factor for the entropy, $W_{EP} = 0.3$.
25	j	Index of inner ring pixels, $j \in [1, \ldots, 8]$.	52	W_{HP}	Weight factor for the mean histogram of the gradient orientation at the vessel edges, $W_{HP} = 0.3$.
26	K_m	Feature point of index m.	53	W_{TG}	Weight factor for the total candidate feature points, $W_{TG} = 0.4$.
27	$K_{m,p,q}$	Feature point of index m in the coordinate system at the respective octave p and level q.	54	W_{UG}	Weight factor for the peak deviation nonuniformity, $W_{UG} = 0.3$.

Appendix B

Table A2. Characteristics of retinal vessels and noises in blue squares. Red lines in (ii) and (iv) are cross-sectional lines to extract intensity profiles in (iii) and (v).

Table A2. *Cont.*

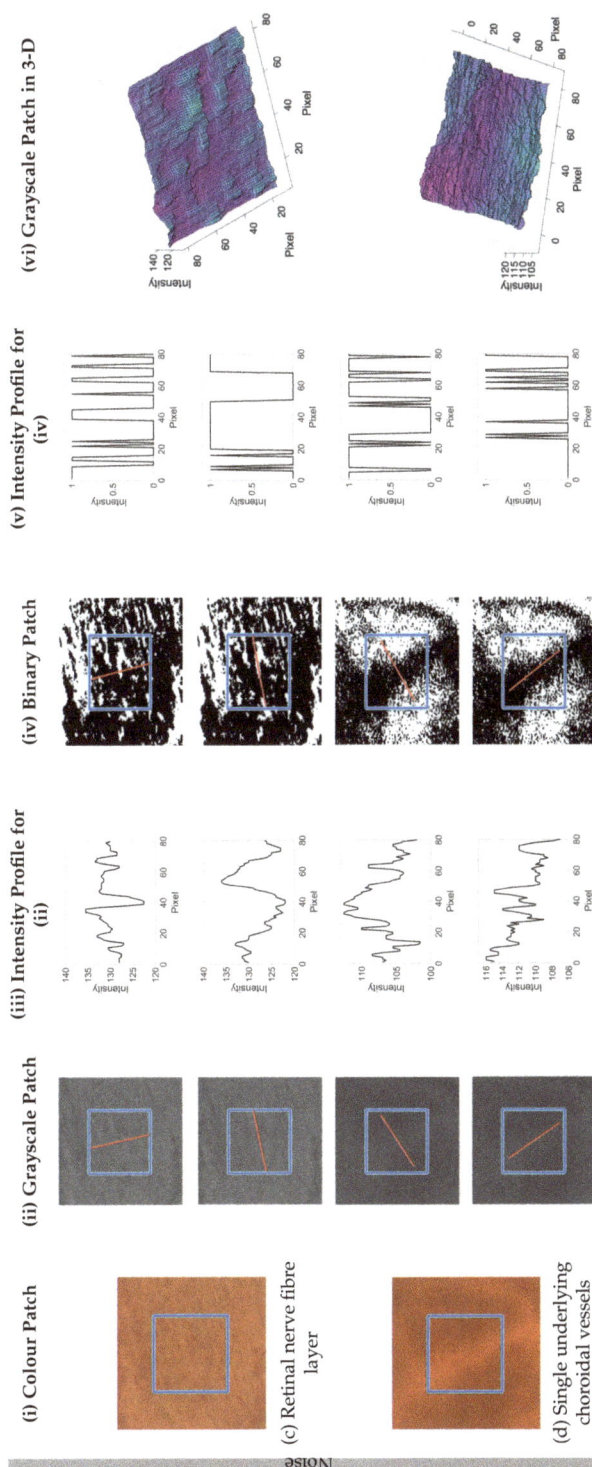

Table A2. *Cont.*

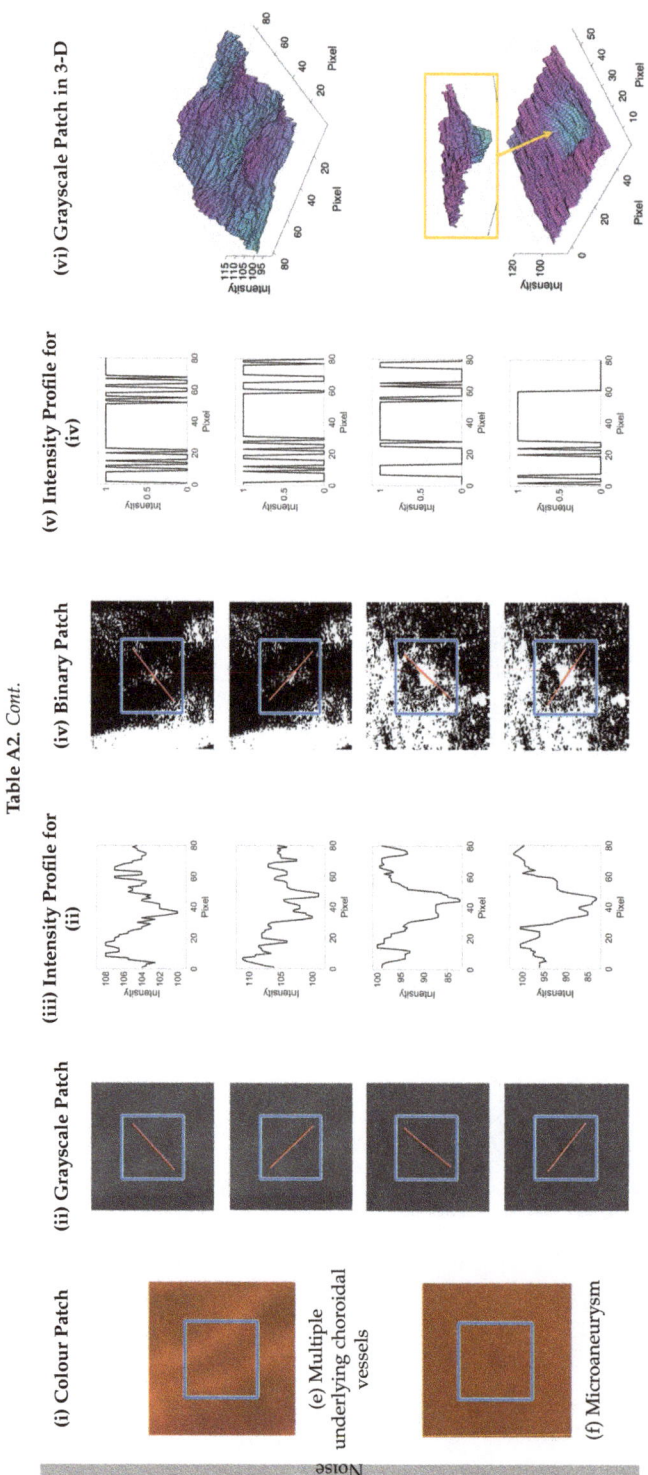

Table A2. *Cont.*

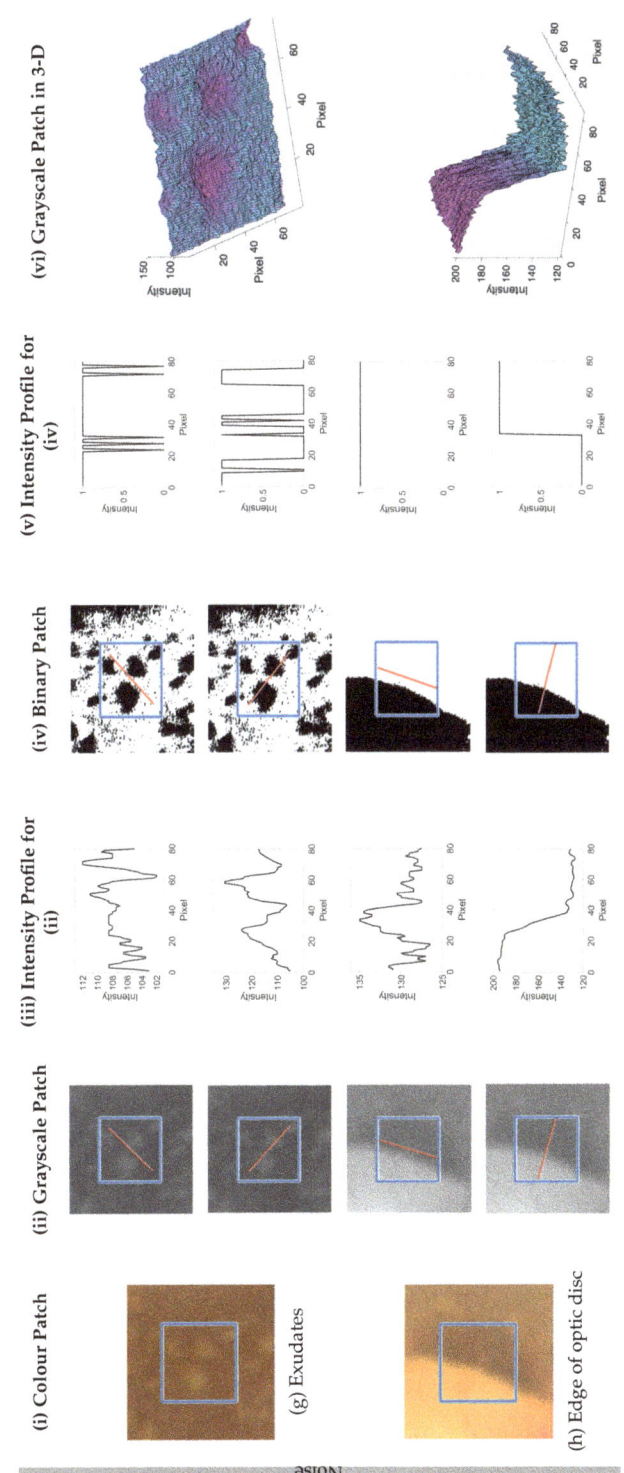

References

1. Hernandez-Matas, C.; Zabulis, X.; Argyros, A.A. Retinal image registration as a tool for supporting clinical applications. *Comp. Meth. Prog. Biomed.* **2021**, *199*, 105900. [CrossRef] [PubMed]
2. Legg, P.A.; Rosin, P.L.; Marshall, D.; Morgan, J.E. Improving accuracy and efficiency of mutual information for multi-modal retinal image registration using adaptive probability density estimation. *Comput. Med. Imaging. Graph.* **2013**, *37*, 597–606. [CrossRef] [PubMed]
3. Nakagawa, T.; Suzuki, T.; Hayashi, Y.; Mizukusa, Y.; Hatanaka, Y.; Ishida, K.; Hara, T.; Fujita, H.; Yamamoto, T. Quantitative depth analysis of optic nerve head using stereo retinal fundus image pair. *J. Biomed. Opt.* **2008**, *13*, 064026. [CrossRef] [PubMed]
4. Kolar, R.; Sikula, V.; Base, M. Retinal Image Registration using Phase Correlation. *Anal. Biomed. Signals Images* **2010**, *20*, 244–252. [CrossRef]
5. Kolar, R.; Harabis, V.; Odstrcilik, J. Hybrid retinal image registration using phase correlation. *Imaging Sci. J.* **2013**, *61*, 369–384. [CrossRef]
6. Chanwimaluang, T.; Fan, G.L.; Fransen, S.R. Hybrid Retinal Image Registration. *IEEE Trans. Inf. Technol. Biomed.* **2006**, *10*, 129–142. [CrossRef]
7. Zitova, B.; Flusser, J. Image registration methods: A survey. *Image Vis. Comput.* **2003**, *21*, 977–1000. [CrossRef]
8. Ghassabi, Z.; Shanbehzadeh, J.; Mohammadzadeh, A.; Ostadzadeh, S.S. Colour retinal fundus image registration by selecting stable extremum points in the scale–Invariant feature transform detector. *IET Image Process.* **2015**, *9*, 889–900. [CrossRef]
9. Hernandez-Matas, C.; Zabulis, X.; Argyros, A.A. An Experimental Evaluation of the Accuracy of Keypoints-Based Retinal Image Registration. In Proceedings of the 39th Annual International Conference of the IEEE Engineering in Medicine and Biology Society (EMBC), Seogwipo, Korea, 11–15 July 2017; pp. 377–381.
10. Chen, J.; Chen, J.; Tian, J.; Lee, N.; Zheng, J.; Smith, R.T.; Laine, A.F. A Partial Intensity Invariant Feature Descriptor for Multimodal Retinal Image Registration. *IEEE Trans. Biomed. Eng.* **2010**, *57*, 1707–1718. [CrossRef]
11. Ghassabi, Z.; Shanbehzadeh, J.; Sedaghat, A.; Fatemizadeh, E. An efficient approach for robust multimodal retinal image registration based on UR-SIFT features and PIIFD descriptors. *Eurasip. J. Image Video Process.* **2013**, *2013*, 25. [CrossRef]
12. Ramli, R.; Idris, M.Y.I.; Hasikin, K.; Karim, N.K.A. Histogram-Based Threshold Selection of Retinal Feature for Image Registration. In Proceedings of the 3rd International Conference on Information Technology & Society (IC-ITS), Penang, Malaysia, 31 July–1 August 2017; pp. 105–114.
13. Yang, G.; Stewart, C.V.; Sofka, M.; Tsai, C.-L. Registration of challenging image pairs: Initialization, estimation, and decision. *IEEE Trans. Pattern Anal. Mach. Intell.* **2007**, *29*, 1973–1989. [CrossRef] [PubMed]
14. Ramli, R.; Idris, M.Y.I.; Hasikin, K.; Karim, N.K.A.; Abdul Wahab, A.W.; Ahmedy, I.; Ahmedy, F.; Kadri, N.A.; Arof, H. Feature-Based Retinal Image Registration Using D-Saddle Feature. *J. Healthc. Eng.* **2017**, *2017*, 1489524. [CrossRef] [PubMed]
15. Lowe, D.G. Distinctive image features from scale-Invariant keypoints. *Int. J. Comput. Vis.* **2004**, *60*, 91–110. [CrossRef]
16. Hernandez-Matas, C.; Zabulis, X.; Argyros, A.A. Retinal image registration through simultaneous camera pose and eye shape estimation. In Proceedings of the 38th Annual International Conference of the IEEE Engineering in Medicine and Biology Society (EMBC), Orlando, FL, USA, 16–20 August 2016; pp. 3247–3251.
17. Hernandez-Matas, C.; Zabulis, X.; Triantafyllou, A.; Anyfanti, P.; Argyros, A.A. Retinal image registration under the assumption of a spherical eye. *Comput. Med. Imaging Graph.* **2017**, *55*, 95–105. [CrossRef] [PubMed]
18. Tsai, C.; Li, C.; Yang, G.; Lin, K. The Edge-Driven Dual-Bootstrap Iterative Closest Point Algorithm for Registration of Multimodal Fluorescein Angiogram Sequence. *IEEE Trans. Med. Imaging.* **2010**, *29*, 636–649.
19. Sedaghat, A.; Mokhtarzade, M.; Ebadi, H. Uniform robust scale-Invariant feature matching for optical remote sensing images. *IEEE Trans. Geosci. Remote. Sens.* **2011**, *49*, 4516–4527. [CrossRef]
20. Frangi, A.F.; Niessen, W.J.; Vincken, K.L.; Viergever, M.A. Multiscale vessel enhancement filtering. In Proceedings of the International Conference on Medical Image Computing and Computer-Assisted Intervention (MICCAI'98), Cambridge, MA, USA, 11–13 October 1998.
21. Vonikakis, V.; Chrysostomou, D.; Kouskouridas, R.; Gasteratos, A. A biologically inspired scale-Space for illumination invariant feature detection. *Meas. Sci. Technol.* **2013**, *24*, 074024. [CrossRef]
22. Lee, J.A.; Cheng, J.; Hai Lee, B.; Ping Ong, E.; Xu, G.; Wing Kee Wong, D.; Liu, J.; Laude, A.; Han Lim, T. A low-Dimensional step pattern analysis algorithm with application to multimodal retinal image registration. In Proceedings of the IEEE Conference on Computer Vision and Pattern Recognition (CVPR), Boston, MA, USA, 7–12 June 2015; pp. 1046–1053.
23. Wang, G.; Wang, Z.C.; Chen, Y.F.; Zhao, W.D. Robust point matching method for multimodal retinal image registration. *Biomed. Signal Process. Control.* **2015**, *19*, 68–76. [CrossRef]
24. Hernandez-Matas, C.; Zabulis, X.; Argyros, A.A. Retinal image registration based on keypoint correspondences, spherical eye modeling and camera pose estimation. In Proceedings of the 37th Annual International Conference of the IEEE Engineering in Medicine and Biology Society (EMBC), Milan, Italy, 25–29 August 2015; pp. 5650–5654.
25. Lee, J.A.; Lee, B.H.; Xu, G.; Ong, E.P.; Wong, D.W.K.; Liu, J.; Lim, T.H. Geometric corner extraction in retinal fundus images. In Proceedings of the 2014 36th Annual International Conference of the IEEE Engineering in Medicine and Biology Society, Chicago, IL, USA, 26–30 August 2014; pp. 158–161.

26. Harris, C.; Stephens, M. A combined corner and edge detector. In Proceedings of the 4th Alvey Vision Conference, Manchester, UK, 31 August–2 September 1988; pp. 147–151.
27. Bay, H.; Tuytelaars, T.; van Gool, L. SURF: Speeded up Robust Features. In Proceedings of the 9th European Conference on Computer Vision (ECCV), Graz, Austria, 7–13 May 2006; pp. 404–417.
28. Bay, H.; Ess, A.; Tuytelaars, T.; Van Gool, L. Speeded-Up Robust Features (SURF). *Comput. Vis. Image Underst.* **2008**, *110*, 346–359. [CrossRef]
29. International Telecommunication Union. Studio encoding parameters of digital television for standard 4:3 and wide-Screen 16: 9 aspect ratios. In *Recommendation ITU-R BT.601–7*; ITU: Geneva, Switzerland, 2017; pp. 1–8.
30. Kanan, C.; Cottrell, G.W. Color-to-Grayscale: Does the Method Matter in Image Recognition? *PLoS ONE* **2012**, *7*, e29740. [CrossRef]
31. Burger, W.; Burge, M.J. SIFT—Scale-Invariant Local Features. In *Principles of Digital Image Processing: Advanced Methods*; Springer: London, UK, 2013; pp. 229–295.
32. Aldana-Iuit, J.; Mishkin, D.; Chum, O.; Matas, J. In the Saddle: Chasing Fast and Repeatable Features. In Proceedings of the 23rd International Conference on Pattern Recognition, Cancun, Mexico, 4–8 December 2016.
33. CHASE_DB1 Retinal Image Database. Available online: https://blogs.kingston.ac.uk/retinal/chasedb1/ (accessed on 10 December 2017).
34. Fraz, M.M.; Remagnino, P.; Hoppe, A.; Uyyanonvara, B.; Rudnicka, A.R.; Owen, C.G.; Barman, S.A. An ensemble classification-Based approach applied to retinal blood vessel segmentation. *IEEE Trans. Biomed. Eng.* **2012**, *59*, 2538–2548. [CrossRef] [PubMed]
35. Staal, J.; Abràmoff, M.D.; Niemeijer, M.; Viergever, M.A.; Van Ginneken, B. Ridge-Based vessel segmentation in color images of the retina. *IEEE Trans. Med. Imaging* **2004**, *23*, 501–509. [CrossRef]
36. DRIVE: Digital Retinal Images for Vessel Extraction. Available online: http://www.isi.uu.nl/Research/Databases/DRIVE/ (accessed on 10 December 2017).
37. HRF: High-Resolution Fundus Image Database. Available online: https://www5.cs.fau.de/research/data/fundus-images/ (accessed on 10 December 2017).
38. Budai, A.; Bock, R.; Maier, A.; Hornegger, J.; Michelson, G. Robust vessel segmentation in fundus images. *Int. J. Biomed. Imaging* **2013**, *2013*, 154860. [CrossRef]
39. STARE: Structured Analysis of the Retina. Available online: http://cecas.clemson.edu/~{}ahoover/stare/ (accessed on 10 December 2017).
40. Hoover, A.; Kouznetsova, V.; Goldbaum, M. Locating blood vessels in retinal images by piecewise threshold probing of a matched filter response. *IEEE Trans. Med. Imaging* **2000**, *19*, 203–210. [CrossRef] [PubMed]
41. Hernandez-Matas, C.; Zabulis, X.; Triantafyllou, A.; Anyfanti, P.; Douma, S.; Argyros, A.A. FIRE: Fundus Image Registration dataset. *J. Modeling Ophthalmol.* **2017**, *1*, 16–28. [CrossRef]
42. Saha, S.K.; Xiao, D.; Frost, S.; Kanagasingam, Y. A Two-Step Approach for Longitudinal Registration of Retinal Images. *J. Med. Syst.* **2016**, *40*, 277. [CrossRef]
43. Gonzalez, R.C.; Woods, R.E.; Eddins, S.L. Representation and Description. In *Digital Image Processing Using MATLAB*; Prentice Hall: Hoboken, NJ, USA, 2009.
44. Goerner, F.L.; Duong, T.; Stafford, R.J.; Clarke, G.D. A comparison of five standard methods for evaluating image intensity uniformity in partially parallel imaging MRI. *Med. Phys.* **2013**, *40*, 082302-1–082302-10. [CrossRef]
45. Brown, M.; Lowe, D.G. Invariant Features from Interest Point Groups. In Proceedings of the British Machine Vision Conference (BMVC), Cardiff, UK, 2–5 September 2002.
46. Vedaldi, A.; Fulkerson, B. VLFeat: An open and portable library of computer vision algorithms. In Proceedings of the 18th ACM international conference on Multimedia, Firenze, Italy, 25–29 October 2010; pp. 1469–1472.
47. Torr, P.H.; Zisserman, A. MLESAC: A new robust estimator with application to estimating image geometry. *Comput. Vis. Image Underst.* **2000**, *78*, 138–156. [CrossRef]
48. Goshtasby, A. Image registration by local approximation methods. *Image Vis. Comput.* **1988**, *6*, 255–261. [CrossRef]
49. Pauli, T.W.; Gangaputra, S.; Hubbard, L.D.; Thayer, D.W.; Chandler, C.S.; Peng, Q.; Narkar, A.; Ferrier, N.J.; Danis, R.P. Effect of Image Compression and Resolution on Retinal Vascular Caliber. *Investig. Ophthalmol. Vis. Sci.* **2012**, *53*, 5117–5123. [CrossRef]
50. Brown, D.M.; Ciardella, A. Mosaic Fundus Imaging in the Diagnosis of Retinal Diseases. *Investig. Ophthalmol. Vis. Sci.* **2005**, *46*, 2581.
51. Bontala, A.; Sivaswamy, J.; Pappuru, R.R. Image mosaicing of low quality neonatal retinal images. In Proceedings of the 9th IEEE International Symposium on Biomedical Imaging (ISBI), Barcelona, Spain, 2–5 May 2012; pp. 720–723.
52. Lee, B.H.; Xu, G.; Gopalakrishnan, K.; Ong, E.P.; Li, R.; Wong, D.W.K.; Lim, T.H. AEGIS-Augmented Eye Laser Treatment with Region Guidance for Intelligent Surgery. In Proceedings of the 11th Asian Conference on Computer Aided Surgery (ACCAS 2015), Singapore, 9–11 July 2015.
53. Adal, K.M.; van Etten, P.G.; Martinez, J.P.; van Vliet, L.J.; Vermeer, K.A. Accuracy Assessment of Intra-and Intervisit Fundus Image Registration for Diabetic Retinopathy ScreeningAccuracy Assessment of Fundus Image Registration. *Investig. Ophthalmol. Vis. Sci.* **2015**, *56*, 1805–1812. [CrossRef] [PubMed]

54. Matsopoulos, G.K.; Asvestas, P.A.; Mouravliansky, N.A.; Delibasis, K.K. Multimodal registration of retinal images using self organizing maps. *IEEE Trans. Med. Imaging.* **2004**, *23*, 1557–1563. [CrossRef]
55. Dalal, N.; Triggs, B. Histograms of oriented gradients for human detection. In Proceedings of the IEEE Computer Society Conference on Computer Vision and Pattern Recognition (CVPR), San Diego, CA, USA, 20–25 June 2005; pp. 886–893.
56. Patel, M.I.; Thakar, V.K.; Shah, S.K. Image Registration of Satellite Images with Varying Illumination Level Using HOG Descriptor Based SURF. *Procedia Comput. Sci.* **2016**, *93*, 382–388. [CrossRef]
57. Grabner, M.; Grabner, H.; Bischof, H. Fast approximated SIFT. In Proceedings of the Asian Conference on Computer Vision, Hyderabad, India, 13–16 January 2006.
58. Rashid, M.; Khan, M.A.; Sharif, M.; Raza, M.; Sarfraz, M.M.; Afza, F. Object detection and classification: A joint selection and fusion strategy of deep convolutional neural network and SIFT point features. *Multimed. Tools Appl.* **2019**, *78*, 15751–15777. [CrossRef]
59. Andrei Dmitri, G.; Alex, J.; Maya, V.; Jack, D. Preventing Model Overfitting and Underfitting in Convolutional Neural Networks. *Int. J. Softw. Sci. Comput. Intell. (IJSSCI)* **2018**, *10*, 19–28.

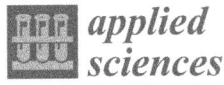

Article

Hardware Optimizations of the X-ray Pre-Processing for Interventional Computed Tomography Using the FPGA

Daniele Passaretti *, Mukesh Ghosh, Shiras Abdurahman, Micaela Lambru Egito and Thilo Pionteck

Institute for Information Technology and Communications, Otto von Guericke University Magdeburg, 39106 Magdeburg, Germany; mukesh.gosh@ovgu.de (M.G.); shiras.abdurahman@ovgu.de (S.A.); micaela.lambru@ovgu.de (M.L.E.); thilo.pionteck@ovgu.de (T.P.)
* Correspondence: daniele.passaretti@ovgu.de

Abstract: In computed tomography imaging, the computationally intensive tasks are the preprocessing of 2D detector data to generate total attenuation or line integral projections and the reconstruction of the 3D volume from the projections. This paper proposes the optimization of the X-ray pre-processing to compute total attenuation projections by avoiding the intermediate step to convert detector data to intensity images. In addition, to fulfill the real-time requirements, we design a configurable hardware architecture for data acquisition systems on FPGAs, with the goal to have a "on-the-fly" pre-processing of 2D projections. Finally, this architecture was configured for exploring and analyzing different arithmetic representations, such as floating-point and fixed-point data formats. This design space exploration has allowed us to find the best representation and data format that minimize execution time and hardware costs, while not affecting image quality. Furthermore, the proposed architecture was integrated in an open-interface computed tomography device, used for evaluating the image quality of the pre-processed 2D projections and the reconstructed 3D volume. By comparing the proposed solution with the state-of-the-art pre-processing algorithm that make use of intensity images, the latency was decreased $4.125\times$, and the resources utilization of $\sim 6.5\times$, with a mean square error in the order of 10^{-15} for all the selected phantom experiments. Finally, by using the fixed-point representation in the different data precisions, the latency and the resource utilization were further decreased, and a mean square error in the order of 10^{-1} was reached.

Keywords: computed tomography; image pre-processing; high-level synthesis; X-ray pre-processing; pipelined architecture

Citation: Passaretti, D.; Ghosh, M.; Abdurahman, S.; Egito, L.M.; Pionteck, T. Hardware Optimizations of the X-ray Pre-Processing for Interventional Computed Tomography Using the FPGA. *Appl. Sci.* **2022**, *12*, 5659. https://doi.org/10.3390/app12115659

Academic Editor: Qi-Huang Zheng

Received: 28 February 2022
Accepted: 28 May 2022
Published: 2 June 2022

Publisher's Note: MDPI stays neutral with regard to jurisdictional claims in published maps and institutional affiliations.

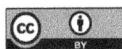

Copyright: © 2022 by the authors. Licensee MDPI, Basel, Switzerland. This article is an open access article distributed under the terms and conditions of the Creative Commons Attribution (CC BY) license (https://creativecommons.org/licenses/by/4.0/).

1. Introduction

Computed tomography (CT) is an X-ray 3D cross-sectional imaging technology and is heavily used for medical and industrial applications. The X-ray source and the 2D detector are the major components of a CT system. The X-ray source generates photons of various energies, which pass through the patient body. The photons undergo the process of attenuation, where a fraction of them are either absorbed or scattered. The unattenuated or transmitted photons are detected by a 2D array of detector cells generating a 2D shadow or projection image of the patient body. The X-ray source–detector pair rotates around the patient and acquires projection images at various angles. The 2D cross-sectional images or 3D volumes of the patient can be generated from the 2D projections using state-of-the-art reconstruction algorithms [1]. The advent of hardware accelerators and efficient algorithms has made real-time volumetric imaging feasible by fast image processing and reconstruction. Clinical CT images have been used for patient diagnosis (diagnostic CT), such as detecting tumors and aneurysms [1]. In addition, the CT scanners (interventional CT) have also been employed for intra-operative guidance (e.g., instrument or needle tracking) and the assessment of interventional procedures, such as tumor ablation [2].

The main objective of the diagnostic CT is the accurate reconstruction of the patient's anatomy with the highest image quality possible (e.g., high spatial resolution, and reduced noise). By contrast, the main challenge of interventional CT is to display the reconstructed images in real time with an acceptable image quality necessary for the smooth functioning of interventional procedures. To overcome the constraints induced by image quality, X-ray dose reduction, and real-time capability, the development of efficient algorithms and their implementation utilizing task and/or data parallelism in hardware accelerators such as graphics processing units (GPU), digital signal processors (DSP) and field programmable gate arrays (FPGA) is an active research area [3–7]. Alcaín et al. [7] published a survey about the different usage of various hardware accelerators in real-time medical imaging. They also discussed interventional CT and the advantage of using hardware accelerators, compared to CPUs.

These accelerators implement specific math co-processors, able to process different data formats. The main standard used for real numbers is the single-precision floating-point format (IEEE 754) [8], which allows a wide range of numerical values. By contrast, due to the hardware complexity of the math co-processor (also known as floating point unit, FPU) to represent and process the IEEE 754 data format, new math co-processors for real number operations are explored in the literature. These are often based on approximate computing techniques [9,10]. For example, tensor core processing units [11,12] enhance the performance of real number operations by using the Bfloat16 format. This format is defined by a custom 16-bit floating point representation [13].

Due to the complexity of the algorithms and the amount of data needed to be processed, the various hardware accelerators are often not capable of running the projection pre-processing and the volume reconstruction in real time [7]. Hence, apart from the investigation of novel algorithms and architectures, the utilization of novel custom number representations and data formats are also explored [12,14]. In fact, in CT image processing, real numbers are involved that can be represented with various data representations and formats. For instance, Maaß et al. [14] employed 32-bit (float) and 16-bit (half) floating-point data formats to represent the projection pixel values. As per their results, the half data format halved the required memory bandwidth without compromising the accuracy of reconstruction.

For the best of our knowledge, in CT image processing, the exploration of the design space (with the different data representations and formats) is a complex task in which there are no systematic solutions which guide the designer to select either a custom or a standard data format. All proposed solutions implement the CT pre-processing and reconstruction algorithm with a pre-selected data format without considering which data format is optimal for the image quality, the real-time requirements, and the hardware realization, at the same time. Maaß et al. [14] compared 32-bit and 16-bit floating-point data formats without considering the impact of these in terms of hardware cost and additional data representation, such as fixed point. For exploring new custom co-processors, FPGAs are well-suitable platforms. In contrast to CPUs, GPUs, and DSPs that have a fixed instruction-set architecture (ISA) and data representations, FPGAs allow designers to define custom hardware architectures and to explore custom data representations [6]. Therefore, they can be used for exploring the design space, where different custom and standard data formats are defined and selected.

Contributions. In this article, we propose various hardware optimizations of the X-ray pre-processing step in interventional CT. It involves the optimization of the numerical computation of total attenuation values and its hardware acceleration. This pre-processing step is also called *I0-correction*. First, we apply the pre-processing algorithm on the digital detector signals without the intermediate step to convert them to intensity images. Consequently, the total attenuation computation formula is simplified in terms of arithmetic and hardware complexity. Second, we implement a custom hardware accelerator as dataflow architecture, called the CT pre-processing core, that pre-processes the raw sensor data on the fly, without storing data in external memory. Furthermore, this core is designed using high-level synthesis (HLS), and it is configurable for various encoding and data widths of fixed-point and floating-point representations. In addition to the proposed pre-processing optimization, we integrated the implementation of the CT pre-processing core in an open-interface CT assembled in our laboratory. The proposed core implemented on FPGA can be integrated directly with the data acquisition system (DAS), which collects the detector signals and forwards the pre-processed data to the reconstruction system.

Finally, we perform a design space exploration (DSE) to find which real number representation and data format better fits the pre-processing step for interventional CT applications. The DSE considers the different data representations as input variables and the qualitative and quantitative metrics, such as image quality, execution time, and the X-ray dose as decision variables. We systematically pre-select the input data formats based on the raw sensor and the reconstruction data formats. In addition, we pre-select specific metrics for estimating hardware costs, such as execution time, data width, and memory bandwidth required per pixel. Apart from that, we use image quality metrics, such as mean square error (MSE) of the 2D image and *low contrast*, *noise* and *uniformity* of the 3D volume. The image quality is analyzed after reconstructing the images of a dedicated CT image quality phantom known as CATPHAN® 500 [15] phantom [15].

Structure. This paper is organized as follows: Section 2 describes the CT scanner, the difference between attenuation and intensity projection images, and the computing theory for real number representations; Section 3 explains the related works; Sections 4 and 5 present the optimization of projection pre-processing and the CT pre-processing core; Section 6 illustrates the implementation and the CT integration; Section 7 introduces the DSE for the different real number representations; Section 8 describes the phantom modules, the image quality metrics, and CT settings utilized for the DSE; Sections 9 and 10 show the results of the X-ray pre-processing for various real number representations.

2. Background

This section describes the CT scanner, how FPGAs are used in CT, and the theory of the computation of total attenuation required during the pre-processing steps of the CT reconstruction. In addition, we describe the different data representations for real numbers used in our design space exploration.

2.1. Computed Tomography Scanner

The word tomography is derived from the Greek words tomos (slice or section) and graphein (to write or draw) [16]. Therefore, CT can be defined as the depiction of the cross-sectional images or slices of a patient's body [17]. The multiple slices can be stacked together to form a three-dimensional image or volume [17].

As shown in Figure 1, the CT scanner consists of an X-ray tube or source, a gantry module, a detector system (DMS), collimators, a motorized patient's table, and an image reconstruction unit. For controlling and synchronizing all these components, different FPGAs are used in the CT scanner [18]. The X-ray tube system, collimators, and detector are fixed on the rotating disk, mounted on the gantry; the rest of the components are fixed on the stationary side. The communication between the rotating and stationary sides is done through slip-ring technology consisting of brushes that permit the electrical connection between the rotating and stationary sides.

The CT scanner works by moving the patient table to the space inside the gantry module, and when the patient's body goes through it, the X-ray tube system and the DMS rotates around the object's body with a frequency of about 170 rpm [16]. In the meantime, the X-ray tube system shoots a narrow beam of photons through the object's body. The attenuated beam photons of the object's body are acquired by detector sensors on the opposite side of the X-ray tube system [16]. The data are acquired as pixels of 2D images, called projections. Usually, modern CT scanners collect over 1160 projections per round [18]. These data are transferred to the image reconstruction unit, where the volume of the object's body is reconstructed as volume.

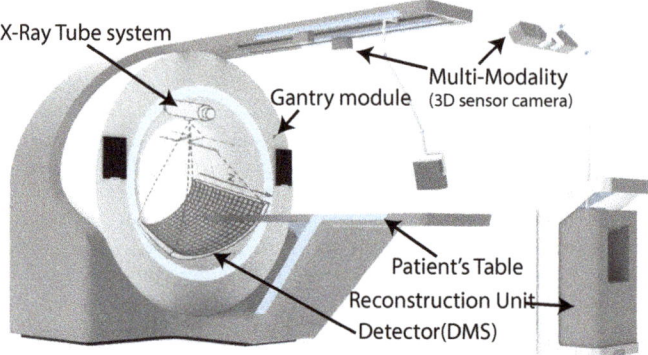

Figure 1. CT scanner components. Reprinted/adapted with permission from Ref. [18]. Copyright 2019, IEEE.

The image formation in CT involves pre-processing acquired detector data, reconstructing the volume from the processed projections, and post-processing the reconstructed volume. CT reconstruction from the processed projections (total attenuation values or line integrals) is an inverse problem [19]; it means that input values (3D volumes) are estimated from the output values (2D images). Numerous solutions can be found for this problem in the literature, including the filtered back-projection (FBP) and iterative reconstruction [20–23]. Our article focuses on the X-ray pre-processing step to compute the total attenuation values from the digitized detector data. In interventional CT, it has to be executed in real time.

2.2. Pre-Processing: X-ray I0-Correction

During CT data acquisition, the patient body is irradiated with the photons emanating from the X-ray source. Some of the photons are attenuated during the photon–matter interaction. An X-ray detector detects the unattenuated or transmitted photons generating projection images. X-ray detection involves the two-level conversion process, where the X-ray photons are converted to light, and the photo-diode array converts them to electrical signals. Analog-to-digital converters (ADCs) of the acquisition system will transform electric signals into digital signals and store them in a compressed format. These 2D images are called detector data projections and are denoted by $d(u,v)$, where u and v are the detector row and column indices. Conventionally, the detector data projections are transformed into X-ray intensity projections as per the following equation:

$$I(u,v) = c \cdot e^{-d(u,v)} \qquad (1)$$

where c is a scaling factor. $I(u,v)$ is the intensity image data. The exponential decay of the X-ray intensity during X-ray transmission through the patient body is given by the Beer–Lambert law [20,23]. The total attenuation values along the X-ray path are given by

$$P(u,v) = ln\left(\frac{I_0(u,v)}{I(u,v)}\right) \qquad (2)$$

where I_0 projections are stored in the CT system during the calibration of the scanner by acquiring the intensity projections without any object. Formula (2) is also called *I0-correction*. A CT 3D volume is reconstructed from the attenuation projections using state-of-the-art reconstruction algorithms.

From the detector, the DAS collects the raw sensor data which must be multiplied with a factor of f to obtain the detector data projections, as given by

$$d(u,v) = f \cdot Raw(u,v) \qquad (3)$$

Commercial CTs usually do not provide the projections as detector data projections, but they convert them to intensity image data. In fact, pre-processing algorithms usually process projections in intensity image data and then apply the *I0-correction* for the reconstruction step.

In Section 4, we propose a mathematical optimization of the *I0-correction* that uses directly the raw sensor data, instead of using the converted intensity image data.

2.3. Real Number Representations

As mentioned above, the CT reconstruction algorithms use real numbers. In computing, real numbers are usually represented by the float or the double format. These formats are two different encodings of the standard for floating-point arithmetic (IEEE 754) [8]. This standard specifies conversions and arithmetic representations, and methods for binary and decimal floating-point arithmetic. As shown in Figure 2, the floating-point numbers are represented by their sign (S), exponent (E), and mantissa (M) bits. The floating-point value can be represented as a function of S, E and M, as follows:

$$f(S, E, M) = \begin{cases} (-)^S \cdot 2^{E+1-2^{e-1}} \cdot (1 + M \cdot 2^{-m}) & \text{for } 0 < E < 2^{e-1} \quad (4) \\ (-)^S \cdot (1 + M \cdot 2^{-m}) & \text{else} \quad (5) \end{cases}$$

In the formula above, m represents the amount of mantissa bits (e.g., in single precision, floating-point m is equal to 23).

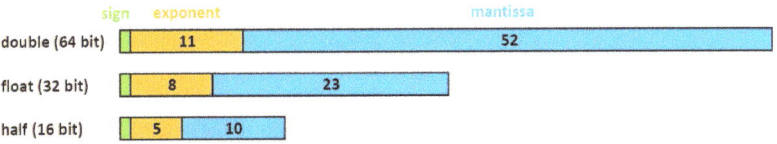

Figure 2. Encodings of the floating-point standard.

According to IEEE 754 standard, there are four different formats of encoding for the floating-point, with 16, 32, 64 and 128 bits, and they are called half-precision, single-precision, double-precision and quad-precision respectively. E and M have different data widths, based on the selected encoding, as shown in Figure 2.

The various encodings determine number representations with different accuracy. In addition, they use different arithmetic processing units, which have different performance in terms of power consumption, execution time, memory utilization, and chip area. For example, the single-precision floating point represents numbers in the range between 2^{-149} and 2^{128}, with a relative error of 2^{-23}, caused by truncating digits.

As the target data to process are limited in a small range of values, and the accuracy of the IEEE 754 representation is not required for the target application, new custom and approximate representations have been proposed in literature, with the aim to optimize hardware resources, data resources, and execution time. A proposed solution in the literature is the **fixed-point** representation [24].

As shown in Figure 3, this representation is composed of three parts: *sign* (S), *integer* (I) and *fraction* (F) fields. There is no fixed encoding for this representation, but the hardware designer sets the size of the *data width* (W), that is equal to S + I + F. The size of I and F depends on the values to represent, and the desired accuracy. Furthermore, math co-processors for fixed-point operations are usually faster than the respective for the IEEE-754 standard, because the same operation implemented in fixed-point precision use fewer logic gates and hardware resources than floating-point precision, but usually it has a lower accuracy and can represent a smaller range of numbers. In Section 7, we explore different settings of the parameters S, I and F for finding the optimal configuration of these parameters with an acceptable accuracy of the CT dataset.

Figure 3. Fixed-point representation.

3. Related Works

In the literature, there are a lot of algorithms and hardware accelerators for CT pre-processing and reconstruction. Most of them use FPGAs [25–31], and GPUs [32–36] as a target platform because these offer a high level of flexibility and parallelism. Here, we do not compare the different architectures for FPGAs with the proposed CT pre-processed core because it is not possible to compare them and it is also out of the scope of our article. Instead, we are interested in optimizing the pre-processing step and investigating the impact of data formats on the reconstructed image; we only consider the different data formats used in these works. In addition, we report the related works, where the authors analyzed and compared different data formats in CT reconstruction, and point out the difference with our work that aim to find the best data format in interventional CT.

Dandekar et al. in [4] presented a reconfigurable architecture for the real-time pre-processing of interventional CT. They proposed a streaming architecture that optimizes latency. They implemented a median filtering and anisotropic diffusion filtering based on neighborhood voxels (3D pixels). This property was used for implementing a custom brick-caching schema that improves the memory performance. They describe their architecture in VHDL with different fixed-data formats: 8, 12 and 16 bits. With the custom implementation of these optimizations, they achieve a processing rate of 46 frames per second for images of size $256 \times 256 \times 64$ voxels.

Another important work comes from Korcyl et al. in [37]. They built real-time tomographic data processing on FPGA SoC devices. They designed the whole system from detector's scanner to the reconstruction unit. The reconstruction system is implemented on a single FPGA board that processes the image in real-time. The architecture is composed of 8 parallel pipelines that acquire data from the scan. Inside, they de-couple the data, process them and display the images to the doctor, without using any external memory access. These FPGA accelerators for real-time CT pre-processing and reconstruction have different architectures, which use custom and standard data formats. Even if they optimize the architectures with a custom data format, they do not investigate the impact of the data format on the pre-processed and reconstructed image. They select a data format which fulfills the hardware requirements of their specific solution. In our work, we investigate the impact of the data formats on the pre-processed and reconstructed image. In addition, the CT pre-processing core can be configured at the synthesis time for using different data formats for raw sensor data, pre-processing data and reconstructed data.

For the best of our knowledge, in the literature, only Clemens Maaß et al. in [14] investigated the impact of data formats on the reconstructed image. They worked with different encodings of the IEEE-754 standard and they showed that the half-precision floating-point can enable a fast image reconstruction process without declining image quality [14]. So, instead of 32-bit single precision, 16-bit half precision is used as data format, and it reduces the traffic on the memory bus [14]. Due to arithmetic complexity, the back-projection needs to access the external memory multiple times [14]. By choosing the half-representation data format, they can reduce the data traffic and can increase the throughput of the memory bus. This work focuses on the difference between half- and single-precision floating point representation, but does not consider fixed-point representation and custom data representation, which also are used in CT image processing.

For example, Nourazar and Goossens [12] proposed an iterative CT reconstruction algorithm optimized for tensor cores of NVidia GPUs. To enhance the performance, they performed the reconstruction algorithm with a mixed-precision computation; the error of the mixed-precision computation was almost equal to single-precision (32-bit) floating-point computation [12]. Using a mixed-precision computation means that different data formats are used in the reconstruction algorithm for representing the same real value.

In our work, through a DSE, we systematically search in the design space the best data format for interventional CT. Different from Clemens Maaß et al. [14], we use a DSE in our methodology and we do not only consider the image error as the MSE and *noise*, but we also consider hardware cost metrics and image quality metrics, such as *low contrast* and *uniformity*. In addition, we do not limit our study to the floating-point representation, but we also consider fixed-point representation. Furthermore, with the proposed CT pre-processing core, custom data formats can be investigated.

4. X-ray I0-Correction Optimization

In this section, we describe the proposed method and formulas for performing the I0-correction directly on the acquired raw sensor data, without converting them to intensity domain images.

As explained in Section 2.2, most of the commercial CT scanners provide the projections, directly converted in the intensity domain, as real or integer number values, and the total attenuation correction is applied with Formula (2). This formula is computationally complex to implement because the logarithm operation usually is not a primitive operation in the math co-processors. In addition, for using this formula, the collected data must be converted from raw sensor data to intensity data inside the CT scanner; the conversion determines an additional latency between the DMS and the reconstruction system. In fact, for converting data from raw sensor data to intensity data, Formulas (1) and (3) are used. Formula (1) comprises an exponential operation, which is also not a primitive operation in most of math co-processors.

In our proposed optimization, we consider raw sensor data as input for the I0-correction. In this way, we have merged Formulas (1)–(3) which are usually separated and implemented in the CT data acquisition system and the reconstruction system. By merging them, we obtain the following formula:

$$P(u,v) = \log_e \left(\frac{c \cdot exp(-(f \cdot Raw_0(u,v)))}{c \cdot exp(-(f \cdot Raw(u,v)))} \right) \tag{6}$$

If we implement Formula (6) as is, the logarithm and the power operations should be implemented. However, since we implement it inside the data acquisition system of the CT, we apply the mathematical simplification that results in the equivalent formula, shown in (7).

$$P(u,v) = \log_{10}(2) \cdot f \cdot (Raw_0(u,v) - Raw(u,v)) \tag{7}$$

Therefore, as shown in Formula (7), the I0-correction can be performed directly on raw sensor data with basic operations provided by most of the math co-processors. This mathematical optimization determines the decreasing of the resource utilization and execution time, compared to the implementation of Formula (6).

Furthermore, to perform the I0-correction and the whole pre-processing step on the fly, we propose the implementation of the algorithm in a dataflow architecture. To describe how Formulas (6) and (7) were implemented in the dataflow architecture, we used the data flow graph representation [38], as shown in Figures 4 and 5. In the data flow graph the square boxes represent the input/output data and constants, the circular boxes, the operation and the arrows the flow of data. The dataflow graph shows the flow and the data and dependency of the operations. The various operations in the boxes have different latency and hardware costs in a math co-processor. The values of these metrics depend on the implemented operation and the selected data format. In the next sections, we focus on the hardware implementation of the dataflow architecture, its integration in the data acquisition system of the open-interface CT and how different data formats influence performance.

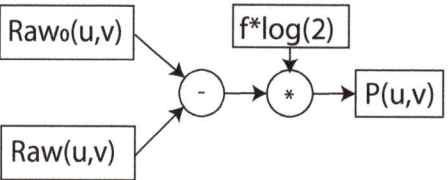

Figure 4. Data flow graph representation for the optimized I0-correction.

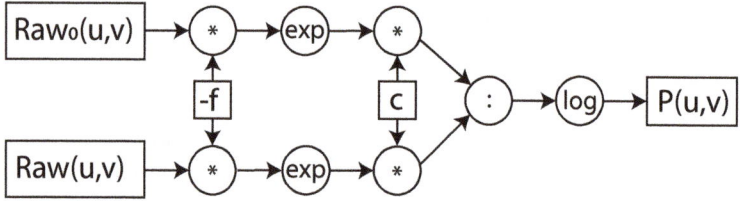

Figure 5. Data flow graph representation for the standard I0-correction.

5. CT Pre-Processing Core Architecture

In this section, we describe our CT pre-processing core, which implements the I0-correction. For fulfilling the real-time requirements, the CT pre-processing core is designed as a dataflow architecture, which has a constant delay and throughput. Furthermore, to process data with high clock frequency and to reduce the critical path of the arithmetic operations, the dataflow architecture is pipelined. The depth of the pipeline depends on the data format and prepossessing algorithm, as explained in Section 9.

The CT pre-processing core, as shown in Figure 6, has the following three main stages:

- **Sensor-data conversion stage**: This stage obtains the pixel raw sensor data of the I0-image and the current image collected by the data acquisition system (DAS). In this stage, each pixel is converted to the selected pre-processing data format. At synthesis time, a custom configuration for floating-point or fixed-point representation must be selected.
- **Image-processing stage**: In this stage, pixel data are ready to be pre-processed in the selected data representation. This stage has multiple internal stages, and it is scalable for additional pre-processing steps. In this article, we focus on the pre-processing step, based on Formulas (6) and (7).
- **Reconstruction conversion stage**: This stage obtains the pre-processed data (attenuation image) and converts them in the reconstruction data format, defined at the synthesis time. The output results are ready for the reconstruction, and they are forwarded to the data stream unit, which is responsible either for storing or sending them to the reconstruction system.

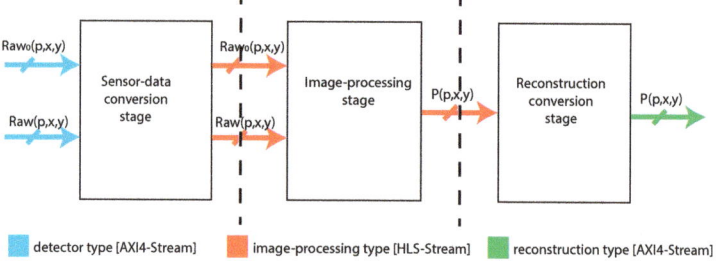

Figure 6. CT pre-processing core.

For communicating, the CT pre-processing core uses the AXI4-Stream interface. This flexible interface can be configured with different data widths, so it can be easily used for different data representations, and integrated in any system that uses the AXI4-Stream standard.

The CT pre-processing core is designed for processing one pixel per clock cycle. If the DAS collects multiple pixels per clock cycle, multiple instances of this core must be added; in this way, all the collected pixels are processed in parallel. For example, in the integration with the DAS of our open-interface CT, we have four instances because the DAS collects four pixels per clock cycle, as is explained in the following Section 6.

Furthermore, the CT processing core is designed and implemented to be configurable for custom data representations that are defined at synthesis time. In this way, the architecture can be easily used for DSE, as it is explained in Section 7.

6. CT Pre-Processing Core Implementation and Integration

In this section, we describe the implementation of the CT pre-processing core and its integration in the DAS of a running open-interface CT. This DAS component is implemented by a ZC706 evaluation board with the XC7Z045 MPSoC-FPGA model from Xilinx [39]. An MPSoC-FPGA is a system on chip (SoC) containing an FPGA part and a processing system (PS) part with multiple CPUs and a GPU.

6.1. IP Block Design

For implementing the CT pre-processing core on the Xilinx board, we used Vitis™ HLS, which is the Xilinx high-level synthesis tool that allows C, C++, and OpenCL™ functions to become hardwired onto the device logic fabric and RAM/DSP blocks. The HSL implementation results in a register transfer level (RTL) block design, also called IP block design, which can be implemented on FPGA. Moreover, by describing our hardware components with Vitis™ HLS, we do not have to describe the arithmetic hardware components at the logic gate level. In fact, Vitis™ HLS utilizes optimized arithmetic hardware components, provided by Xilinx as a library.

The CT pre-processing core is described with C++ source code. Each stage of the dataflow architecture is encapsulated in a C++ function. The arguments of each function describe the input/output ports of the stage. In synthesis, to obtain the pipelined dataflow architecture, we use the directives "`#pragma HLS DATAFLOW`" and "`#pragma HLS PIPELINE dataflow`" provided by Vitis™ HLS. These directives allow to implement C++ loops and C++ functions as a pipelined dataflow RTL block design.

Externally, the CT pre-processing core communicates via AXI4-STREAM interfaces. These are defined by using the data format "`hls::axis`" and the directive "`#pragma HLS INTERFACE axis`", which can be only used for the external interfaces of the core. As a result, for interconnecting the three internal stages of the CT pre-processing with a stream interface, the "hls::stream" template type and the directive "`#pragma HLS STREAM variable=data format`" are used.

Furthermore, we define three primitive data formats, which allow to parameterize the core for different data formats in the three main stages of the CT pre-processing core:

- `Detector format`: This format refers to the raw-sensor data that are generated by the DMS and collected by the data-flow module in the DAS. It defines the input data format of the *sensor-data conversion stage*.
- `Image-processing format`: This format refers to the desired data format for the pre-processing steps. It defines the output data format of the *sensor-data conversion stage*, the data format for the *image-processing stage*, and the input data format of the *reconstruction conversion stage*.
- `Reconstruction format`: This format refers to the reconstruction representation. It defines the output data format of the *reconstruction conversion stage*.

The designer in Vitis™ HLS defines the primitive data formats as the C++ class at synthesis time.

For DSE purposes, we configure the CT processing core with different encoding of the floating-point and fixed-point representations. For implementing these representations with the Xilinx arithmetic processing units, we use the provided libraries `hls_math`, `hls_half`, and `ap_fixed`. These allow us to use *double, float, single, half and ap_fixed<W,I>* formats. In fixed format, W refers to the data width and I the integer part of the real value number. In Section 9, the implementation results of the different configurations used in the DSE are discussed.

6.2. Open-Interface CT

Before describing the integration of the CT pre-processing core within the DAS, we introduce our open-interface CT architecture, as well as the DAS architecture, which is the central control unit of the system, the flow of data from the DMS to the reconstruction system.

Our open-interface CT, as shown in Figure 7, consists of the following components: a 64 row DMS and an X-ray tube system, a gantry module from Schleifring [40], a patient table, and a reconstruction system. As shown in Figure 8, all these components are controlled by the DAS, which is fixed in the rotating side and is implemented on the XC7Z045 MPSoC-FPGA.

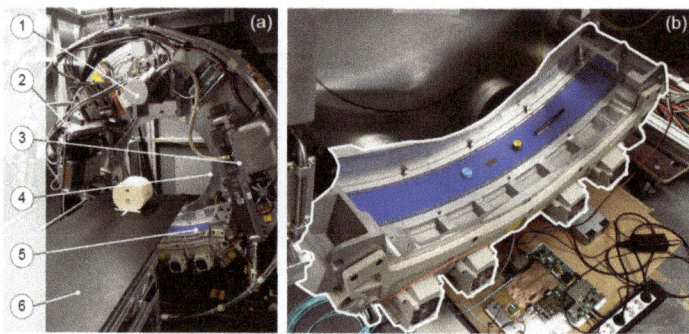

Figure 7. Components of our open-interface CT system. (**a**) Complete experimental CT system with (1) X-ray tube, (2) cooling system, (3) generator, (4) gantry subsystem with bore, (5) multiline DMS, (6) patient table. (**b**) Detailed view of the DMS and CCU implemented on the Xilinx ZC706 Evaluation Kit.

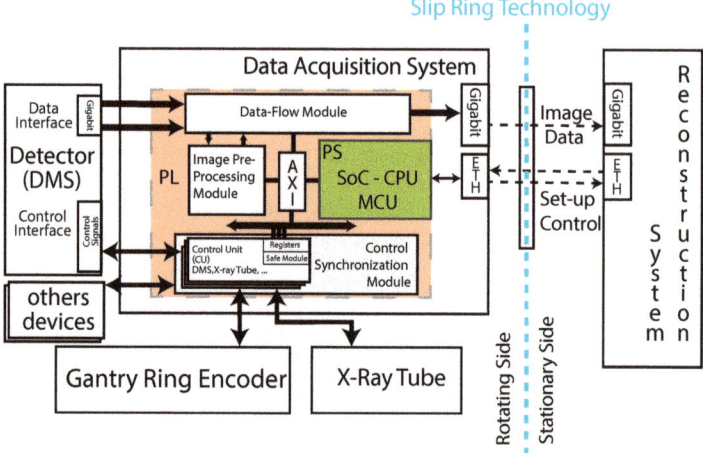

Figure 8. System architecture of the open-interface CT, Reprinted with permission from Ref. [41]. Copyright 2020, IEEE.

From the hardware designer prospective, the design of the open-interface CT is based on the system architecture shown in Figure 8, where the the DAS and the reconstruction systems are the components responsible for controlling and reconstructing tasks, respectively. The DAS has three main modules on the FPGA part of the MPSoC-FPGA and has a software stack on the PS part for controlling them [41].

The DAS system has the following modules, which are implemented in the FPGA part and controlled by the PS part:

- **Control-synchronization module**: This module is responsible for controlling and synchronizing all the external components on the stationary and the rotating sides. It is scalable, allowing an easy integration of other components in the open-interface CT, such as additional DMSs, X-ray tube systems and other sensors for multi-modality CT.
- **Data-flow module**: This module is responsible for collecting projections from the DMS, to manage eventually transmitting errors and to forward them to the *image pre-processing module*. After the pre-processing steps, it sends all the pre-processed data to the reconstruction system. It is implemented with a pipelined datapath that collects and forwards data in real time, without buffering them in external memory [42].
- **Image pre-processing module**: This module represents the proposed CT pre-processing core.

During the acquisition, the DMS acquires the raw sensor data and forwards them to the DAS over the gigabit interface. The raw sensor data are collected in the data-flow module of the DAS, which properly merges them and forwards to the image pre-processing module, where our CT pre-processing core is implemented. Here, the raw sensor data are converted to the selected pre-processing data format, pre-processed from raw sensor data to attenuation data and converted to the selected reconstruction data format. After that, the pre-processed attenuation data are forwarded to the reconstruction system, through the data flow module, over the gigabit slip ring connection. In the reconstruction system, the 3D volume is reconstructed.

6.3. Data Acquisition System Integration

The CT pre-processing core is integrated in the image pre-processing module of the DAS. We created the IP block design by Vitis™ HLS, and it was instantiated in the DAS design as the IP core by using Vivado Design Suite.

Based on the DAS, the DMS and the reconstruction algorithm requirements, we set the clock frequency, the input and output data representations of our CT processing core, as follows:

- `clock frequency = 100 MHz`: It is the clock frequency for collecting data.
- `input data = short format`: It is a 16-bit unsigned representation, which is used for the raw sensor data.
- `output data = float format`: It is a 32-bit single-precision floating-point representation, which is used for the reconstruction algorithm.

Due to these requirements, we set these two data formats in the *sensor-data conversion stage* and the *reconstruction conversion stage*, respectively. Yet, in the image-processing stage, we explored different data formats, with the aim to find the optimal data format for interventional CT application.

7. Design Space Exploration

In this section, we explain our approach for the design space exploration of the different data formats and representations, applied on the pre-processing step. In addition, we describe the parameters and the metrics used to find the optimal data format and representation.

The DSE of all possible data representations in CT applications is time consuming. In fact, for each input configuration, the 3D volume must be reconstructed, and the image quality analysis must be performed. Due to that, it results in a complex problem, where it is impossible to analyze all configurations for the different representations in the design space. To simplify the exploration process, we define two steps that limit the size of the problem itself. First, we make the *"pre-selection of data formats and representations"* for the input parameters, and after that the *"pre-selection of metrics"*. In this way, we reduce the set of input parameters and decrease the evaluation time of each solution. As input parameter, we also have the clock frequency, but it does not affect the image quality, so we set it at 100 MHz. The value of the set frequency is based on the data-rate of the collected data. In this way, we decrease the design space because different clock frequencies can generate different design performances in resource utilization and latency.

7.1. Pre-Selection of Data Formats and Representations

To pre-select the data formats and reduce the size of the design space, we use a top–down approach. At the beginning, we decided to explore only standardized data formats that are also implemented in the new commercial architectures, such as GPUs, and TPUs. In this way, we focused on floating-point and fixed-point representations.

For interventional CT applications, the goal is to minimize latency while maintaining high accuracy for having a real-time reconstruction. For this reason, in the second step, from the pre-selected data representations, we considered only formats with data widths in the range from 16 to 32. The values of this range are related to the data widths of raw sensor data and reconstructed data. In fact, raw sensor data are usually represented with short format (16-bit data width), and reconstructed data with float format (16-bit data width). In addition, we considered the double format (64-bit data width), which we used as a reference point in the image quality analysis. Therefore, for the floating-point representation, we limited our study to three different encodings: *half*, *single* and *double* precision.

By contrast, regarding the fixed-point representation with a fixed-rounding configuration, if all possible formats in the range from 16 to 32 bits are considered, 408 configuration formats are possible. Therefore, we considered only the upper bound and lower bound configurations, which are 16 and 32 bits. For these two data widths, there are 16 plus 32 possible configurations as fixed-point representation. Therefore, to reduce our DSE from these 48 to the desired 2 configurations, we analyzed the raw sensor data and selected one configuration for 32-bit fixed-point and one for 16 bit fixed point. The raw sensor data are represented as 16-bit unsigned, so we configured the 32-bit fixed-point with I and F both equal to 16 bits. In this way, the 32-bit fixed-point does not approximate any values in the *sensor data conversion stage*.

Due to the fractional part of the fixed-point representation, the 16-bit fixed point cannot contain the 16-bit unsigned, without approximation. Therefore, to find the best configuration, we started from the 16-bit fixed-point configuration that has 8 bits for integer and fractional, and we estimated the MSE. The MSE is the mean squared difference between a reference value and an approximated value [43]. This is often used to measure the image quality between two images [44]. To find other configurations, we analyzed the multiplication factor of Formula (7), which can be approximated with a shift of the dot in the number. So, we removed the multiplication and shifted the dot by decreasing/increasing the integer and fractional parts, respectively, to reach the lowest MSE. In this way, we reached the best configuration of 16-bit fixed-point with 4-bit and 12-bit for the integer and fraction parts, respectively.

With this methodology, we pre-selected four data representations for the DSE, which are half-precision and single-precision floating-point, and 16-bit and 32-bit fixed point, where I and F are equal to 16 and 16 bits, and equal to 4 and 12 bits, respectively.

7.2. Selection of Metrics

To reduce the time involved in the DSE for generating the different results, we also selected metrics that are significant for the hardware performance and the image quality analysis in the case of interventional CT.

For the hardware performance evaluation, we considered the resource utilization of the FPGA and the execution time of the different solutions. In our case, we only analyzed the execution time of the CT pre-processing core, which is expressed as latency from the Vitis™ HLS tool. For analyzing the resource utilization of the FPGA, we considered the configurable blocks and memories mostly used for image processing applications. These are digital signal processing (DSP) blocks, flip-flop registers (FF), BRAM memory, and look-up tables (LUTs) for the combinatorial logic [45].

For the image quality analysis, of the different solutions, we considered the following metrics: MSE of the 2D projections, and *noise*, *low contrast* and *uniformity* of the reconstructed 3D volume. The MSE was applied on the 2D projections for measuring if the collected data have an acceptable accuracy for the reconstruction. In this way, we only reconstructed and performed the image quality analysis on acceptable configurations. The other selected metrics for the image quality analysis are useful for interventional CT applications. The *uniformity* and *noise* metrics are important to identify the eventual image degradation, caused by the arithmetic approximation of the different data formats. The *low contrast* metric is important for tumor detection [15], useful in tumor ablation, during surgery.

8. Image Quality Analysis

For performing the image quality analysis, we considered three elements: the CT acquisition configuration, the significant metrics, and a representative phantom. Usually, most of the work in the literature considers different CT scanners and/or acquisition configurations to research how these elements influence the image quality [46–48]. However, in our research, we are interested in comprehending the influence of the data formats on the image quality, independently by the CT scanner and acquisition configuration. Therefore for our experiments, we used one scanner with a single configuration for the CT acquisition. Additionally, we used the CATPHAN® 500 [15], which is a representative phantom. In fact, this provides the complete characterization for maximizing the image quality.

8.1. CATPHAN® 500

The CATPHAN® 500 [15], as shown in Figure 9, has four modules enclosed in a 20 cm housing. Each module is used for performing different image quality metrics, such as geometry alignment, *uniformity*, *noise* and *low contrast*. Before describing the modules, we introduce the Hounsfield unit (HU), also referred as the "*CT number*". It is the relative quantitative measurement of radio density [49]. Radiologists uses it in the interpretation of CT images because different body tissues have different densities.

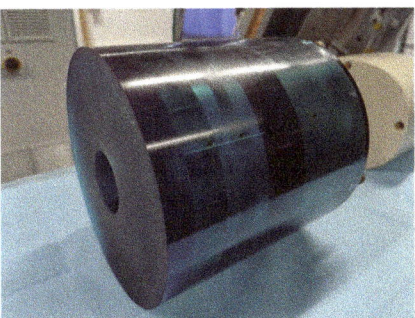

Figure 9. CATPHAN® 500.

We scanned the different modules with the same CT scanner configuration. Based on the pre-selected metrics, we used the three following modules:

- **CTP515 Low Contrast Module**: This module consists of a series of cylindrical rods of various diameters and three contrast levels to measure low contrast performance [15]. The roads, as shown in Figure 10, are provided on z-axis positions, for avoiding any volume-averaging errors [50]. The different low contrast are useful for identifying small low contrast objects, such as tumors. Subslice targets have a nominal 1.0% contrast and z-axis lengths of 3, 5, and 7 mm. For each of these lengths, there are targets with diameters of 3, 5, 7 and 9 mm [50]. We acquired this phantom section to perform the *low contrast* image quality for the different data formats.

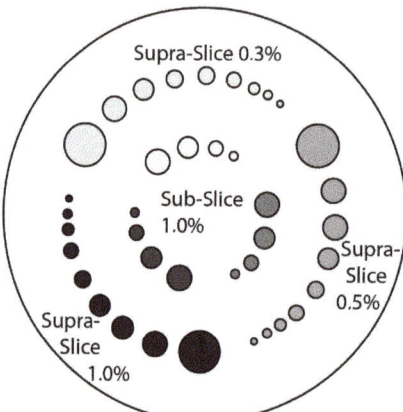

Figure 10. Section of the CTP515 low contrast module.

- **CTP486 Uniformity Module**: This module is cast from a uniform material with a "*CT number*" designed to be within 2% of water's density under standard scanning protocols [15]. This module is used for measurements of spatial uniformity, which means CT number and noise value. As shown in Figure 11, this module has a different region of interest (ROI) that can be targeted for measuring the *uniformity* of the different areas of a phantom section. In fact, the mean CT number and standard deviation of a large number of points, in a given ROI of the scan, is determined for central and peripheral locations within the scan image for each format of the scanning protocol [50].

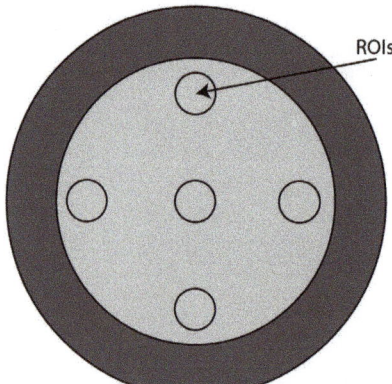

Figure 11. CTP486 uniformity module.

- **CTP401 Slice Geometry and Sensitometry Module**: This module is used to verify the phantom position. The module, as shown in Figure 12, includes four sensitometry targets (Teflon, Acrylic, LDPE and Air) to measure the CT number linearity [15]. The module also contains five acrylic spheres to evaluate the scanner's imaging of subslice spherical volumes. The diameters of the acrylic spheres are 2 mm, 4 mm, 6 mm, 8 mm, and 10 mm. We used this phantom for a human visual analysis of the CT images, in relation to the different materials and the size of the spheres.

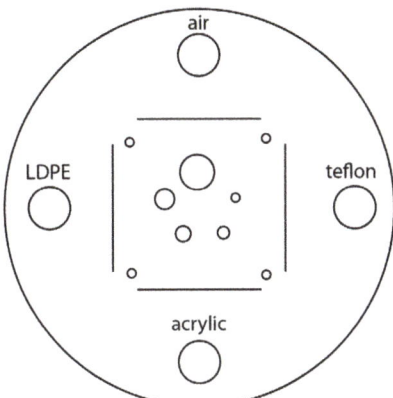

Figure 12. CTP401 slice geometry and sensitometry module.

8.2. CT Acquisition Configuration

In the open-interface CT, we manually set-up the components with the following parameters:

- X-ray tube system
  - Voltage: 120 KV
  - Intensity: 250 mA
- Detector system
  - Number of row slices: 64
  - x and y slice width: 0.625 mm
  - Number of projections per round: 1160
  - Size of the projection matrix in pixel: 672 × 64
- Gantry system
  - Number of rounds per second: 1
- Reconstruction system
  - Reconstruction algorithm: Feldkamp (FDK) algorithm [21]
  - z slice width: 1 mm
  - Size of the reconstructed matrix in pixel: 512 × 512

Furthermore, we pre-acquired and stored the I0-images, which are the projections without phantom of one round. Figure 13 shows one of these projections stored as a *short* data format.

Figure 13. I0-image: 2D projection without object.

Since, the I0-images are in the original raw sensor data, we only acquired it once, when we started our experiments.

8.3. Image Quality Metrics Calculation

For each image quality parameter, we used a mathematical estimation of it. For the pixel error of the 2D projections, we calculated the MSE, which gives the error interpretation of the approximated image [44]. The formula of MSE is the following:

$$MSE = \frac{1}{V}\sum_{j=1}^{V}(A_j - S_j)^2 \quad (8)$$

Here, A_j is the pixel value of the main image and S_j is the pixel value of the estimated image [43]. As the main image, we selected the pre-processed image with *double* format.

For calculating the values of the *noise*, *uniformity* and *low contrast* from the reconstructed volume, we considered a different ROI per module, as suggested by the CATPHAN® 500 Manual [15]. For selecting the ROI, we used the reconstructed images shown with red and blue circles in Figure 14, where the pre-processing was done with the double format. For the *noise* analysis, we calculated the standard deviation of the CT number for each of the ROIs, placed on the uniformity module and shown in Figure 14.

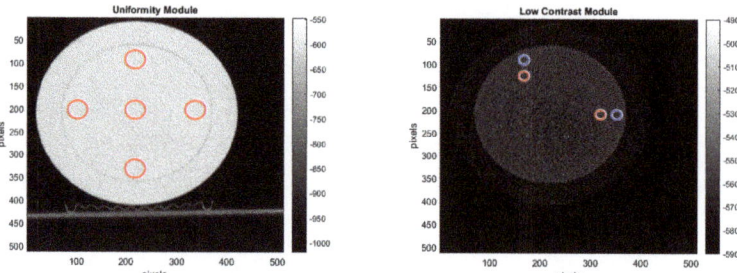

Figure 14. Uniformity module, placements of the ROIs.

For the uniformity analysis, five ROIs with 40 pixels in diameter are placed on the module, four peripheral ROIs and one central ROI. The average CT number, in HU, is obtained for each of these ROIs, and the uniformity is measured as the maximum difference between the mean value of the center ROI and one of the peripheral ROIs.

For the *low contrast* analysis, we calculated the contrast noise ratio (CNR) by placing a ROI of 20 pixels in diameter in the larger targets of both the supra-slice 1.0% and supra-slice 0.5%, and in the background area right beside it. The CNR was calculated using Formula (9) and averaged over 32 reconstructed slices.

$$CNR = \frac{|S_T - S_B|}{\sigma_B} \quad (9)$$

In Formula (9), S_A and S_B are the signal intensity of the supra-slice target and the background region, respectively, and σ_B is the standard deviation of the background.

9. Results and Discussion

This section shows and discusses the results of the proposed optimized method with the different data formats used in the DSE. First, we compare the proposed method and the standard method presented in Section 2.2. Second, we compare and discuss the results of the pre-processing step and reconstruction image for the different data format configurations selected within the DSE. Finally, we define which data format seems to be the best for the pre-processing step in interventional CT.

We used Vitis™ HLS for the hardware performance analysis in terms of hardware cost. In this article, we focus on the resource utilization and execution time of the CT pre-processing core, which is configured to process one pixel per clock cycle. If the DAS collects multiple pixels per clock cycle, multiple instances of the CT pre-processing core must be added to the design. Due to the data parallelism, the resource utilization increases linearly, while the overall execution time remains constant. In the reported results, we selected the XC7Z045 MPSoC-FPGA model from Xilinx [39] as the FPGA target platform.

9.1. Standard and Optimized Methods

As explained in Section 4, the standard method for I0-correction and the optimized method were implemented in the CT pre-processing core. The two versions, shown in Figures 4 and 5, were implemented with pipelining. In the optimized version, the logarithm operation is pre-calculated because its argument is constant. The algorithm executes only subtraction and multiplication operations. By contrast, the standard method executes an additional power operation and logarithm operations, which are expensive in terms of execution time and resource utilization. To compare and quantify the two methods independently by the data format, we selected the same *image-processing format* (single-precision floating point), and synthesized both with Vitis™ HLS. Furthermore, we analyzed the MSE of the 2D pre-processed projections. The estimated MSE is 3.21×10^{-15}, which is almost 0. With the reported low MSE, we also validated our solution and we can confirm that the two methods are equivalent, as expected from the mathematical simplification. In fact, both methods generate the same output projections. The MSE is not exactly 0 because the two methods evolve different operations and math co-processors components that approximate the values in different ways.

As expected, the two methods differ in terms of hardware performance. The optimized method, as reported in Table 1, does not use any BRAM and requires about 10 times less DSP, FF and LUT resources, the standard method to perform a complex operation, as logarithm and power need to buffer data; for this reason, BRAM is utilized. In addition, these complex operations determine the higher LUT, FF and DSP utilization. FPGAs have a small limited number of DSPs, and therefore, their utilization should be minimized, when it is possible. Moreover, the low required resource utilization for our solution allows to implement and integrate the pre-processing core directly in the DMS, closest to the sensor.

Table 1. Hardware report for CT pre-processing core (instance for 1 pixel per clock cycle).

Precision Name	BRAM 18K	DSP	FF	LUT	Latency
Standard method (float)	2	30	3497	6881	660 ns
Optimized method (float)	0	5	527	785	160 ns

Due to the real-time requirements, the most important metric is the execution time/latency. In this case, we analyzed the latency of the single operations for the two methods; the results are also shown in Table 1. The standard method has a latency of 660 ns, while the optimized method has a latency of 160 ns. In the standard method, there are power, division and logarithm operations that are much slower operations than subtraction and multiplication operations. In fact, the optimized method has only one multiplication and one subtraction, which have low latency, as shown in Table 2 and discussed in Section 9.2. For this reason, our solution achieves a speed-up of about 4.125× compared to the standard method with the same data format. We see that in the optimized method configured with the 32 bit-fixed point data format, we reach a speed-up of about 16.5× compared to the standard method. This latency enhancement is a significant improvement for the real-time requirements of the interventional CT application.

Table 2. Timing analysis of the standard method.

1st Stage			2nd Stage					3rd Stage
Buffer	Conv.	Mul.	Exp.	Div.	Div.	Log.	Muls	Buffer
10 ns	50 ns	40 ns	140 ns	120 ns	120 ns	130 ns	40 ns	10 ns

By using the dataflow architecture, both solutions make it possible to pre-process a new pixel each clock cycle. It was not possible to compare the optimized methods with the related works, in terms of hardware implementation, due to the lack of information.

Related works provide the whole execution time, without considering the pre-processing step and its impact on reconstruction.

9.2. Comparison of the Data Formats

Before analyzing the results of the different data format configurations with the pre-selected metrics, we performed a human visual analysis of the CTP401 module. In the human visual analysis, we observed that the pre-processing step was well performed and the grid between sensors was removed. Figure 15 shows the 2D projections pre- and post-processing with the different data format configurations. Yet, we did not observe differences between the different configurations with the human visual analysis.

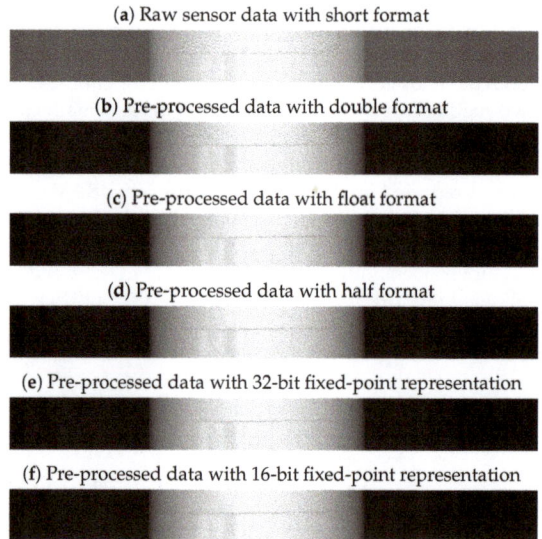

Figure 15. Single projection of module CTP401, before and after the pre-processing.

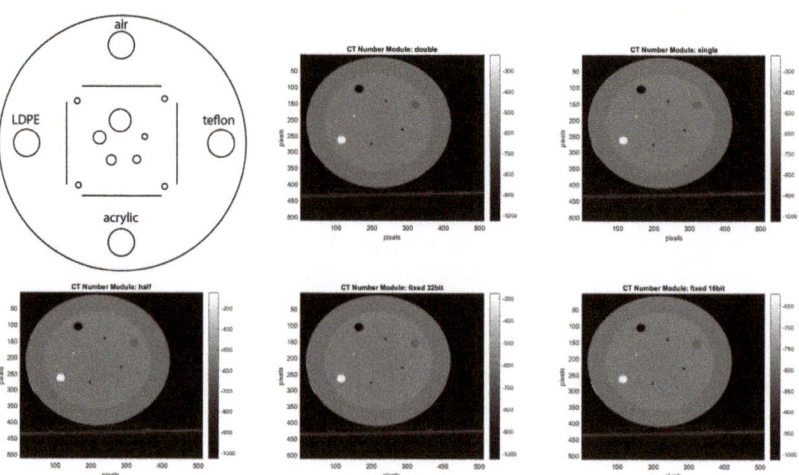

Figure 16. Reconstructed image of the CTP401 module for human visual analysis.

The human visual analysis was conducted also for the reconstructed images, shown in Figure 16. We observed that all target materials can be distinguished independently by the data format configuration utilized in the pre-processing step. This means that the image quality does not seem to change in terms of human visual analysis.

Since with the human visual analysis, it is not possible to compare the accuracy and the information lost between the different data formats, we estimated the MSE of the projections. The MSE, as explained in Section 7, is the key point used for reducing the eligible data formats for the DSE. It was crucial to select the two data format configurations of the 16-bit and 32-bit fixed-point; we reduced from 48 to 2 possible data format configurations. The MSE is a reasonable metric in this step because it can be applied to 2D projections before the reconstruction. In addition, we noticed that it is in the same order of magnitude for the different phantoms. However, the MSE does not consider all image quality metrics, which are significant to understanding how data formats influence the quality of reconstructed images. Therefore, we performed the measurement of *low contrast*, *noise* and *uniformity* for the reconstructed images. For calculating these metrics, we acquired, pre-processed with different data format configurations, and reconstructed the modules shown in Figures 17 and 18.

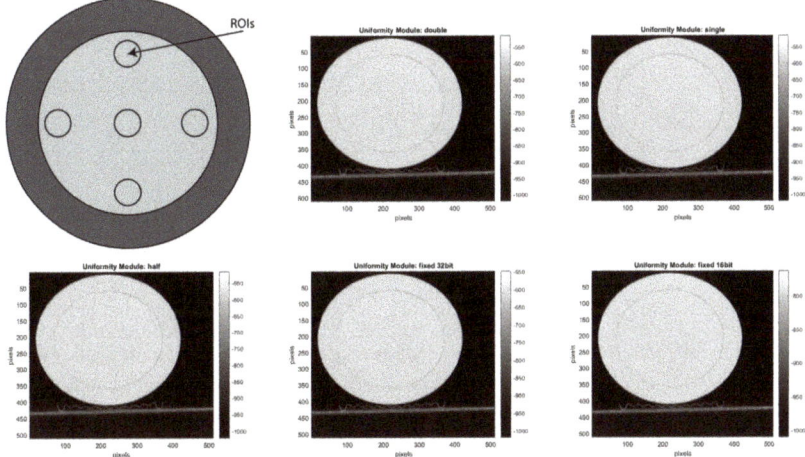

Figure 17. Reconstructed image of the CTP486 module, for noise and uniformity analysis.

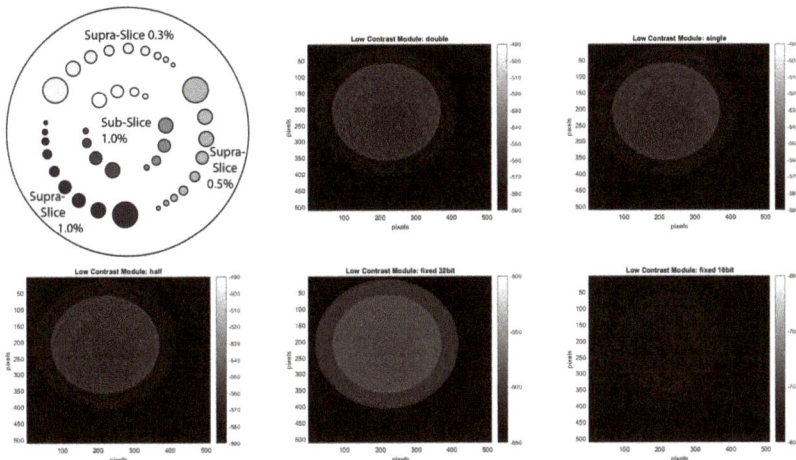

Figure 18. Reconstructed image of the CTP515 module, for low contrast analysis.

The results of the image quality analysis are shown in Table 3. We observed that the MSE of all configurations is lower than 1. This value is very good in terms of image quality since the MSE is usually between 2.36 and 2.37 also in medical image compression [51]. By comparing the other image quality metrics of all data formats with the double format, the values were judged to be good in most of the cases. In fact, these are in the same order of magnitude as shown in Table 3. The only data format where the approximation of the pre-processing has slightly influenced the reconstructed images is the 16-bit fixed point. Due to the approximation made and the bit truncation involved for converting the raw sensor data from 16-bit unsigned to 16-bit fixed point, the low contrast pixels are blurred. Therefore, the contrast noise ratio (CNR) is about 0.2 lower than the double configuration. By contrast, due to the blurred low contrast pixels of the 16-bit fixed-point configuration, a lower *noise* and a better *uniformity* was estimated for this configuration, compared to other data formats. In fact, in images with blurred pixels, the pixel values are similar, and therefore, there is a lower *noise* and a better *uniformity*. From this image quality analysis, we can conclude that all data formats result in an acceptable pre-processed and reconstructed image quality. The 16-bit fixed point has some problems that would make sense to choose it only if the hardware cost has much advantages, compared to other solutions.

Table 3. Image quality estimation of different data format configurations.

Resource Name	Half	Float	Double	Fixed 16	Fixed 32
MSE	2.39×10^{-7}	3.21×10^{-15}	0	0.22	0.0039
CNR Supra-Slice 1.0% [ΔHU]	0.555	0.566	0.566	0.335	0.536
Noise [HU]	5.8	5.7	5.7	2.7	5.3
Uniformity [ΔHU]	3.54	3.57	3.57	2.44	3.5

To define the hardware costs of the different data types, we compared the resource utilization and the latency of the various data format configurations. As shown in Table 4, the utilization of all FPGA resources decreases from floating-point to fixed-point representations, independently of the data width. In fact, DSPs are minimized from 14 of the double configurations to 0 and 1 of the 32-bit fixed-point and 16-bit fixed-point configurations, respectively. In FPGA, the number of DSPs is crucial because they are in the order of hundreds, while LUTs and FFs are in the order of hundreds of thousands. Therefore, the low utilization of resources in fixed-point representations allows the FPGA to implement additional pre-processing steps on the fly. The best result comes from the 32-bit fixed point; this configuration is the only one that utilizes 0 DSPs and implements all operations with LUTs and FFs. Therefore, even if it utilizes more LUTs than 16-bit fixed-point, we can confirm that 32-bit fixed-point is the data format with the best performance in terms of resource utilization concerning the FPGA available resources. The 32-bit fixed-point has better performance than the 16-bit fixed-point due to the fact that Vitis™ HLS optimizes the 32-bit fixed-point format in the provided libraries.

Table 4. Resource utilization of different data format configurations.

Resource Name	Half	Float	Double	Fixed 16	Fixed 32
BRAM 18k	0	0	0	0	0
DSP	4	5	14	1	0
FF	382	527	1292	167	309
LUT	223	785	1796	941	1245

Finally, we analyzed the execution time in the different cases. The results in Table 5 show the advantage of using fixed-point representation compared to floating-point representation. In fact, 16-bit and 32-bit fixed-point configurations are 2.2× and 4× faster than the single-precision floating-point configuration, respectively. The conversion between the collected data and fixed-point representation is faster than floating-point representation because it is implemented with a combinatorial shift, which is implemented in hardware with a bitwise assignment. Due to that, the conversion is implemented together with the subtraction, which is also implemented with combinatorial logic. For this reason, the reported conversion execution time is close to 0.

As mentioned above, due to the Vitis™ HLS optimization and the DSP optimization, 32-bit fixed-point configuration implements all operations with FFs and LUTs; therefore, it has also lower latency than 16-bit fixed-point configuration. In fact, the former configuration does not use DSPs for the multiplication, so its execution time is 10 ns (1 clock cycles). By contrast, as shown in Table 5, due to the DSPs latency, the latter configuration spent 30 ns (3 clock cycles) for the multiplication, which is the time required by DSP to process one operation.

Table 5. Timing analysis of different data format configurations; all values are expressed in *ns*.

		1st Stage		2nd Stage			3rd Stage	
Configuration	Total	Read	Conv.	Buffer	Sub.	Mul.	Conv.	Write
Half	190	10	50	20	50	40	10	10
Float	160	10	50	0	50	40	0	10
Double	220	10	50	0	70	60	20	10
Fixed 16-bit	70	0	0	0	10	30	20	10
Fixed 32-bit	40	0	0	0	10	10	10	10

To compare all the metrics of various configurations, we used the radar graphs shown in Figure 19. Since the values have different units and scales, the min-max normalization is used [52]. Double configuration has the maximum quality and hardware performance, so it has most of the values equal to 1. By analyzing and comparing all results, we found that the 32-bit fixed-point configuration is optimal for interventional CT pre-processing in terms of image quality and resource utilization.

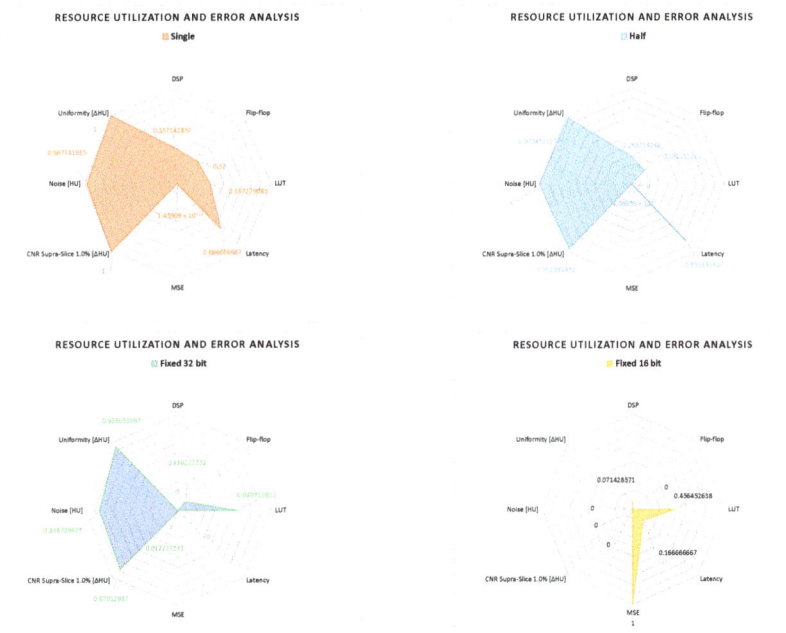

Figure 19. *Cont.*

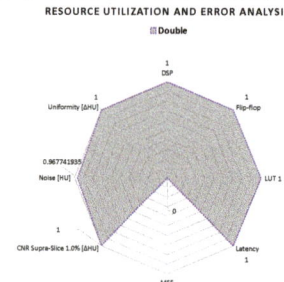

Figure 19. Metrics analysis of the data format configurations; a good value of resource utilization, latency, noise, and MSE should be close to 0; by contrast, a good value of low contrast and uniformity should be close to 1.

The 32-bit fixed point is the best compromise between image quality and hardware preference. It maximizes the hardware performance, and the image quality after the reconstruction decreases only 7% in comparison with the double format. In contrast to [14], we do not consider the required external memory bandwidth for the different configurations because we are interested in finding only the best data format configuration in the pre-processing step. In this step, our CT pre-processing core processes projections on the fly and does not use any external memory, which usually is the main bottleneck GPU and CPU solutions.

10. Summary

In this article, we proposed a hardware acceleration of the pre-processing step for interventional CT. By performing this algorithm on the raw sensor data, we reduced the number of operations and their complexity. In addition, with this optimization, we achieved a speed-up of about $4.125\times$ compared to the standard method. Furthermore, we have implemented the algorithm in the proposed CT pre-processing core. This FPGA accelerator pre-processes CT projections on the fly and can be configured for pre-processing pixels with different data formats. In addition, we performed a design space exploration of the different data formats between double, float, half floating point, and the different configurations of 16-bit and 32-bit fixed point. Among them, we found out that 32-bit fixed point is the optimal data format for pre-processing steps in interventional CT. In fact, with 32-bit fixed point, we achieve a speed-up of $16.5\times$ compared to the standard method, and it utilizes less FPGA resources. Additionally, with 32-bit fixed point, the image quality of the reconstructed image decreases only about 7% compared to the double format. In future works, we aim to extend this exploration also to the reconstruction step, where mixed-precision data formats could be used.

Author Contributions: Conceptualization, D.P. and T.P.; methodology, D.P.; software, D.P., M.G. and M.L.E.; validation, D.P., S.A. and M.L.E.; formal analysis, D.P. and S.A.; investigation, D.P. and M.G.; resources, S.A.; data curation, M.G.; writing—original draft preparation, D.P., M.G. and M.L.E.; writing—review and editing, D.P., S.A. and T.P.; visualization, M.G., S.A. and M.L.E.; supervision, T.P.; project administration, T.P.; funding acquisition, T.P. All authors have read and agreed to the published version of the manuscript.

Funding: This research was partly funded by Ministry of Economics, Science and Digitization of Saxony-Anhalt within the Forschungscampus STIMULATE under grant number I 117. The Article Processing Charge was funded by the Open Access Publication Fund of Magdeburg University.

Conflicts of Interest: The authors declare no conflict of interest.

References

1. Kalender, W.A. X-ray computed tomography. *Phys. Med. Biol.* **2006**, *51*, R29–R43. [CrossRef] [PubMed]
2. Jones, A.K.; Dixon, R.G.; Collins, J.D.; Walser, E.M.; Nikolic, B. Best practice guidelines for CT-guided interventional procedures. *J. Vasc. Interv. Radiol.* **2018**, *29*, 518–519. [CrossRef] [PubMed]
3. Aggarwal, P.; Mehra, R. High speed CT image reconstruction using FPGA. *Int. J. Comput. Appl.* **2011**, *22*, 7–10. [CrossRef]
4. Dandekar, O.; Castro-Pareja, C.; Shekhar, R. FPGA-based real-time 3D image preprocessing for image-guided medical interventions. *J. Real-Time Image Process.* **2007**, *1*, 285–301. [CrossRef]
5. Després, P.; Jia, X. A review of GPU-based medical image reconstruction. *Phys. Medica* **2017**, *42*, 76–92. [CrossRef]
6. Ravi, M.; Sewa, A.; Shashidhar, T.G.; Sanagapati, S.S.S. FPGA as a Hardware Accelerator for Computation Intensive Maximum Likelihood Expectation Maximization Medical Image Reconstruction Algorithm. *IEEE Access* **2019**, *7*, 111727–111735. [CrossRef]
7. Alcaín, E.; Fernández, P.R.; Nieto, R.; Montemayor, A.S.; Vilas, J.; Galiana-Bordera, A.; Martinez-Girones, P.M.; Prieto-de la Lastra, C.; Rodriguez-Vila, B.; Bonet, M.; et al. Hardware Architectures for Real-Time Medical Imaging. *Electronics* **2021**, *10*, 3118. [CrossRef]
8. *IEEE Std 754-2019*; IEEE Standard for Floating-Point Arithmetic. Revision of IEEE 754-2008. IEEE: Piscataway, NJ, USA, 2019; pp. 1–84. [CrossRef]
9. Xu, Q.; Mytkowicz, T.; Kim, N.S. Approximate Computing: A Survey. *IEEE Des. Test* **2016**, *33*, 8–22. [CrossRef]
10. Jiang, H.; Santiago, F.J.H.; Mo, H.; Liu, L.; Han, J. Approximate Arithmetic Circuits: A Survey, Characterization, and Recent Applications. *Proc. IEEE* **2020**, *108*, 2108–2135. [CrossRef]
11. Markidis, S.; Chien, S.W.D.; Laure, E.; Peng, I.B.; Vetter, J.S. NVIDIA Tensor Core Programmability, Performance amp; Precision. In Proceedings of the 2018 IEEE International Parallel and Distributed Processing Symposium Workshops (IPDPSW), Vancouver, BC, Canada, 21–25 May 2018; pp. 522–531. [CrossRef]
12. Nourazar, M.; Goossens, B. Accelerating iterative CT reconstruction algorithms using Tensor Cores. *J. Real-Time Image Process.* **2021**, *18*, 1979–1991. [CrossRef]
13. Google. BFloat16: The Secret to High Performance on Cloud TPUs. Available online: https://cloud.google.com/blog/products/ai-machine-learning/bfloat16-the-secret-to-high-performance-on-cloud-tpus (accessed on 23 January 2022).
14. Maaß, C.; Baer, M.; Kachelrieß, M. CT image reconstruction with half precision floating-point values. *Med. Phys.* **2011**, *38*, S95–S105. [CrossRef] [PubMed]
15. Laboratory, T.P. Catphan 500. Available online: https://www.phantomlab.com/catphan-500 (accessed on 23 January 2022).
16. for Devices, C.; Health, R. What Is Computed Tomography? 2020. Available online: https://www.fda.gov/radiation-emitting-products/medical-x-ray-imaging/what-computed-tomography (accessed on 21 June 2021).
17. Webb, A.G. *Introduction to Biomedical Imaging*; John Wiley & Sons: Hoboken, NJ, USA, 2017.
18. Passaretti, D.; Joseph, J.M.; Pionteck, T. Survey on FPGAs in Medical Radiology Applications: Challenges, Architectures and Programming Models. In Proceedings of the 2019 International Conference on Field-Programmable Technology (ICFPT), Tianjin, China, 9–13 December 2019; pp. 279–282.
19. Kimura, M.; Yamaguchi, Y.; Al-Ola, A.; Omar, M.; Yoshinaga, T. Tomographic Inverse Problem with Estimating Missing Projections. *Math. Probl. Eng.* **2019**, *2019*, 7932318. [CrossRef]
20. Kinahan, P.E.; Hasegawa, B.H.; Beyer, T. X-ray-based attenuation correction for positron emission tomography/computed tomography scanners. In *Seminars in Nuclear Medicine*; Elsevier: Amsterdam, The Netherlands, 2003; Volume 33, pp. 166–179.
21. Feldkamp, L.A.; Davis, L.C.; Kress, J.W. Practical cone-beam algorithm. *J. Opt. Soc. Am. A* **1984**, *1*, 612–619. [CrossRef]
22. Wang, A.S.; Stayman, J.W.; Otake, Y.; Kleinszig, G.; Vogt, S.; Gallia, G.L.; Khanna, A.J.; Siewerdsen, J.H. Soft-tissue imaging with C-arm cone-beam CT using statistical reconstruction. *Phys. Med. Biol.* **2014**, *59*, 1005. [CrossRef] [PubMed]
23. Hsieh, J. *Computed Tomography: Principles, Design, Artifacts, and Recent Advances*; SPIE Press: Bellingham, WA, USA, 2003; Volume 114.
24. Omondi, A.R. *Computer Arithmetic Systems: Algorithms, Architecture and Implementation*; Prentice Hall International (UK) Ltd.: Hemel Hempstead, UK, 1994.
25. Coric, S.; Leeser, M.; Miller, E.; Trepanier, M. Parallel-beam backprojection: An FPGA implementation optimized for medical imaging. In Proceedings of the 2002 ACM/SIGDA Tenth International Symposium on Field-Programmable Gate Arrays, Monterey, CA, USA, 24–26 February 2002; pp. 217–226.
26. Goddard, I.; Trepanier, M. High-speed cone-beam reconstruction: An embedded systems approach. In *Medical Imaging 2002: Visualization, Image-Guided Procedures, and Display*; SPIE: Bellingham, WA, USA, 2002; Volume 4681, pp. 483–491.
27. Heigl, B.; Kowarschik, M. High-speed reconstruction for C-arm computed tomography. In Proceedings of the 9th International Meeting on Fully Three-Dimensional Image Reconstruction in Radiology and Nuclear Medicine, Lindau, Germany, 9–13 July 2007; pp. 25–28.
28. Deng, J.; Yan, B.; Li, J.; Li, L. Parallel no-waiting pipelining accelerating CT image reconstruction based on FPGA. In Proceedings of the 2010 3rd International Conference on Biomedical Engineering and Informatics, Yantai, China, 16–18 October 2010; Volume 1, pp. 451–455.
29. Qiao, L.; Luo, G.; Zhang, W.; Jiang, M. FPGA Acceleration of Ray-Based Iterative Algorithm for 3D Low-Dose CT Reconstruction. In Proceedings of the 2020 30th International Conference on Field-Programmable Logic and Applications (FPL), Gothenburg, Sweden, 31 August–4 September 2020; pp. 98–102.

30. Choi, Y.k.; Cong, J. Acceleration of EM-based 3D CT reconstruction using FPGA. *IEEE Trans. Biomed. Circuits Syst.* **2015**, *10*, 754–767. [CrossRef]
31. Windisch, D.; Knodel, O.; Juckeland, G.; Hampel, U.; Bieberle, A. FPGA-based Real-Time Data Acquisition for Ultrafast X-Ray Computed Tomography. *IEEE Trans. Nucl. Sci.* **2021**, *68*, 2779–2786. [CrossRef]
32. Wang, B.; Zhu, L.; Jia, K.; Zheng, J. Accelerated cone beam CT reconstruction based on OpenCL. In Proceedings of the 2010 International Conference on Image Analysis and Signal Processing, Trois-Rivières, QC, Canada, 30 June–2 July 2010; pp. 291–295.
33. Chen, J.; Cong, J.; Vese, L.A.; Villasenor, J.; Yan, M.; Zou, Y. A hybrid architecture for compressive sensing 3-D CT reconstruction. *IEEE J. Emerg. Sel. Top. Circuits Syst.* **2012**, *2*, 616–625. [CrossRef]
34. Scherl, H.; Keck, B.; Kowarschik, M.; Hornegger, J. Fast GPU-based CT reconstruction using the common unified device architecture (CUDA). In Proceedings of the 2007 IEEE Nuclear Science Symposium Conference Record, Honolulu, HI, USA, 28 October–3 November 2007; Volume 6, pp. 4464–4466.
35. Zhao, X.; Bian, J.; Sidky, E.Y.; Cho, S.; Zhang, P.; Pan, X. GPU-based 3D cone-beam CT image reconstruction: Application to micro CT. In Proceedings of the 2007 IEEE Nuclear Science Symposium Conference Record, Honolulu, HI, USA, 28 October–3 November 2007; Volume 5, pp. 3922–3925.
36. Shi, B.; Chen, S.; Huang, F.; Wang, C.; Bi, K. The parallel processing based on CUDA for convolution filter FDK reconstruction of CT. In Proceedings of the 2010 3rd International Symposium on Parallel Architectures, Algorithms and Programming, Dalian, China, 18–20 December 2010; pp. 149–153.
37. Korcyl, G.; Białas, P.; Curceanu, C.; Czerwiński, E.; Dulski, K.; Flak, B.; Gajos, A.; Głowacz, B.; Gorgol, M.; Hiesmayr, B.C.; et al. Evaluation of single-chip, real-time tomographic data processing on FPGA SoC devices. *IEEE Trans. Med. Imaging* **2018**, *37*, 2526–2535. [CrossRef]
38. Orailoglu, A.; Gajski, D.D. Flow graph representation. In Proceedings of the 23rd ACM/IEEE Design Automation Conference, Las Vegas, NV, USA, 29 June–2 July 1986; pp. 503–509.
39. *ZC706 Evaluation Board for the Zynq-7000 XC7Z045 SoC*; Xilinx: San Jose, CA, USA, 2019.
40. Schleifring. Gantry. Available online: https://www.schleifring.de/wp-content/uploads/2019/09/CT-Applications_January18.pdf (accessed on 25 December 2021).
41. Passaretti, D.; Pionteck, T. Hardware/Software Co-Design of a control and data acquisition system for Computed Tomography. In Proceedings of the 2020 9th International Conference on Modern Circuits and Systems Technologies (MOCAST), Bremen, Germany, 7–9 September 2020; pp. 1–4. [CrossRef]
42. Passaretti, D.; Pionteck, T. Configurable Pipelined Datapath for Data Acquisition in Interventional Computed Tomography. In Proceedings of the 2021 IEEE 29th Annual International Symposium on Field-Programmable Custom Computing Machines (FCCM), Orlando, FL, USA, 9–12 May 2021; p. 257. [CrossRef]
43. Fomby, T. *Scoring Measures for Prediction Problems*; Department of Economics, Southern Methodist University: Dallas, TX, USA, 2008.
44. Measures of Image Quality. Available online: https://homepages.inf.ed.ac.uk/rbf/CVonline/LOCAL_COPIES/VELDHUIZEN/node18.html (accessed on 25 February 2022).
45. Xilinx. 7 Series FPGAs Configurable Logic Block, UG474 (v1.8). 2016. Available online: https://www.xilinx.com/support/documentation/user_guides/ug474_7Series_CLB.pdf (accessed on 27 December 2021).
46. Roa, A.M.A.; Andersen, H.K.; Martinsen, A.C.T. CT image quality over time: Comparison of image quality for six different CT scanners over a six-year period. *J. Appl. Clin. Med. Phys.* **2015**, *16*, 350–365. [CrossRef]
47. Gulliksrud, K.; Stokke, C.; Martinsen, A.C.T. How to measure CT image quality: Variations in CT-numbers, uniformity and low contrast resolution for a CT quality assurance phantom. *Phys. Med.* **2014**, *30*, 521–526. [CrossRef]
48. Husby, E.; Svendsen, E.D.; Andersen, H.K.; Martinsen, A.C.T. 100 days with scans of the same Catphan phantom on the same CT scanner. *J. Appl. Clin. Med/ Phys.* **2017**, *18*, 224–231. [CrossRef] [PubMed]
49. DenOtter, T.D.; Schubert, J. *Hounsfield Unit*; StatPearls Publishing: Treasure Island, FL, USA, 2021.
50. Laboratory, T.P. Catphan 500 and 600 Product Guide. Available online: https://static1.squarespace.com/static/5367b059e4b05a1adcd295c2/t/615ef40255dbd2709cd9cfbd/1633612803610/CTP500600ProductGuide20211006.pdf (accessed on 23 January 2022).
51. Fidler, A.; Skaleric, U.; Likar, B. The impact of image information on compressibility and degradation in medical image compression. *Med. Phys.* **2006**, *33*, 2832–2838. [CrossRef] [PubMed]
52. Suarez-Alvarez, M.M.; Pham, D.T.; Prostov, M.Y.; Prostov, Y.I. Statistical approach to normalization of feature vectors and clustering of mixed datasets. *Proc. R. Soc. A Math. Phys. Eng. Sci.* **2012**, *468*, 2630–2651. [CrossRef]

MDPI
St. Alban-Anlage 66
4052 Basel
Switzerland
Tel. +41 61 683 77 34
Fax +41 61 302 89 18
www.mdpi.com

Applied Sciences Editorial Office
E-mail: applsci@mdpi.com
www.mdpi.com/journal/applsci

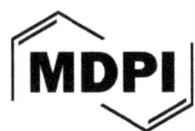

www.ingramcontent.com/pod-product-compliance
Lightning Source LLC
LaVergne TN
LVHW070415100526
838202LV00014B/1461